Basic Immunology

Basic Immunology
Functions and Disorders
of the Immune System

FOURTH EDITION

Abul K. Abbas, MBBS

Distinguished Professor in Pathology
Chair, Department of Pathology
University of California San Francisco
San Francisco, California

Andrew H. Lichtman, MD, PhD

Professor of Pathology
Harvard Medical School
Brigham and Women's Hospital
Boston, Massachusetts

Shiv Pillai, MBBS, PhD

Professor of Medicine and Health Sciences
   and Technology
Harvard Medical School
Massachusetts General Hospital
Boston, Massachusetts

Illustrations by

David L. Baker, MA
Alexandra Baker, MS, CMI
DNA Illustrations, Inc.

ELSEVIER
SAUNDERS

1600 John F. Kennedy Blvd.
Ste 1800
Philadelphia, PA 19103-2899

Notices

Knowledge and best practice in this field are constantly changing. As new research and experience broaden our understanding, changes in research methods, professional practices, or medical treatment may become necessary.

Practitioners and researchers must always rely on their own experience and knowledge in evaluating and using any information, methods, compounds, or experiments described herein. In using such information or methods they should be mindful of their own safety and the safety of others, including parties for whom they have a professional responsibility.

With respect to any drug or pharmaceutical products identified, readers are advised to check the most current information provided (i) on procedures featured or (ii) by the manufacturer of each product to be administered, to verify the recommended dose or formula, the method and duration of administration, and contraindications. It is the responsibility of practitioners, relying on their own experience and knowledge of their patients, to make diagnoses, to determine dosages and the best treatment for each individual patient, and to take all appropriate safety precautions.

To the fullest extent of the law, neither the Publisher nor the authors, contributors, or editors, assume any liability for any injury and/or damage to persons or property as a matter of products liability, negligence or otherwise, or from any use or operation of any methods, products, instructions, or ideas contained in the material herein.

Library of Congress Cataloging-in-Publication Data

978-1-4557-0707-2

Senior Content Strategist: James Merritt
Content Development Manager: Rebecca Gruliow
Publishing Services Manager: Patricia Tannian
Senior Project Manager: Sarah Wunderly
Design Direction: Steven Stave

Printed in China

Last digit is the print number: 9 8 7 6 5 4 3 2 1

To Our Students

PREFACE

The fourth edition of *Basic Immunology* has been thoroughly revised to include recent important advances in our understanding of the immune system and to organize and present information in order to maximize its usefulness to students and teachers. The previous three editions of *Basic Immunology* have been enthusiastically received by students in the many courses that we and our colleagues teach, and we have not wavered from the guiding principles on which the book has been based through all the past editions. Our experience as immunology teachers and course directors has helped us to judge the right amount of detailed information that can be usefully included in introductory medical school and undergraduate courses, and the value of presenting the principles of immunology in a succinct and clear manner. We believe a concise and modern consideration of immunology is now a realistic goal, largely because immunology has matured as a discipline and has now reached the stage when the essential components of the immune system, and how they interact in immune responses, are understood quite well. As a result, we can now teach our students, with reasonable confidence, how the immune system works. In addition, we are better able to relate experimental results, using simple models, to the more complex, but physiologically relevant, issue of host defense against infectious pathogens. There has also been exciting progress in applying basic principles to understanding and treating human diseases.

This book has been written to address the perceived needs of both medical school and undergraduate curricula and to take advantage of the new understanding of immunology. We have tried to achieve several goals. First, we have presented the most important principles governing the function of the immune system by synthesizing key concepts from the vast amount of experimental data that emerge in the field of immunology. The choice of what is most important is based largely on what is most clearly established by scientific investigation and what has the most relevance to human health and disease. We also have realized that in any concise discussion of complex phenomena it is inevitable that exceptions and caveats cannot be discussed in any detail. Second, we have focused on immune responses against infectious microbes, and most of our discussions of the immune system are in this context. Third, we have made liberal use of illustrations to highlight important principles, but have reduced factual details that may be found in more comprehensive textbooks. Fourth, we have also discussed immunologic diseases from the perspective of principles, emphasizing their relation to normal immune responses and avoiding details of clinical syndromes and treatments. We have added selected clinical cases in an appendix to illustrate how the principles of immunology may be applied to common human diseases. Finally, in order to make each chapter readable on its own, we have repeated key ideas in different places in the book. We feel such repetition will help students to grasp the most important concepts.

We hope that students will find this new edition of *Basic Immunology* clear, cogent, manageable, and enjoyable to read. We hope the book will convey our sense of wonder about the immune system and excitement about how the field has evolved and how it continues to grow in relevance to human health and disease. Finally, although we were spurred to tackle this project because of our associations with medical school courses, we hope the book will be valued by students of allied health and biology as well. We will have succeeded if the book can answer many of the questions these students have about the immune system and, at the same time, encourage them to delve even more deeply into immunology.

Several individuals played key roles in the writing of this book. Our new editor, James Merritt, has been an enthusiastic source of encouragement and advice. Our two talented illustrators, David and Alexandra Baker of DNA Illustrations, have revamped all the artwork for this new edition, and have transformed our ideas into pictures that are informative and aesthetically pleasing. Sarah Wunderly has moved the book through the production process in an efficient and professional manner. Our development editor, Rebecca Gruliow, has kept the project organized and on track despite pressures of time and logistics. To all of them we owe our many thanks. Finally, we owe an enormous debt of gratitude to our families, whose support and encouragement have been unwavering.

Abul K. Abbas
Andrew H. Lichtman
Shiv Pillai

CONTENTS

Introduction to the Immune System
Nomenclature, General Properties, and Components

Immunity is defined as resistance to disease, specifically infectious disease. The collection of cells, tissues, and molecules that mediate resistance to infections is called the **immune system,** and the coordinated reaction of these cells and molecules to infectious microbes is the **immune response. Immunology** is the study of the immune system, including its responses to microbial pathogens and damaged tissues and its role in disease. **The most important physiologic function of the immune system is to prevent infections and to eradicate established infections,** and this is the principal context in which immune responses are discussed throughout this book.

The importance of the immune system for health is dramatically illustrated by the frequent observation that individuals with defective immune responses are susceptible to serious, often life-threatening infections (Fig. 1–1). Conversely, stimulating immune responses against microbes through vaccination is the most effective method for protecting individuals against infections; this approach has led to the worldwide eradication of smallpox, the only disease that has been eliminated from civilization by human intervention (Fig. 1–2). The emergence of acquired immunodeficiency syndrome (AIDS) in the 1980s tragically emphasized the importance of the immune system for defending individuals against infection. The impact of immunology, however, goes beyond infectious disease (see Fig. 1–1). The immune system

Role of the immune system	Implications
Defense against infections	Deficient immunity results in increased susceptibility to infections; exemplified by AIDS
	Vaccination boosts immune defenses and protects against infections
Defense against tumors	Potential for immunotherapy of cancer
The immune system recognizes and responds to tissue grafts and newly introduced molecules	Immune responses are barriers to transplantation and gene therapy
The immune system can injure cells and induce pathologic inflammation	Immune responses are the cause of allergic, autoimmune, and other inflammatory diseases

FIGURE 1–1 Importance of the immune system in health and disease. This table summarizes some of the physiologic functions of the immune system and its role in disease; AIDS, Acquired immunodeficiency syndrome.

prevents the growth of some tumors, and several methods to treat cancers by stimulating immune responses against tumor cells are in development. Immune responses also participate in the clearance of dead cells and in initiating tissue repair.

In contrast to these beneficial roles, abnormal immune responses are the causes of many inflammatory diseases with serious morbidity and mortality. The immune response is the major barrier to successful organ transplantation to treat organ failure. The products of immune

Disease	Maximum number of cases (year)	Number of cases in 2009	Percent change
Diphtheria	206,939 (1921)	0	-99.99
Measles	894,134 (1941)	61	-99.99
Mumps	152,209 (1968)	982	-99.35
Pertussis	265,269 (1934)	13,506	-94.72
Polio (paralytic)	21,269 (1952)	0	-100.0
Rubella	57,686 (1969)	4	-99.99
Tetanus	1,560 (1923)	14	-99.10
Hemophilus influenza type B	~20,000 (1984)	25	-99.88
Hepatitis B	26,611 (1985)	3,020	-87.66

FIGURE 1–2 Effectiveness of vaccination for some common infectious diseases. This table illustrates the striking decrease in the incidence of selected infectious diseases for which effective vaccines have been developed. For some infections, such as hepatitis B, a vaccine has become available recently, and the incidence of the disease is continuing to decline. *(Modified from Orenstein WA, Hinman AR, Bart KJ, Hadler SC: Immunization. In Mandell GL, Bennett JE, Dolin R, editors: Principles and practices of infectious diseases, ed 4, New York, 1995, Churchill Livingstone; and MMWR 58:1458-1469, 2010.)*

cells are also of great practical use. For example, antibodies, which are proteins made by certain cells of the immune system, are used in clinical laboratory testing and in research as highly specific reagents for detecting a wide variety of molecules in the circulation and in cells and tissues. Antibodies designed to block or eliminate potentially harmful molecules and cells are in widespread use for the treatment of immunologic diseases, cancers, and other types of disorders. For all these reasons, the field of immunology has captured the attention of clinicians, scientists, and the lay public.

This chapter introduces the nomenclature of immunology, important general properties of all immune responses, and the cells and tissues that are the principal components of the immune system. In particular, the following questions are addressed:

- What types of immune responses protect individuals from infections?
- What are the important characteristics of immunity, and what mechanisms are responsible for these characteristics?

- How are the cells and tissues of the immune system organized to find and respond to microbes in ways that lead to their elimination?

We conclude the chapter with a brief overview of immune responses against microbes. The basic principles introduced here set the stage for more detailed discussions of immune responses in later chapters. A glossary of the important terms used in this book is provided in Appendix I.

INNATE AND ADAPTIVE IMMUNITY

Host defense mechanisms consist of innate immunity, which mediates the initial protection against infections, and adaptive immunity, which develops more slowly and provides more specialized and effective defense against infections (Fig. 1–3). **Innate immunity,** also called natural immunity or native immunity, is always present in healthy individuals (hence the term innate), prepared

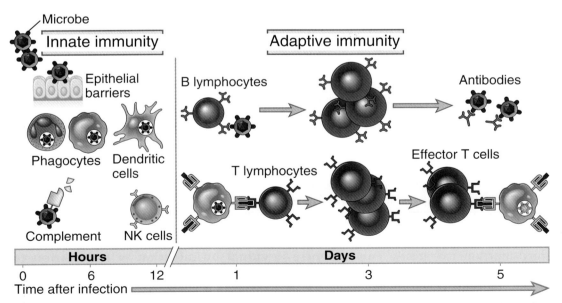

FIGURE 1–3 Principal mechanisms of innate and adaptive immunity. The mechanisms of innate immunity provide the initial defense against infections. Some mechanisms (e.g., epithelial barriers) prevent infections, and other mechanisms (e.g., phagocytes, natural killer [NK] cells, the complement system) eliminate microbes. Adaptive immune responses develop later and are mediated by lymphocytes and their products. Antibodies block infections and eliminate microbes, and T lymphocytes eradicate intracellular microbes. The kinetics of the innate and adaptive immune responses are approximations and may vary in different infections.

to block the entry of microbes and rapidly eliminate microbes that do succeed in entering host tissues. **Adaptive immunity,** also called specific immunity or acquired immunity, requires expansion and differentiation of lymphocytes in response to microbes before it can provide effective defense; that is, it adapts to the presence of microbial invaders. Innate immunity is phylogenetically older, and the more specialized and powerful adaptive immune system evolved later.

The first line of defense in innate immunity is provided by epithelial barriers and by cells and natural antibiotics present in epithelia, all of which function to block the entry of microbes. If microbes do breach epithelia and enter the tissues or circulation, they are attacked by phagocytes, specialized lymphocytes called natural killer cells, and several plasma proteins, including the proteins of the complement system. All these mechanisms of innate immunity specifically recognize and react against microbes. In addition to providing early defense against infections, innate immune responses enhance adaptive immune responses against the infectious agents. The components and mechanisms of innate immunity are discussed in detail in Chapter 2.

Defense against infectious microbes additionally requires adaptive immune responses, especially with microbes that are pathogenic for humans (i.e., capable of causing disease) and may have evolved to resist innate immunity. **The adaptive immune system consists of lymphocytes and their products, such as antibodies.** Whereas the mechanisms of innate immunity recognize structures shared by classes of microbes, the cells of adaptive immunity (lymphocytes) express receptors that specifically recognize a much wider variety of molecules produced by microbes as well as noninfectious substances. These substances are called **antigens.** Adaptive immune responses often use the cells and molecules of the innate immune system to eliminate microbes, and adaptive immunity functions to greatly enhance these antimicrobial mechanisms of innate immunity. For example, antibodies (a component of adaptive immunity) bind to microbes, and these coated microbes avidly bind to and activate phagocytes (a component of innate immunity), which ingest and destroy the microbes. Similar examples of the cooperation between innate and adaptive immunity are discussed in later chapters.

TYPES OF ADAPTIVE IMMUNITY

The two types of adaptive immunity, humoral immunity and cell-mediated immunity, are mediated by different cells and molecules and provide defense against extracellular microbes and intracellular microbes, respectively (Fig. 1–4). **Humoral immunity** is mediated by proteins called **antibodies,** which are produced by cells called **B lymphocytes.** Antibodies are secreted into the circulation and mucosal fluids, and they neutralize and eliminate microbes and microbial toxins that are present outside of host cells, in the blood and in the lumens of mucosal organs, such as the gastrointestinal and respiratory tracts. One of the most important functions of antibodies is to stop microbes that are present at mucosal surfaces and in the blood from gaining access to and colonizing host cells and connective tissues. In this way, antibodies prevent infections from ever being established. Antibodies cannot gain access to microbes that live and divide inside infected cells. Defense against such intracellular microbes is called **cell-mediated immunity** because it is mediated by cells, which are called **T lymphocytes.** Some T lymphocytes activate phagocytes to destroy microbes that have been ingested by the phagocytes into intracellular vesicles. Other T lymphocytes kill any type of host cells that are harboring infectious microbes in the cytoplasm. Thus, the antibodies produced by B lymphocytes recognize extracellular microbial antigens, whereas T lymphocytes recognize antigens produced by intracellular microbes. Another important difference between B and T lymphocytes is that most T cells recognize only protein antigens, whereas B cells and antibodies are able to recognize many different types of molecules, including proteins, carbohydrates, nucleic acids, and lipids.

Immunity may be induced in an individual by infection or vaccination (active immunity) or conferred on an individual by transfer of antibodies or lymphocytes from an actively immunized individual (passive immunity). In **active immunity,** an individual exposed to the antigens of a microbe mounts an active response to eradicate the infection and develops resistance to later infection by that

FIGURE 1–4 Types of adaptive immunity. In humoral immunity, B lymphocytes secrete antibodies that eliminate extracellular microbes. In cell-mediated immunity, different types of T lymphocytes recruit and activate phagocytes to destroy ingested microbes and kill infected cells.

microbe. Such an individual is said to be immune to that microbe, in contrast with a naive individual, not previously exposed to that microbe's antigens. We are concerned mainly with the mechanisms of active immunity. In **passive immunity,** a naive individual receives antibodies or cells (e.g., lymphocytes, feasible only in genetically identical [inbred] animals) from another individual already immune to an infection; for the lifetime of the transferred antibodies or cells, the recipient is able to combat the infection. Passive immunity is therefore useful for rapidly conferring immunity even before the individual is able to mount an active response, but it does not induce long-lived resistance to

the infection. The only physiologic example of passive immunity is seen in newborns, whose immune systems are not mature enough to respond to many pathogens but who are protected against infections by acquiring antibodies from their mothers through the placenta and breast milk.

PROPERTIES OF ADAPTIVE IMMUNE RESPONSES

Several properties of adaptive immune responses are crucial for the effectiveness of these responses in combating infections (Fig. 1–5).

Feature	Functional significance
Specificity	Ensures that distinct antigens elicit responses that target those antigens
Diversity	Enables immune system to respond to a large variety of antigens
Memory	Leads to rapid and enhanced responses to repeated exposures to the same antigens
Clonal expansion	Increases number of antigen-specific lymphocytes to keep pace with microbes
Specialization	Generates responses that are optimal for defense against different types of microbes
Contraction and homeostasis	Allows immune system to respond to newly encountered antigens
Nonreactivity to self	Prevents injury to the host during responses to foreign antigens

FIGURE 1–5 Properties of adaptive immune responses. This table summarizes the important properties of adaptive immune responses and how each feature contributes to host defense against microbes.

Specificity and Diversity

The adaptive immune system is capable of distinguishing among millions of different antigens or portions of antigens. **Specificity** is the ability to distinguish between many different antigens. It implies that the total collection of lymphocyte specificities, sometimes called the **lymphocyte repertoire,** is extremely **diverse.** The basis for this remarkable specificity and diversity is that lymphocytes express clonally distributed receptors for antigens, meaning that the total population of lymphocytes consists of many different clones (each made up of one cell and its progeny), and each clone expresses an antigen receptor that is different from the receptors of all other clones. The **clonal selection hypothesis,** formulated in the 1950s, correctly predicted that clones of lymphocytes specific for different antigens develop before an encounter with these antigens, and each antigen elicits an immune response by selecting and activating the lymphocytes of a specific clone (Fig. 1–6). We now know the molecular basis for how the specificity and diversity of lymphocytes are generated (see Chapter 4).

The **diversity** of the lymphocyte repertoire, which enables the immune system to respond to a vast number and variety of antigens, also means that very few cells, perhaps as few as one in 100,000 or one in 1 million lymphocytes, are specific for any one antigen. The total number of naive (unactivated) lymphocytes that can recognize and react against any one antigen ranges from about 1,000 to 10,000 cells. To mount an effective defense against microbes, these few cells have to give rise to a large number of lymphocytes capable of destroying the microbes. The remarkable effectiveness of immune responses is attributable to several features of adaptive immunity, including (1) marked expansion of the pool of lymphocytes specific for any antigen on exposure to that antigen, (2) positive feedback loops that amplify immune responses, and (3) selection mechanisms that preserve the most useful lymphocytes. These characteristics of the adaptive immune system are described in later chapters.

Memory

The immune system mounts larger and more effective responses to repeated exposures to the same antigen. The response to the first exposure to antigen, called the **primary immune response,** is mediated by lymphocytes called naive lymphocytes that are seeing antigen for the first time (Fig. 1–7). The term naive refers to these cells being immunologically inexperienced, not having previously responded to antigens. Subsequent encounters with the same antigen lead to responses called **secondary immune responses** that usually are more rapid, larger, and better able to eliminate the antigen than primary responses. Secondary responses are the result of the activation of memory lymphocytes, which are long-lived cells that were induced during the primary immune response. **Immunologic memory** optimizes the ability of the immune system to combat persistent and recurrent infections, because each encounter with a microbe generates more memory cells and activates previously generated memory cells. Memory also is one of the reasons why vaccines confer long-lasting protection against infections.

Lymphocyte clones with diverse receptors arise in generative lymphoid organs

Clones of mature lymphocytes specific for many antigens enter lymphoid tissues

Antigen-specific clones are activated ("selected") by antigens

Antigen-specific immune responses occur

Lymphocyte precursor

Mature lymphocytes

Antigen X   Antigen Y

Anti-X antibody   Anti-Y antibody

FIGURE 1–6 Clonal selection. Mature lymphocytes with receptors for many antigens develop before encountering these antigens. A clone refers to a population of lymphocytes with identical antigen receptors and therefore specificities; all these cells are presumably derived from one precursor cell. Each antigen (e.g., X and Y) selects a preexisting clone of specific lymphocytes and stimulates the proliferation and differentiation of that clone. The diagram shows only B lymphocytes giving rise to antibody-secreting cells, but the same principle applies to T lymphocytes. The antigens shown are surface molecules of microbes, but clonal selection also is true for extracellular soluble and intracellular antigens.

Other Features of Adaptive Immunity

Adaptive immune responses have other characteristics that are important for their functions (see Fig. 1–5). When lymphocytes are activated by antigens, they undergo proliferation, generating many thousands of clonal progeny cells, all with the same antigen specificity. This process, called **clonal expansion,** rapidly increases the number of cells specific for the antigen encountered, enabling few antigen-specific lymphocytes to serve their defensive role, and ensures that adaptive immunity keeps pace with rapidly proliferating microbes. Immune responses are specialized, and different responses are designed to defend best against different classes of microbes. All immune responses are self-limited and decline as the infection is eliminated, allowing the system

to return to a resting state, prepared to respond to another infection.

The immune system is able to react against an enormous number and variety of microbes and other foreign antigens, but it normally does not react against the host's own potentially antigenic substances—so-called **self antigens.** This unresponsiveness to self is called **immunological tolerance**, referring to the ability of the immune system to coexist with (tolerate) potentially antigenic self molecules, cells, and tissues.

CELLS OF THE IMMUNE SYSTEM

The cells of the adaptive immune system consist of lymphocytes, antigen-presenting cells that

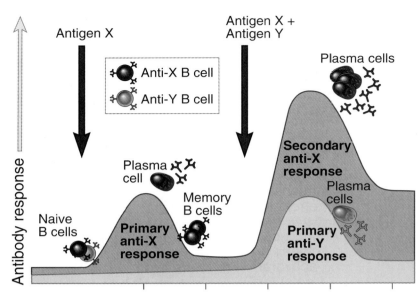

FIGURE 1–7 Primary and secondary immune responses. Antigens X and Y induce the production of different antibodies (a reflection of specificity). The secondary response to antigen X is more rapid and larger than the primary response (illustrating memory) and is different from the primary response to antigen Y (again reflecting specificity). Antibody levels decline with time after each immunization. The level of antibody produced is shown as arbitrary values and varies with the type of antigen exposure. Only B cells are shown, but the same features are seen with T cell responses to antigens. The time after immunization may be 1-3 weeks for a primary response and 2-7 days for a secondary response, but the kinetics vary depending on the antigen and nature of immunization.

capture and display microbial antigens, and effector cells (which include activated lymphocytes and other cells, particularly other leukocytes) that eliminate microbes (Fig. 1–8). This section describes the important functional properties of the major cell populations; a discussion of cellular morphology may be found in histology textbooks. The cells of innate immunity are described in Chapter 2.

Lymphocytes

Lymphocytes are the only cells that produce receptors specific for diverse antigens and are the key mediators of adaptive immunity. Although all lymphocytes are morphologically similar and rather unremarkable in appearance, they are heterogeneous in lineage, function, and phenotype and are capable of complex biologic responses and activities (Fig. 1–9). These cells often are distinguishable by surface proteins that may be identified using panels of monoclonal antibodies. The standard nomenclature for these proteins is the **CD** (cluster of differentiation) numerical designation, which is used to delineate surface proteins that define a particular cell type or stage of cell differentiation and that are recognized by a

cluster or group of antibodies. (A list of CD molecules mentioned in the book is provided in Appendix II.)

As alluded to earlier, B lymphocytes are the only cells capable of producing antibodies; therefore they are the cells that mediate humoral immunity. B cells express membrane forms of antibodies that serve as the receptors that recognize antigens and initiate the process of activation of the cells. Soluble antigens and antigens on the surface of microbes and other cells may bind to these B lymphocyte antigen receptors, initiating the process of B cell activation. This leads to the secretion of soluble forms of antibodies with the same antigen specificity as the membrane receptors.

T lymphocytes are responsible for cell-mediated immunity. The antigen receptors of most T lymphocytes recognize only peptide fragments of protein antigens that are bound to specialized peptide display molecules called major histocompatibility complex (MHC) molecules on the surface of specialized cells called antigen-presenting cells (see Chapter 3). Among T lymphocytes, CD4+ T cells are called **helper T cells** because they help B lymphocytes to produce antibodies and help phagocytes to destroy ingested microbes. CD8+ T lymphocytes

Cell type	Principal function(s)
Lymphocytes: B lymphocytes; T lymphocytes; natural killer cells *Blood lymphocyte*	Specific recognition of antigens: B lymphocytes: mediators of humoral immunity T lymphocytes: mediators of cell-mediated immunity Natural killer cells: cells of innate immunity
Antigen-presenting cells: dendritic cells; macrophages; follicular dendritic cells *Dendritic cell* *Blood monocyte*	Capture of antigens for display to lymphocytes: Dendritic cells: initiation of T cell responses Macrophages: effector phase of cell-mediated immunity Follicular dendritic cells: display of antigens to B lymphocytes in humoral immune responses
Effector cells: T lymphocytes; macrophages; granulocytes *Neutrophil*	Elimination of antigens: T lymphocytes: helper T cells and cytotoxic T lymphocytes Macrophages and monocytes: cells of the mononuclear phagocyte system Granulocytes: neutrophils, eosinophils

FIGURE 1–8 Principal cells of the immune system. This table shows the major cell types involved in immune responses, and the key functions of these cells. Micrographs in the left panels illustrate the morphology of some cells of each type. Note that tissue macrophages are derived from blood monocytes.

are called **cytotoxic T lymphocytes** (CTLs) because they kill cells harboring intracellular microbes. Some CD4$^+$ T cells belong to a special subset that functions to prevent or limit immune responses; these are called **regulatory T lymphocytes.** Another class of lymphocytes is called **natural killer (NK) cells,** which also kill infected host cells, but unlike B and T cells, they do not express clonally distributed antigen receptors. NK cells are components of innate immunity, capable of rapidly attacking infected cells.

All lymphocytes arise from stem cells in the bone marrow (Fig. 1–10). **B lymphocytes mature in the bone marrow, and T lymphocytes mature in an organ called the thymus.** These sites in which mature lymphocytes are produced (generated) are called the **generative lymphoid organs.** Mature lymphocytes leave the generative lymphoid organs and enter the circulation and the **peripheral lymphoid organs,** where they may encounter antigen for which they express specific receptors.

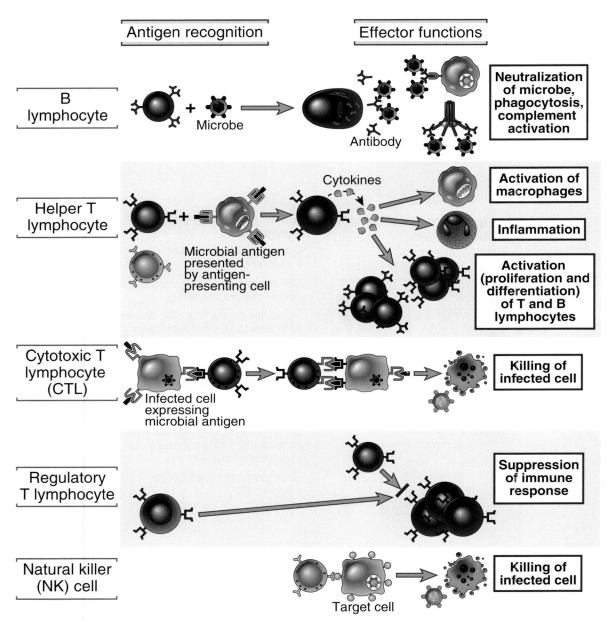

FIGURE 1–9 Classes of lymphocytes. Different classes of lymphocytes recognize distinct types of antigens and differentiate into effector cells whose function is to eliminate the antigens. B lymphocytes recognize soluble or cell surface antigens and differentiate into antibody-secreting cells. Helper T lymphocytes recognize antigens on the surfaces of antigen-presenting cells and secrete cytokines, which stimulate different mechanisms of immunity and inflammation. Cytotoxic T lymphocytes recognize antigens in infected cells and kill these cells. (Note that T lymphocytes recognize peptides that are displayed by MHC molecules, discussed in Chapter 3.) Regulatory T cells limit the activation of other lymphocytes, especially of T cells, and prevent autoimmunity. Natural killer cells recognize changes on the surface of infected cells and kill these cells. NK cells are cells of innate immunity, and all the other lymphocytes are cells of the adaptive immune system.

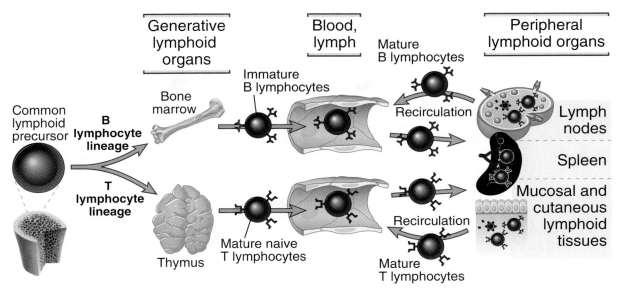

FIGURE 1–10 Maturation of lymphocytes. Lymphocytes develop from precursors in the generative lymphoid organs (bone marrow and thymus). Mature lymphocytes enter the peripheral lymphoid organs, where they respond to foreign antigens and recirculate in the blood and lymph.

When naive lymphocytes recognize microbial antigens and also receive additional signals induced by microbes, the antigen-specific lymphocytes proliferate and differentiate into effector cells and memory cells (Fig. 1–11). **Naive lymphocytes** express receptors for antigens but do not perform the functions that are required to eliminate antigens. These cells reside in and circulate between peripheral lymphoid organs and survive for several weeks or months, waiting to find and respond to antigen. If they are not activated by antigen, naive lymphocytes die by the process of apoptosis and are replaced by new cells that have arisen in the generative lymphoid organs. The differentiation of naive lymphocytes into effector cells and memory cells is initiated by antigen recognition, thus ensuring that the immune response that develops is specific for the antigen. **Effector cells** are the differentiated progeny of naive cells that have the ability to produce molecules that function to eliminate antigens. The effector cells in the B lymphocyte lineage are antibody-secreting cells, called **plasma cells.** Plasma cells develop in response to antigenic stimulation in the peripheral lymphoid organs, where they may stay and produce antibodies. Antibody-secreting cells, called **plasmablasts,** are also

present in the blood. Some of these migrate to the bone marrow, where they mature into long-lived plasma cells and continue to produce small amounts of antibody long after the infection is eradicated, providing immediate protection in case the infection recurs.

Effector $CD4^+$ T cells (helper T cells) produce proteins called **cytokines** that activate B cells, macrophages, and other cell types, thereby mediating the helper function of this lineage. Effector $CD8^+$ T cells (CTLs) have the machinery to kill infected host cells. The development and functions of these effector cells are discussed in later chapters. Effector T lymphocytes are short-lived and die as the antigen is eliminated.

Memory cells, also generated from the progeny of antigen-stimulated lymphocytes, do survive for long periods in the absence of antigen. Therefore, the frequency of memory cells increases with age, presumably because of exposure to environmental microbes. In fact, memory cells make up less than 5% of peripheral blood T cells in a newborn, but 50% or more in an adult. Memory cells are functionally inactive; they do not perform effector functions unless stimulated by antigen. When memory cells encounter the same antigen that induced their development, the cells rapidly respond to initiate secondary immune responses. The signals that

FIGURE 1–11 Stages in the life history of lymphocytes. A, Naive lymphocytes recognize foreign antigens to initiate adaptive immune responses. Naive lymphocytes need signals in addition to antigens to proliferate and differentiate into effector cells; these additional signals are not shown. Effector cells, which develop from naive cells, function to eliminate antigens. The effector cells of the B lymphocyte lineage are antibody-secreting plasma cells (some of which are long-lived). The effector cells of the CD4 T lymphocyte lineage produce cytokines. (The effector cells of the CD8 lineage are CTLs; these are not shown.) Other progeny of the antigen-stimulated lymphocytes differentiate into long-lived memory cells. **B,** The important characteristics of naive, effector, and memory cells in the B and T lymphocyte lineages are summarized. The generation and functions of effector cells, including changes in migration patterns and types of immunoglobulin produced, are described in later chapters.

generate and maintain memory cells are not well understood but include cytokines.

Antigen-Presenting Cells

The common portals of entry for microbes— the skin, gastrointestinal tract, and respiratory tract—contain specialized antigen-presenting cells (APCs) located in the epithelium that capture antigens, transport them to peripheral lymphoid tissues, and display (present) them to lymphocytes. This function of antigen capture and presentation is best understood for a cell type that is called **dendritic cells** because of their long surface membrane processes. Dendritic cells capture protein antigens of microbes entering through the epithelia and transport the antigens to regional lymph nodes, where the antigen-bearing dendritic cells display portions of the antigens for recognition by T lymphocytes. If a microbe has invaded through the epithelium, it may be phagocytosed by macrophages that live in tissues and in various organs. Microbes or their antigens that enter lymphoid organs may be captured by dendritic cells or macrophages that reside in these organs and presented to lymphocytes. Dendritic cells are the most effective APCs for initiating T cell responses. The process of antigen presentation to T cells is described in Chapter 3.

Cells that are specialized to display antigens to T lymphocytes have another important feature that gives them the ability to trigger T cell responses. These specialized cells respond to microbes by producing surface and secreted proteins that are required, together with antigen, to activate naive T lymphocytes to proliferate and differentiate into effector cells. Specialized cells that display antigens to T cells and provide additional activating signals sometimes are called professional APCs. The prototypic professional APCs are dendritic cells, but macrophages, B cells, and a few other cell types may serve the same function in various immune responses.

Less is known about cells that may capture antigens for display to B lymphocytes. B lymphocytes may directly recognize the antigens of microbes (either released or on the surface of the microbes), or macrophages lining lymphatic channels may capture antigens and display them to B cells. A type of cell called the **follicular dendritic cell** resides in the germinal centers of lymphoid follicles in the peripheral lymphoid organs and displays antigens that stimulate the differentiation of B cells in the follicles (see Chapter 7). Follicular dendritic cells (FDCs) do not present antigens to T cells and differ from the dendritic cells described earlier that function as APCs for T lymphocytes.

Effector Cells

The cells that eliminate microbes are called effector cells and consist of lymphocytes and other leukocytes. The effector cells of the B and T lymphocyte lineages were mentioned earlier. The elimination of microbes often requires the participation of other, nonlymphoid leukocytes, such as granulocytes and macrophages. These leukocytes may function as effector cells in both innate immunity and adaptive immunity. In innate immunity, macrophages and some granulocytes directly recognize microbes and eliminate them (see Chapter 2). In adaptive immunity, the products of B and T lymphocytes enhance the activities of macrophages and recruit other leukocytes and activate them to kill microbes.

TISSUES OF THE IMMUNE SYSTEM

The tissues of the immune system consist of the generative lymphoid organs, in which T and B lymphocytes mature and become competent to respond to antigens, and the peripheral lymphoid organs, in which adaptive immune responses to microbes are initiated (see Fig. 1–10). The generative (also called primary or central) lymphoid organs are described in Chapter 4, when we discuss the process of lymphocyte maturation. The following section highlights some of the features of peripheral (or secondary) lymphoid organs that are important for the development of adaptive immunity.

Peripheral Lymphoid Organs

The peripheral lymphoid organs, which consist of the lymph nodes, the spleen, and the mucosal and cutaneous immune systems, are organized to optimize interactions of antigens, APCs, and lymphocytes in a way that promotes the development of adaptive immune responses. T and B lymphocytes must locate microbes that enter at any site in the body, then respond to these microbes and eliminate them. In addition, as previously discussed, in the normal immune system very few of these lymphocytes are specific for any one antigen. It is not possible for the few lymphocytes specific for any antigen to patrol all possible sites of antigen entry. The anatomic organization of peripheral lymphoid organs enables APCs to concentrate antigens in these organs and lymphocytes to locate and respond to the antigens. This organization is complemented by a remarkable ability of lymphocytes to circulate throughout the body in such a way that naive lymphocytes preferentially go to the specialized organs in which antigen is concentrated, and effector cells go to sites of infection where microbes must be eliminated. Furthermore, different types of lymphocytes often need to communicate to generate effective immune responses. For example, helper T cells specific for an antigen interact with and help B lymphocytes specific for the same antigen, resulting in antibody production. An important function of lymphoid organs is to bring these rare cells together so that they interact productively.

Lymph nodes are encapsulated nodular aggregates of lymphoid tissues located along lymphatic channels throughout the body (Fig. 1–12). Fluid constantly leaks out of blood vessels in all epithelia and connective tissues and most parenchymal organs. This fluid, called **lymph,** is drained by lymphatic vessels from the tissues to the lymph nodes and eventually back into the blood circulation. Therefore, the lymph contains a mixture of substances absorbed from epithelia and tissues. As the lymph passes through lymph nodes, APCs in the nodes are able to sample the antigens of microbes that may enter through epithelia into tissues. In addition, dendritic cells pick up antigens of microbes from epithelia and other tissues and transport these antigens to the lymph nodes. The net result of these processes of antigen capture and transport is that the antigens of microbes entering through epithelia or colonizing tissues become concentrated in draining lymph nodes.

The **spleen** is a highly vascularized abdominal organ that serves the same role in immune responses to blood-borne antigens as that of lymph nodes in responses to lymph-borne antigens (Fig. 1–13). Blood entering the spleen flows through a network of channels (sinusoids). Blood-borne antigens are trapped and

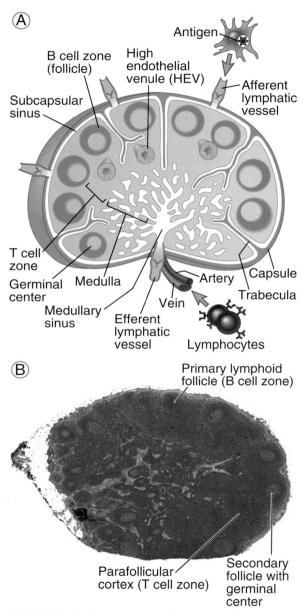

FIGURE 1–12 Morphology of lymph nodes. A, Schematic diagram shows the structural organization of a lymph node. **B,** Light micrograph shows a cross section of a lymph node with numerous follicles in the cortex, some of which contain lightly stained central areas (germinal centers).

FIGURE 1–13 Morphology of the spleen. A, Schematic diagram shows a splenic arteriole surrounded by the periarteriolar lymphoid sheath (PALS) and attached follicle containing a prominent germinal center. The PALS and lymphoid follicles together constitute the white pulp. **B,** Light micrograph of a section of spleen shows an arteriole with the PALS and a follicle with a germinal center. These are surrounded by the red pulp, which is rich in vascular sinusoids.

concentrated by dendritic cells and macrophages in the spleen. The spleen contains abundant phagocytes, which ingest and destroy microbes in the blood.

The **cutaneous immune system** and **mucosal immune system** are specialized collections of lymphoid tissues, APCs, and effector molecules located in and under the epithelia of the skin and the gastrointestinal and respiratory tracts, respectively. Although most of the immune cells in these tissues are diffusely scattered beneath the epithelial barriers, there are discrete collections of lymphocytes and APCs organized in a similar way as in lymph nodes. For example,

pharyngeal tonsils and Peyer's patches of the intestine are two anatomically defined mucosal lymphoid tissues (Fig. 1–14). At any time, at least a quarter of the body's lymphocytes are in the mucosal tissues and skin (reflecting the large size of these tissues), and many of these are memory cells. Cutaneous and mucosal lymphoid tissues are sites of immune responses to antigens that breach epithelia. A challenge for the cutaneous and mucosal immune systems is to be able to respond to pathogens but not react to the enormous numbers of usually harmless commensal microbes present at the epithelial barriers. This is accomplished by several incompletely understood mechanisms, including the action of regulatory T cells and dendritic cells that suppress rather than activate T lymphocytes.

Within the peripheral lymphoid organs, T lymphocytes and B lymphocytes are segregated into different anatomic compartments (Fig. 1–15). In lymph nodes, the B cells are concentrated in discrete structures, called **follicles,** located around the periphery, or cortex, of each node. If the B cells in a follicle have recently responded to an antigen, this follicle may contain a central lightly staining region called a **germinal center.** The role of germinal centers in the production of antibodies is described in Chapter 7. The T lymphocytes are concentrated outside but adjacent to the follicles, in the paracortex. The follicles contain the FDCs described earlier that are involved in the activation of B cells, and the paracortex contains the dendritic cells that present antigens to T lymphocytes. In the spleen, T lymphocytes are concentrated in periarteriolar lymphoid sheaths surrounding small arterioles, and B cells reside in the follicles.

The anatomic organization of peripheral lymphoid organs is tightly regulated to allow immune responses to develop after stimulation by antigens. B lymphocytes are attracted to and retained in the follicles because of the action of a class of cytokines called **chemokines** (chemoattractant cytokines; chemokines and other cytokines are discussed in more detail in later chapters). FDCs in the follicles constantly secrete a particular chemokine for which naive B cells express a receptor, called CXCR5. The chemokine that binds to CXCR5 attracts B cells from the blood into the follicles of lymphoid organs. Similarly, T cells are segregated in the paracortex of lymph nodes and the periarteriolar lymphoid sheaths of the spleen, because naive T lymphocytes express a receptor,

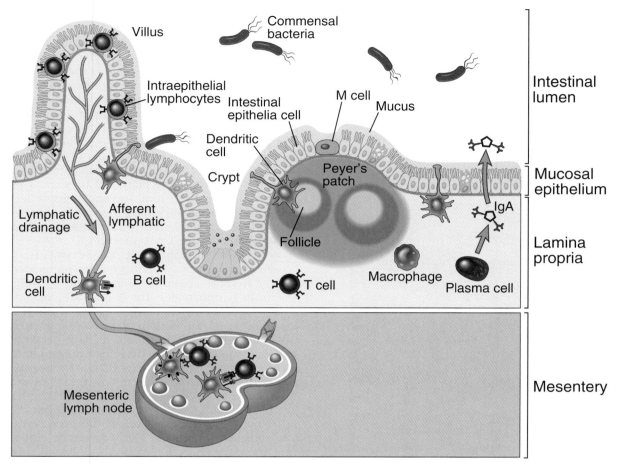

FIGURE 1–14 Mucosal immune system. Schematic diagram of the mucosal immune system uses the small bowel as an example. Many commensal bacteria are present in the lumen. The mucus-secreting epithelium provides an innate barrier to microbial invasion (discussed in Chapter 2). Specialized epithelial cells, such as M cells, promote the transport of antigens from the lumen into underlying tissues. Cells in the lamina propria, including dendritic cells, T lymphocytes, and macrophages, provide innate and adaptive immune defense against invading microbes; some of these cells are organized into specialized structures, such as Peyer's patches in the small intestine. Immunoglobulin A (IgA) is a type of antibody abundantly produced in mucosal tissues that is transported into the lumen, where it binds and neutralizes microbes (Chapter 8).

called CCR7, that recognizes chemokines that are produced in these regions of the lymph nodes and spleen. As a result, T lymphocytes are recruited from the blood into the parafollicular cortex region of the lymph node and the periarteriolar lymphoid sheaths of the spleen. When the lymphocytes are activated by antigens, they alter their expression of chemokine receptors. The B cells and T cells then migrate toward each other and meet at the edge of follicles, where helper T cells interact with and help B cells to differentiate into antibody-producing cells (see Chapter 7). Thus, these lymphocyte populations are kept apart from each other until it is useful for them to interact, after exposure to an antigen. This is an excellent example of how the structure of lymphoid organs ensures that the cells that have recognized and responded to an antigen interact and communicate with one another only when necessary.

Many of the activated lymphocytes, especially the T cells, ultimately exit the node through efferent lymphatic vessels and leave the spleen through veins. These activated lymphocytes end up in the circulation and can go to distant sites of infection.

FIGURE 1–15 Segregation of T and B lymphocytes in different regions of peripheral lymphoid organs. **A,** Schematic diagram illustrates the path by which naive T and B lymphocytes migrate to different areas of a lymph node. Naive B and T lymphocytes enter through a high endothelial venule (HEV), shown in cross section, and are drawn to different areas of the node by chemokines that are produced in these areas and bind selectively to either cell type. Also shown is the migration of dendritic cells, which pick up antigens from epithelia, enter through afferent lymphatic vessels, and migrate to the T cell–rich areas of the node (Chapter 3). **B,** In this histologic section of a lymph node, the B lymphocytes, located in the follicles, are stained green, and the T cells, in the parafollicular cortex, are stained red using immunofluorescence. In this technique, a section of the tissue is stained with antibodies specific for T or B cells coupled to fluorochromes that emit different colors when excited at the appropriate wavelengths. The anatomic segregation of T and B cells also occurs in the spleen (not shown). *(Courtesy Drs. Kathryn Pape and Jennifer Walter, University of Minnesota Medical School, Minneapolis.)*

Lymphocyte Recirculation and Migration into Tissues

Naive lymphocytes constantly recirculate between the blood and peripheral lymphoid organs, where they may be activated by antigens to become effector cells, and the effector lymphocytes migrate from lymphoid tissues to sites of infection, where microbes are eliminated (Fig. 1–16). Thus, lymphocytes at distinct stages of their lives migrate to the different sites where they are needed for their functions. Migration of effector lymphocytes to sites of infection is most relevant for T cells, because effector T cells have to locate and eliminate microbes at these sites. By contrast, plasma cells do not need to migrate to sites of infection; instead, they secrete antibodies, and the antibodies enter the blood, where they may bind blood-borne pathogens or toxins. In addition, antibodies may be carried to tissue sites of infection by the circulation.

Naive T lymphocytes that have matured in the thymus and entered the circulation migrate to lymph nodes, where they can find antigens that enter through lymphatic vessels that drain epithelia and parenchymal organs. These naive T cells enter lymph nodes through specialized postcapillary venules, called **high endothelial venules** (HEVs). The adhesion molecules used by the T cells to bind to the endothelium are described in Chapter 6. Chemokines produced in the T cell zones of the lymph nodes and displayed on HEV surfaces bind to the chemokine receptor CCR7 expressed on naive T cells, which causes the T cells to bind tightly to HEVs. The naive T cells then migrate into the T cell zone, where antigens are displayed by dendritic cells. Naive B cells also enter lymphoid tissues, but then migrate to follicles in response to chemokines that bind CXCR5, the chemokine receptor expressed on these B cells.

In the lymph node, if a T cell specifically recognizes an antigen on a dendritic cell, that T cell forms stable conjugates with the dendritic cell and is activated. Such an encounter between an antigen and a specific lymphocyte is likely to be a random event, but most T cells in the body circulate through some lymph nodes at least once a day. As mentioned earlier and described further in Chapter 3, the likelihood of the correct T cell finding its antigen is increased in peripheral lymphoid organs, particularly lymph nodes,

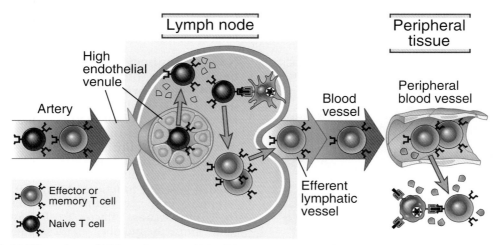

FIGURE 1–16 Migration of T lymphocytes. Naive T lymphocytes migrate from the blood through high endothelial venules into the T cell zones of lymph nodes, where the cells are activated by antigens. Activated T cells exit the nodes, enter the bloodstream, and migrate preferentially to peripheral tissues at sites of infection and inflammation. The adhesion molecules involved in the attachment of T cells to endothelial cells are described in Chapter 6.

because microbial antigens are concentrated in the same regions of these organs through which naive T cells circulate. Thus, T cells find the antigen they can recognize, and these T cells are activated to proliferate and differentiate. Naive cells that have not encountered specific antigens leave the lymph nodes and reenter the circulation. The effector cells that are generated upon T cell activation preferentially migrate into the tissues infected by microbes, where the T lymphocytes perform their function of eradicating the infection. Specific signals control these precise patterns of migration of naive and activated T cells (see Chapter 6).

B lymphocytes that recognize and respond to antigen in lymph node follicles differentiate into antibody-secreting cells, which either remain in the lymph nodes or migrate to the bone marrow (see Chapter 7).

Memory T cells consist of different populations; some cells recirculate through lymph nodes, where they can mount secondary responses to captured antigens, and other cells migrate to sites of infection, where they can respond rapidly to eliminate the infection.

We know less about lymphocyte circulation through the spleen or other lymphoid tissues. The spleen does not contain HEVs, but the general pattern of naive lymphocyte migration through this organ probably is similar to migration through lymph nodes.

OVERVIEW OF IMMUNE RESPONSES TO MICROBES

Now that we have described the major components of the immune system, it is useful to summarize the key features of immune responses to microbes. The focus here is on the physiologic function of the immune system—defense against infections. In subsequent chapters, each of these features is discussed in more detail.

Early Innate Immune Response to Microbes

The principal barriers between the host and the environment are the epithelia of the skin and the gastrointestinal and respiratory tracts. Infectious microbes usually enter through these routes and attempt to colonize the host. Epithelia serve as physical and functional barriers to infections, simultaneously impeding the entry of microbes and interfering with their growth through production of natural antimicrobial agents. If microbes are able to traverse these epithelia and enter tissues and the circulation, they encounter the defense mechanisms of innate immunity, which are designed to react rapidly against microbes and their products. Phagocytes, including neutrophils and macrophages, ingest microbes into vesicles and destroy them by producing microbicidal substances in these vesicles. Macrophages and dendritic cells that encounter microbes also secrete cytokines, which serve numerous functions.

The two major cellular reactions of innate immunity are **inflammation,** which is induced by cytokines and other molecules and serves to bring leukocytes and plasma proteins to the site of infection or injury, and **antiviral defense,** which is mediated by type I interferons (a particular family of cytokines) and NK cells. Many plasma proteins are involved in host defense, including the proteins of the complement system, which are activated by microbes, and whose products kill microbes and coat (opsonize) them for phagocytosis by macrophages and neutrophils. In addition to combating infections, innate immune responses stimulate subsequent adaptive immunity, providing signals that are essential for initiating the responses of antigen-specific T and B lymphocytes. The combined actions of the mechanisms of innate immunity can eradicate some infections and keep other pathogens in check until the more powerful adaptive immune response is activated.

Adaptive Immune Response

The adaptive immune system uses the following strategies to combat the majority of microbes:

- Secreted antibodies bind to extracellular microbes, block their ability to infect host cells, and promote their ingestion and subsequent destruction by phagocytes.
- Phagocytes ingest microbes and kill them, and helper T cells enhance the microbicidal abilities of the phagocytes.
- Helper T cells recruit leukocytes to destroy microbes and enhance epithelial barrier function to expel microbes.
- Cytotoxic T lymphocytes destroy cells infected by microbes that are inaccessible to antibodies.

Adaptive immune responses develop in steps, each of which corresponds to particular reactions of lymphocytes (Fig. 1–17).

Capture and Display of Microbial Antigens
Microbes that enter through epithelia, as well as their protein antigens, are captured by dendritic cells residing in these epithelia, and the cell-bound antigens are transported to draining lymph nodes. Protein antigens are processed in the dendritic cells to generate peptides that are displayed on the surface of the APCs bound to MHC molecules. Naive T cells recognize these peptide-MHC complexes, and this is the first step in the initiation of T cell responses. Protein antigens also are recognized by B lymphocytes in the lymphoid follicles of the peripheral lymphoid organs. Polysaccharides and other nonprotein antigens are captured in the lymphoid organs and are recognized by B lymphocytes but not by T cells.

As part of the innate immune response, the dendritic cells that present the antigen to naive T cells are activated to express molecules called costimulators and to secrete cytokines, both of which are needed, in addition to the antigen, to stimulate the proliferation and differentiation of T lymphocytes. The innate immune response to some microbes and polysaccharide antigens also results in the activation of the complement system, which generates cleavage products of proteins that have various immune functions. Some complement-generated products enhance the proliferation and differentiation of B lymphocytes. Thus, antigen (often referred to as signal 1) and molecules produced during innate immune responses (signal 2) function cooperatively to activate antigen-specific lymphocytes. The requirement for microbe-triggered signal 2 ensures that the adaptive immune response is induced by microbes and not by harmless substances. Signals generated in lymphocytes by the engagement of antigen receptors and receptors for costimulators lead to the transcription of various genes, which encode cytokines, cytokine receptors, effector molecules, and proteins that control cell survival and cycling. All these molecules are involved in the responses of the lymphocytes.

Cell-Mediated Immunity: Activation of T Lymphocytes and Elimination of Cell-Associated Microbes
When activated by antigen and costimulators in lymphoid organs, naive T cells secrete cytokines that function as growth factors and respond to other cytokines secreted by APCs. The combination of signals (antigen, costimulation, and cytokines) stimulates the proliferation of the T cells and their differentiation into effector T cells. The effector T cells generated in the lymphoid organ may migrate back into the blood and then into any site where the antigen (or microbe) is present. These effector cells are reactivated by

FIGURE 1–17 Phases of adaptive immune response. An adaptive immune response consists of distinct phases; the first three are recognition of antigen, activation of lymphocytes, and elimination of antigen (effector phase). The response declines as antigen-stimulated lymphocytes die by apoptosis, restoring the baseline steady state called homeostasis, and the antigen-specific cells that survive are responsible for memory. The duration of each phase may vary in different immune responses. These principles apply to both humoral immunity (mediated by B lymphocytes) and cell-mediated immunity (mediated by T lymphocytes).

antigen at sites of infection and perform the functions responsible for elimination of the microbes. Different classes of T cells differentiate into effector cells with distinct functional properties. Helper T cells secrete cytokines and express surface molecules that mediate their functions. Some of these activated helper T cells function to recruit neutrophils and other leukocytes to sites of infection; other helper cells activate macrophages to kill ingested microbes; and still other helper T cells stay in the lymphoid organs and help B lymphocytes. CTLs directly kill cells harboring microbes in the cytoplasm. These microbes may be viruses that infect many cell types or bacteria that are ingested by macrophages but have learned to escape from phagocytic vesicles into the cytoplasm (where they are inaccessible to the

killing machinery of phagocytes, which is largely confined to vesicles). By destroying the infected cells, CTLs eliminate the reservoirs of infection.

Humoral Immunity: Activation of B Lymphocytes and Elimination of Extracellular Microbes

On activation, B lymphocytes proliferate and then differentiate into plasma cells that secrete different classes of antibodies with distinct functions. Many polysaccharide and lipid antigens have multiple identical antigenic determinants (epitopes) that are able to engage many antigen receptor molecules on each B cell and initiate the process of B cell activation. Typical globular protein antigens are not able to bind to many antigen receptors, and the full response of B cells to protein antigens requires help from CD4[+] T cells. B cells ingest protein antigens, degrade them, and display peptides bound to MHC molecules for recognition by helper T cells. The helper T cells express cytokines and cell surface proteins, which work together to activate the B cells.

Some of the progeny of the expanded B cell clones differentiate into antibody-secreting cells. Each B cell secretes antibodies that have the same antigen-binding site as the cell surface antibodies (B cell antigen receptors) that first recognized the antigen. Polysaccharides and lipids stimulate secretion mainly of a class of antibody called immunoglobulin M (IgM). Protein antigens stimulate helper T cells, which induce the production of antibodies of different classes (IgG, IgA, and IgE). This production of different antibodies, all with the same specificity, is called **heavy-chain class (or isotype) switching;** it increases the defensive capability of the antibody response, enabling antibodies to serve many functions. Helper T cells also stimulate the production of antibodies with higher and higher affinity for the antigen. This process, called **affinity maturation,** improves the quality of the humoral immune response.

The humoral immune response defends against microbes in many ways. Antibodies bind to microbes and prevent them from infecting cells, thereby neutralizing the microbes. Antibodies coat (opsonize) microbes and target them for phagocytosis, because phagocytes (neutrophils and macrophages) express receptors for the antibodies. Additionally, antibodies activate the complement system, generating protein fragments that promote phagocytosis and destruction of microbes. Specialized types of antibodies and specialized transport mechanisms for antibodies serve distinct roles at particular anatomic sites, including the lumens of the respiratory and gastrointestinal tracts or the placenta and fetus.

Decline of Immune Responses and Immunologic Memory

The majority of effector lymphocytes induced by an infectious pathogen die by apoptosis after the microbe is eliminated, thus returning the immune system to its basal resting state, called **homeostasis.** This occurs because microbes provide essential stimuli for lymphocyte survival and activation and effector cells are short-lived.

Therefore, as the stimuli are eliminated, the activated lymphocytes are no longer kept alive. The initial activation of lymphocytes generates long-lived memory cells, which may survive for years after the infection and mount rapid and robust responses to a repeat encounter with the antigen.

SUMMARY

* The physiologic function of the immune system is to protect individuals against infections.
* Innate immunity is the early line of defense, mediated by cells and molecules that are always present and ready to eliminate infectious microbes.
* Adaptive immunity is mediated by lymphocytes stimulated by microbial antigens, requires clonal expansion and differentiation of the lymphocytes before it is effective, and responds more effectively against each successive exposure to a microbe.
* Lymphocytes are the cells of adaptive immunity and are the only cells with clonally distributed receptors with fine specificities for different antigens.
* Adaptive immunity consists of humoral immunity, in which antibodies neutralize and eradicate extracellular microbes and toxins, and cell-mediated immunity, in which T lymphocytes eradicate intracellular microbes.
* Adaptive immune responses consist of sequential phases: antigen recognition by lymphocytes, activation of the lymphocytes to proliferate and to differentiate into effector and memory cells, elimination of the microbes, decline of the immune response, and long-lived memory.
* Different populations of lymphocytes serve distinct functions and may be distinguished by the surface expression of particular membrane molecules.
* B lymphocytes are the only cells that produce antibodies. B lymphocytes express membrane antibodies that recognize antigens, and the progeny of activated B cells, called plasma cells, secrete the antibodies that neutralize and eliminate the antigen.
* T lymphocytes recognize peptide fragments of protein antigens displayed on

other cells. Helper T lymphocytes produce cytokines that activate phagocytes to destroy ingested microbes, recruit leukocytes, and activate B lymphocytes to produce antibodies. Cytotoxic T lymphocytes (CTLs) kill infected cells harboring microbes in the cytoplasm.

* Antigen-presenting cells (APCs) capture antigens of microbes that enter through epithelia, concentrate these antigens in lymphoid organs, and display the antigens for recognition by T cells.

* Lymphocytes and APCs are organized in peripheral lymphoid organs, where immune responses are initiated and develop.

* Naive lymphocytes circulate through peripheral lymphoid organs searching for foreign antigens. Effector T lymphocytes migrate to peripheral sites of infection, where they function to eliminate infectious microbes. Plasma cells remain in lymphoid organs and the bone marrow, where they secrete antibodies that enter the circulation and find and eliminate microbes.

REVIEW QUESTIONS

1. What are the two types of adaptive immunity, and what types of microbes do these adaptive immune responses combat?
2. What are the principal classes of lymphocytes, and how do they differ in function?
3. What are the important differences among naive, effector, and memory T and B lymphocytes?
4. Where are T and B lymphocytes located in lymph nodes, and how is their anatomic separation maintained?
5. How do naive and effector T lymphocytes differ in their patterns of migration?

Answers to and discussion of the Review Questions are available at studentconsult.com.

Innate Immunity
The Early Defense Against Infections

As multicellular organisms such as plants, invertebrates, and vertebrates arose during evolution, they had to develop mechanisms for defending themselves against microbial infections and for eliminating damaged and necrotic cells. The defense mechanisms that evolved first are always present in the organism, ready to recognize and eliminate microbes and dead cells; therefore, this type of host defense is known as **innate immunity,** also called natural immunity or native immunity. The cells and molecules that are responsible for innate immunity make up the innate immune system.

Innate immunity is the critical first step in host defense against infections. It efficiently targets microbes and is capable of controlling and even eradicating infections. The innate immune response is able to combat microbes immediately on infection; in contrast, the adaptive immune response needs to be induced by antigen and therefore is delayed. The innate immune response also instructs the adaptive immune system to respond to different microbes in ways that are effective for combating these microbes. Innate immunity is also a key participant in the clearance of dead tissues and the initiation of repair.

Before we consider adaptive immunity, the main topic of this book, we discuss the early defense reactions of innate immunity in this chapter. The discussion focuses on the following three questions:

1. How does the innate immune system recognize microbes and damaged cells?

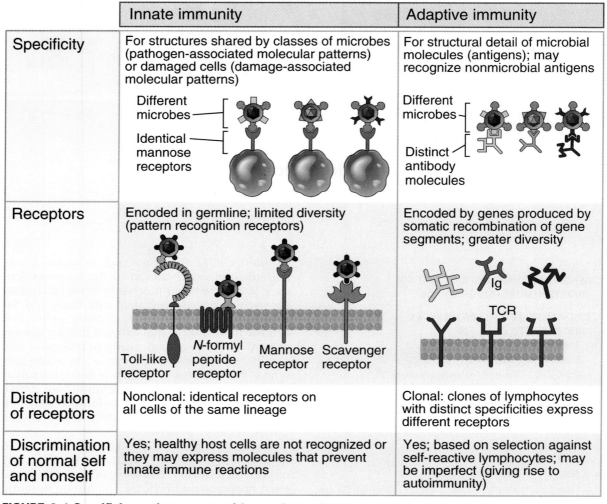

	Innate immunity	Adaptive immunity
Specificity	For structures shared by classes of microbes (pathogen-associated molecular patterns) or damaged cells (damage-associated molecular patterns)	For structural detail of microbial molecules (antigens); may recognize nonmicrobial antigens
Receptors	Encoded in germline; limited diversity (pattern recognition receptors)	Encoded by genes produced by somatic recombination of gene segments; greater diversity
Distribution of receptors	Nonclonal: identical receptors on all cells of the same lineage	Clonal: clones of lymphocytes with distinct specificities express different receptors
Discrimination of normal self and nonself	Yes; healthy host cells are not recognized or they may express molecules that prevent innate immune reactions	Yes; based on selection against self-reactive lymphocytes; may be imperfect (giving rise to autoimmunity)

FIGURE 2–1 Specificity and receptors of innate immunity and adaptive immunity. This table summarizes the important features of the specificity and receptors of innate and adaptive immunity, with select examples illustrated. Ig, Immunoglobulin (antibody); TCR, T cell receptor.

2. How do the different components of innate immunity function to combat different types of microbes?

3. How do innate immune reactions stimulate adaptive immune responses?

GENERAL FEATURES AND SPECIFICITY OF INNATE IMMUNE RESPONSES

The innate immune system performs its defensive functions with a restricted set of reactions, which are more limited than the more varied and specialized responses of adaptive immunity. The specificity of innate immunity is also different in several respects from the specificity of lymphocytes, the recognition systems of adaptive immunity (Fig. 2–1).

The two principal types of reactions of the innate immune system are inflammation and antiviral defense. Inflammation consists of the accumulation and activation of leukocytes and plasma proteins at sites of infection or tissue injury. These cells and proteins act together to kill mainly extracellular microbes and to eliminate damaged tissues. Innate immune defense against intracellular viruses is mediated mainly by natural killer (NK) cells, which kill virus-infected cells, and by cytokines called type I interferons, which block viral replication within host cells.

The innate immune system usually responds in the same way to repeat encounters with a microbe, whereas the adaptive immune system responds more efficiently to each successive encounter with a microbe. In other words, the innate immune system does not remember prior encounters with microbes and resets to baseline after each such encounter, whereas the adaptive immune system does remember encounters with microbes and reacts more strongly after each encounter. This phenomenon of immunologic memory in the adaptive immune system ensures that host defense reactions are highly effective against repeated or persistent infections, and memory is a basis for how vaccines work.

The innate immune system recognizes structures that are shared by various classes of microbes and are not present on normal host cells. The mechanisms of innate immunity recognize and respond to a limited number of microbial molecules, much less than the almost unlimited number of microbial and nonmicrobial antigens that are recognized by the adaptive immune system. Each component of innate immunity may recognize many bacteria, viruses, or fungi. For example, phagocytes express receptors for bacterial endotoxin, also called lipopolysaccharide (LPS), and other receptors for peptidoglycans, each of which is present in the cell walls of many bacterial species but is not produced by mammalian cells. Other receptors of phagocytes recognize terminal mannose residues, which are typical of bacterial but not mammalian glycoproteins. Mammalian cells recognize and respond to double-stranded ribonucleic acid (dsRNA), which is found in many viruses but not in mammalian cells, and to unmethylated CG-rich (CpG) oligonucleotides, which are common in microbial DNA but are not abundant in mammalian DNA. The microbial molecules that stimulate innate immunity are often called **pathogen-associated molecular patterns** (PAMPs), to indicate that they are present in infectious agents (pathogens) and shared by microbes of the same type (i.e., they are molecular patterns). The receptors of innate immunity that recognize these shared structures are called **pattern recognition receptors.**

The components of innate immunity have evolved to recognize structures of microbes that are often essential for the survival and infectivity of these microbes. This characteristic of innate immunity makes it a highly effective defense mechanism because a microbe cannot evade innate immunity simply by mutating or not expressing the targets of innate immune recognition: Microbes that do not express functional forms of these structures lose their ability to infect and colonize the host. In contrast, microbes frequently evade adaptive immunity by mutating the antigens that are recognized by lymphocytes, because these antigens are usually not required for the life of the microbes.

The innate immune system also recognizes molecules that are released from damaged or necrotic cells. Such molecules are called **damage-associated molecular patterns** (DAMPs). The subsequent responses to DAMPs serve to eliminate the damaged cells and to initiate the processes of tissue repair.

The receptors of the innate immune system are encoded in the germline and are not produced by somatic recombination of genes. These germline-encoded pattern recognition receptors have evolved as a protective adaptation of multicellular organisms against potentially harmful microbes. In contrast, the antigen receptors of lymphocytes, namely, antibodies and T cell receptors, are produced by somatic recombination of receptor genes during the maturation of these cells (see Chapter 4). Gene recombination can generate many more structurally different receptors than can be produced from inherited germline genes, but these different receptors cannot have a predetermined specificity for microbes. Therefore, the specificity of adaptive immunity is much more diverse than that of innate immunity, and the adaptive immune system is capable of recognizing many more chemically distinct structures. It is estimated that the total population of lymphocytes can recognize as many as a billion different antigens; in other words, these lymphocytes express as many as a billion antigen receptors, each with a unique specificity. By contrast, all the receptors of innate immunity probably recognize less than a thousand microbial patterns. Furthermore, the receptors of the adaptive immune system are clonally distributed, meaning that each clone of lymphocytes (B cells and T cells) has a different receptor specific for a particular antigen. In contrast, in the innate immune system the receptors are nonclonally distributed; that is, identical receptors are expressed on all the cells of a particular type, such as macrophages. Therefore, many cells of innate immunity may recognize and respond to the same microbe.

The innate immune system does not react against the host. This inability of the innate immune system to react against an individual's own, or self, cells and molecules results partly from the inherent specificity of innate immunity for microbial structures and partly from mammalian cell expression of regulatory molecules that prevent innate immune reactions. The adaptive immune system also discriminates between self and nonself; in the adaptive immune system, lymphocytes capable of recognizing self antigens are produced, but they die or are inactivated on encounter with self antigens.

The innate immune response can be considered as a series of reactions that provide defense at the following stages of microbial infections:

- At the portals of entry for microbes: Most microbial infections are acquired through the epithelia of the skin and gastrointestinal and respiratory systems. The earliest defense mechanisms active at these sites are epithelia providing physical barriers and antimicrobial molecules and lymphoid cells in these epithelia.
- In the tissues: Microbes that breach epithelia, as well as dead cells in tissues, are detected by resident macrophages, dendritic cells, and other sentinel cells. Some of these cells react mainly by secreting cytokines, which initiate the process of inflammation, and phagocytes destroy the microbes and eliminate the damaged cells.
- In the blood: Plasma proteins, including proteins of the complement system, react against microbes and promote their destruction.
- Viruses elicit special reactions, including the production of interferons from infected cells that inhibit infection of other cells and the killing of infected cells by NK cells.

We will return to a more detailed discussion of these components of innate immunity and their reactions later in the chapter. We start with a consideration of how microbes, damaged cells, and other foreign substances are detected, and how innate immune responses are triggered.

CELLULAR RECEPTORS FOR MICROBES AND DAMAGED CELLS

The receptors used by the innate immune system to react against microbes and damaged cells are expressed on phagocytes, dendritic cells, and many other cell types, including lymphocytes and epithelial and endothelial cells. These receptors are expressed in different cellular compartments where microbes may be located. Some are present on the cell surface; others are present in the endoplasmic reticulum and are rapidly recruited to vesicles (endosomes) into which microbial products are ingested; and still others are in the cytosol, where they function as sensors of cytoplasmic microbes (Fig. 2–2). Some of these same receptors respond to the products of damaged cells and a variety of foreign substances, such as crystals deposited in cells and tissues. These receptors for PAMPs and DAMPs belong to several protein families.

Toll-Like Receptors

Toll-like receptors (TLRs) are homologous to a *Drosophila* protein called *Toll*, which was discovered for its role in the development of the fly and later shown to be essential for protecting flies against infections. Different TLRs are specific for different components of microbes (Fig. 2–3). TLR-2 recognizes several bacterial lipoglycans; TLRs 3, 7, and 8 are specific for viral nucleic acids (e.g., dsRNA); TLR-4 is specific for bacterial LPS (endotoxin), TLR-5 for a bacterial flagellar protein called flagellin, and TLR-9 for unmethylated CpG oligonucleotides, which are more abundant in microbial DNA than in mammalian DNA. Some TLRs are present on the cell surface, where they recognize products of extracellular microbes, and other TLRs are in endosomes, into which microbes are ingested.

Signals generated by engagement of TLRs activate transcription factors that stimulate expression of genes encoding cytokines, enzymes, and other proteins involved in the antimicrobial functions of activated phagocytes and other cells (Fig. 2–4). Among the most important

FIGURE 2–2 Cellular locations of receptors of the innate immune system. Some receptors, such as certain Toll-like receptors (TLRs) and lectins, are located on cell surfaces; other TLRs are in endosomes. Some receptors for viral nucleic acids, bacterial peptides, and products of damaged cells are in the cytoplasm. NOD and RIG refer to the founding members of families of structurally homologous cytosolic receptors for bacterial and viral products, respectively. (Their full names are historical and do not reflect their functions.) There are four major families of cellular receptors in innate immunity: TLRs, CLRs (C-type lectin receptors), NLRs (NOD-like receptors) and RLRs (RIG-like receptors).

transcription factors activated by TLR signals are nuclear factor κB (NF-κB), which promotes expression of various cytokines and endothelial adhesion molecules, and interferon regulatory factors (IRFs), which stimulate production of the antiviral cytokines, type I interferons.

Rare inherited mutations of signaling molecules downstream of TLRs are associated with recurrent and severe infections, particularly bacterial pneumonia, highlighting the importance of these pathways in host defense against microbes.

NOD-Like Receptors and the Inflammasome

The **NOD-like receptors** (NLRs) are a large family of cytosolic receptors that sense DAMPs and PAMPs in the cytoplasm. All NLRs share structural features, including a domain called NOD (nucleotide oligomerization domain). Some NLRs recognize a wide variety of structurally unrelated substances and use a special signaling mechanism (Fig. 2–5). One of the

best-characterized and prototypic NLRs, called NLRP-3 (NOD-like receptor family, pyrin domain containing 3), senses the presence of microbial products; substances that indicate cell damage and death, including released adenosine triphosphate (ATP), uric acid crystals derived from nucleic acids, and changes in intracellular potassium ion (K^+) concentration; and endogenous substances that are deposited in cells and tissues in excessive amounts (e.g., cholesterol crystals, free fatty acids).

After recognition of these varied substances, or perhaps some common chemical alteration induced by these substances, NLRP-3 oligomerizes with an adaptor protein and an inactive (pro) form of the enzyme caspase-1. Once recruited, caspase-1 is activated and cleaves a precursor form of the cytokine interleukin-1β (IL-1β) to generate biologically active IL-1β. As discussed later, IL-1 induces acute inflammation and causes fever; thus the name pyrin domain in the NLRP-3 protein (Greek, pyro = burn). This

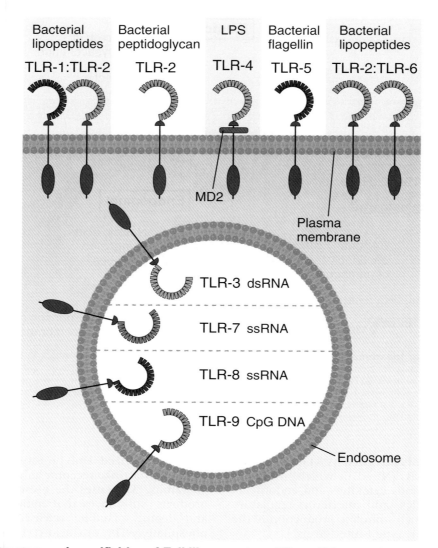

FIGURE 2–3 Structure and specificities of Toll-like receptors. Different TLRs respond to many different, structurally diverse products of microbes. Endosomal TLRs respond only to nucleic acids. All TLRs contain a ligand-binding domain composed of leucine-rich motifs and a cytoplasmic signaling, Toll-like interleukin-1 (IL-1) receptor (TIR) domain. ds, Double-stranded; LPS, lipopolysaccharide; ss, single-stranded.

cytosolic complex of NLRP-3 (the sensor), an adaptor, and caspase-1 is known as the **inflammasome.** The inflammasome is important not only for host defense but also because of its role in several diseases. Gain-of-function mutations in the sensor components of the inflammasome are the cause of rare but severe diseases, called **autoinflammatory syndromes,** characterized by uncontrolled and spontaneous inflammation. IL-1 antagonists are effective treatments for these

diseases. The common joint disease gout is caused by deposition of urate crystals, and the subsequent inflammation is thought to be mediated by inflammasome recognition of the crystals and IL-1β production. The inflammasome may also contribute to atherosclerosis, in which inflammation caused by cholesterol crystals may play a role, and obesity-associated type 2 diabetes, in which IL-1 produced on recognition of lipids may contribute to insulin resistance of tissues.

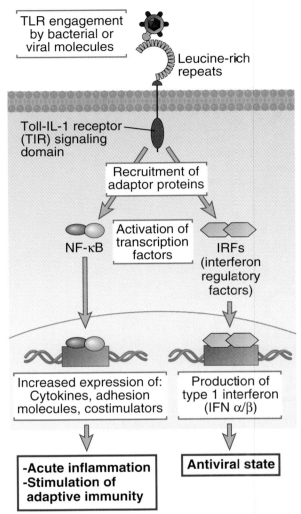

FIGURE 2–4 Signaling functions of Toll-like receptors. TLRs activate similar signaling mechanisms, which involve adaptor proteins and lead to the activation of transcription factors. These transcription factors stimulate the production of proteins that mediate inflammation and antiviral defense. NF-κB, Nuclear factor κB.

NOD-2 is an NLR specific for bacterial peptides that have entered the cytosol. It activates the NF-κB transcription factor but does not signal through the inflammasome. Some polymorphisms of the *NOD2* gene are associated with inflammatory bowel disease; the underlying mechanisms remain poorly understood. Less is known about other members of the NLR family.

Other Cellular Receptors of Innate Immunity

Many other receptor types are involved in innate immune responses to microbes (see Fig. 2–2). Several cytoplasmic receptors recognize viral nucleic acids or bacterial peptides; for example, the RIG-like receptor (RLR) family recognizes viral RNA. A cell surface receptor expressed mainly on phagocytes recognizes peptides that begin with *N*-formylmethionine, which is specific to bacterial proteins, and promotes the migration as well as the antimicrobial activities of the phagocytes. Lectin (carbohydrate-recognizing) receptors are specific for fungal glycans (these receptors are called dectins) and for terminal mannose residues (called mannose receptors); they are involved in the phagocytosis of fungi and bacteria and in inflammatory responses to these pathogens.

Although our emphasis thus far has been on cellular receptors, the innate immune system also contains several circulating molecules that recognize and provide defense against microbes, as discussed later.

COMPONENTS OF INNATE IMMUNITY

The components of the innate immune system include epithelial cells, sentinel cells in tissues (macrophages, dendritic cells, and others), NK cells, and a number of plasma proteins. We next discuss the properties of these cells and soluble proteins and their roles in innate immune responses.

Epithelial Barriers

The common portals of entry of microbes—the skin, gastrointestinal tract, and respiratory tract—are protected by continuous epithelia that provide physical and chemical barriers against infection (Fig. 2–6). The three major interfaces between the body and the external environment are the skin and the gastrointestinal and respiratory tracts. Microbes may enter hosts from the external environment through these interfaces by external physical contact, ingestion, and inhalation. All three portals of entry are lined by continuous epithelia that physically interfere with the entry of

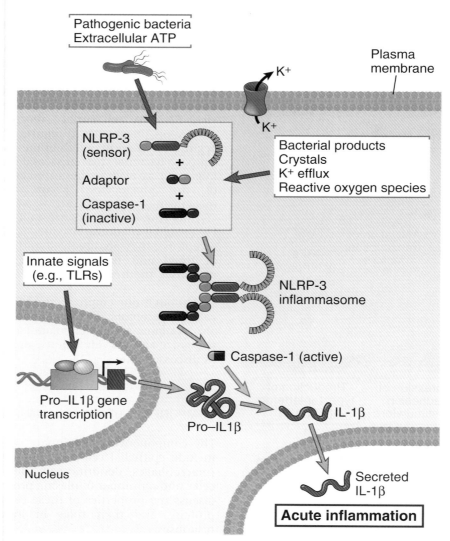

FIGURE 2–5 The inflammasome. Shown is the activation of the NLRP-3 inflammasome, which processes pro–interleukin-1β (pro–IL-1β) to active IL-1. The synthesis of pro-IL-1β is induced by various PAMPs or DAMPs through pattern recognition receptor signaling. Subsequent production of biologically active IL-1β is mediated by the inflammasome. Note that the inflammasome consists of several molecules of NLRP-3, the adaptor, and caspase-1; only one of each is shown. ATP, Adenosine triphosphate; NLRP-3, NOD-like receptor family, pyrin domain containing 3; TLRs, Toll-like receptors.

microbes. Epithelial cells also produce peptide antibiotics, called defensins and cathelicidins, which kill bacteria. In addition, epithelia contain lymphocytes called intraepithelial T lymphocytes that belong to the T cell lineage but express antigen receptors of limited diversity. Some of these T cells express receptors composed of two chains, γ and δ, that are similar but not identical to the highly diverse αβ T cell receptors expressed on the majority of T lymphocytes (see Chapters 4 and 5). Intraepithelial lymphocytes, including γδ T cells, often recognize microbial lipids and other structures that are shared by microbes of the same type. Intraepithelial T lymphocytes presumably react against infectious agents that attempt to breach the epithelia, but the specificity and functions of these cells are still poorly understood.

Physical barrier
to infection

Peptide
antibiotics

Killing of microbes
by locally produced
antibiotics

Intraepithelial
lymphocyte

Killing of microbes
and infected cells
by intraepithelial
lymphocytes

FIGURE 2–6 Functions of epithelia in innate immunity. Epithelia present at the portals of entry of microbes provide physical barriers formed by keratin (in the skin) or secreted mucus (in the gastrointestinal and bronchopulmonary systems), and by tight junctions between epithelial cells. Epithelia also produce antimicrobial substances (e.g., defensins) and harbor lymphocytes that kill microbes and infected cells.

Phagocytes: Neutrophils and Monocytes/Macrophages

The two types of circulating phagocytes, neutrophils and monocytes, are blood cells that are recruited to sites of infection, where they recognize and ingest microbes for intracellular killing. Neutrophils, also called polymorphonuclear leukocytes (PMNs), are the most abundant leukocytes in the blood, numbering 4000 to 10,000 per milliliter (Fig. 2–7, A). In response to infections, the production of neutrophils from the bone marrow increases rapidly, and their number may rise to 20,000 per mL of blood. The production of neutrophils is stimulated by cytokines, known as colony-stimulating factors (CSFs), which are secreted by many cell types in response to infections and act on hematopoietic stem cells to stimulate proliferation and maturation of neutrophil precursors. Neutrophils are the first cell type to respond to most infections, particularly bacterial and fungal infections, and thus are the dominant cells of

acute inflammation, as discussed later. Neutrophils ingest microbes in the circulation, and they rapidly enter extravascular tissues at sites of infection, where they also ingest and destroy microbes. These cells are also recruited to sites of tissue damage in the absence of infection, where they initiate the clearance of cell debris. Neutrophils live for only a few hours in tissues, so they are the early responders, but they do not provide prolonged defense.

Monocytes are less abundant than neutrophils, numbering 500 to 1000 per mL of blood (Fig. 2–7, B). They also ingest microbes in the blood and in tissues. Monocytes that enter extravascular tissues differentiate into cells called **macrophages**, which, unlike neutrophils, survive in these sites for long periods. Blood monocytes and tissue macrophages are two stages of the same cell lineage, which often is called the mononuclear phagocyte system (Fig. 2–8). (This is also called the reticuloendothelial system, for historical reasons, but this name is a misnomer and should be avoided.) Resident macrophages are found in healthy connective tissue and all organs in the body.

Macrophages serve several important roles in host defense—they produce cytokines that initiate and regulate inflammation, they ingest and destroy microbes, and they clear dead tissues and initiate the process of tissue repair (Fig. 2–9). Microbes and products of damaged cells activate macrophages to perform these functions by binding to pattern recognition receptors discussed earlier, including TLRs and NLRs. The phagocytic

A   B

FIGURE 2–7 Morphology of neutrophils and monocytes. A, Light micrograph of blood neutrophil shows the multilobed nucleus, which is why these cells are also called polymorphonuclear leukocytes, and the faint cytoplasmic granules, most of which are lysosomes. **B,** Light micrograph of blood monocyte shows the typical horseshoe-shaped nucleus.

FIGURE 2–8 Stages in maturation of mononuclear phagocytes. Mononuclear phagocytes arise from precursors in the bone marrow. The circulating blood stage is the monocyte. In the tissues, these cells become macrophages; they may be activated by microbes and may differentiate into specialized forms that reside in different tissues. CNS, Central nervous system.

functions of macrophages are mediated by cell surface receptors, such as mannose receptors and scavenger receptors, which directly bind microbes (and other particles), and receptors for products of complement activation and antibodies that coat microbes. Neutrophils use many of the same receptors to recognize and ingest microbes. The complement and antibody receptors also

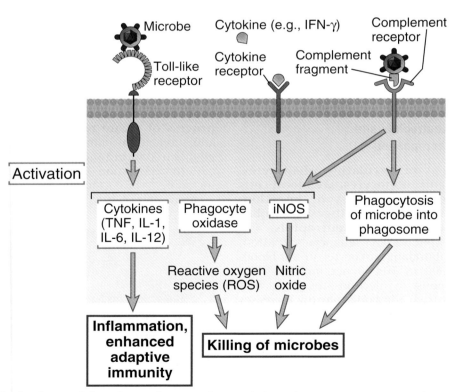

FIGURE 2–9 Activation and functions of macrophages. In innate immune responses, macrophages are activated by microbial products binding to TLRs and by cytokines, such as NK cell–derived interferon-γ (IFN-γ), which lead to the production of proteins that mediate inflammatory and microbicidal functions of these cells. Cell surface complement receptors promote the phagocytosis of complement-coated microbes as well as activation of the macrophages. (Macrophage Fc receptors for IgG [not shown] bind antibody-coated microbes and perform similar functions as the complement receptors.) IL, Interleukin; iNOS, inducible nitric oxide synthase; TNF, tumor necrosis factor.

transduce activating signals that enhance the ability of the phagocytes to kill ingested microbes. The process of phagocytosis and microbial killing is described later, in the context of inflammation.

Macrophages may be activated by two different pathways that serve distinct functions (Fig. 2–10). These pathways of activation have been called classical and alternative. **Classical macrophage activation** is induced by innate immune signals, such as from TLRs, and by the cytokine IFN-γ, which may be produced in both innate and adaptive immune responses. Classically activated macrophages, also called M1, are involved in destroying microbes and in triggering inflammation. **Alternative macrophage activation** occurs in the absence of strong TLR signals and is induced by the cytokines IL-4 and IL-13; these macrophages, called M2, appear to be more important for tissue repair and to control inflammation. The relative abundance of these two forms of activated macrophages may influence the outcome of host reactions and contribute to various disorders. We will return to the functions of these macrophage populations in Chapter 6, when we discuss cell-mediated immunity.

Although our discussion has been limited to the role of phagocytes in innate immunity, macrophages are also important effector cells in both the cell-mediated arm and the humoral arm of

FIGURE 2–10 Classical and alternative macrophage activation. Classically activated (M1) macrophages are induced by microbial products binding to TLRs and cytokines, particularly interferon-γ (IFN-γ), and are microbicidal and proinflammatory. Alternatively activated (M2) macrophages are induced by interleukin-4 (IL-4) and IL-13 (produced by certain subsets of T lymphocytes and other leukocytes) and are important in tissue repair and fibrosis. NO, Nitric oxide; ROS, reactive oxygen species; TGF-β, transforming growth factor β.

adaptive immunity, as discussed in Chapters 6 and 8, respectively.

Dendritic Cells

Dendritic cells respond to microbes by producing numerous cytokines that serve two main functions: they initiate inflammation and they stimulate adaptive immune responses. By sensing microbes and interacting with lymphocytes, especially T cells, dendritic cells constitute an important bridge between innate and adaptive immunity. We discuss the properties and functions of these cells further in Chapter 3, in the context of antigen display, which is a major function of dendritic cells.

Mast Cells

Mast cells are bone marrow–derived cells with abundant cytoplasmic granules that are present in the skin and mucosal epithelium. Mast cells can be activated by microbial products binding to TLRs, as part of innate immunity, or by a special antibody-dependent mechanism. Mast cell granules contain vasoactive amines such as histamine that cause vasodilation and increased capillary permeability as well as proteolytic enzymes that can kill bacteria or inactivate microbial toxins. Mast cells also synthesize and secrete lipid mediators (e.g., prostaglandins) and cytokines (e.g., TNF), which stimulate inflammation. Mast cell products also provide defense against helminths and are responsible for symptoms of allergic diseases (see Chapter 11).

Natural Killer Cells

Natural killer (NK) cells are a class of lymphocytes that recognize infected and stressed cells and respond by killing these cells and by secreting the macrophage-activating cytokine IFN-γ (Fig. 2–11). NK cells make up approximately 10% of the lymphocytes in the blood and peripheral lymphoid organs. NK cells contain abundant cytoplasmic granules and express some unique surface proteins, but do not express immunoglobulins or T cell receptors, the antigen receptors of B and T lymphocytes, respectively.

On activation by infected cells, NK cells empty the contents of their cytoplasmic granules into the extracellular space at the point of contact

FIGURE 2–11 Functions of natural killer (NK) cells. A, NK cells kill host cells infected by intracellular microbes, thus eliminating reservoirs of infection. **B,** NK cells respond to interleukin-12 (IL-12) produced by macrophages and secrete interferon-γ (IFN-γ), which activates the macrophages to kill phagocytosed microbes.

with the infected cell. The granule proteins then enter infected cells and activate enzymes that induce apoptosis. The cytotoxic mechanisms of NK cells, which are the same as the mechanisms used by cytotoxic T lymphocytes (CTLs; see Chapter 6), result in the death of infected cells. Thus, as with CTLs, NK cells function to eliminate cellular reservoirs of infection and eradicate infections by obligate intracellular microbes, such as viruses.

Activated NK cells also synthesize and secrete the cytokine interferon-γ. IFN-γ activates macrophages to become more effective at killing phagocytosed microbes. Cytokines secreted by macrophages and dendritic cells that have encountered microbes enhance the ability of NK cells to protect against infections. Three of these NK cell–activating cytokines are interleukin-15 (IL-15), type I interferons (type I IFNs), and interleukin-12 (IL-12). IL-15 is important for the development and maturation of NK cells,

FIGURE 2–12 Activating and inhibitory receptors of natural killer (NK) cells. A, Healthy host cells express self class I major histocompatibility complex (MHC) molecules, which are recognized by inhibitory receptors, thus ensuring that NK cells do not attack normal host cells. Note that healthy cells may express ligands for activating receptors (as shown) or may not express such ligands, but they are not attacked by NK cells because they engage the inhibitory receptors. **B,** NK cells are activated by infected cells in which ligands for activating receptors are expressed (often at high levels) and class I MHC expression is reduced so that the inhibitory receptors are not engaged. The result is that the infected cells are killed.

and type I IFNs and IL-12 enhance the killing functions of NK cells. Thus, NK cells and macrophages are examples of two cell types that function cooperatively to eliminate intracellular microbes: Macrophages ingest microbes and produce IL-12, IL-12 activates NK cells to secrete IFN-γ, and IFN-γ in turn activates the macrophages to kill the ingested microbes. As discussed in Chapter 6, essentially the same sequence of reactions involving macrophages and T lymphocytes is central to the cell-mediated arm of adaptive immunity.

The activation of NK cells is determined by a balance between engagement of activating and inhibitory receptors (Fig. 2–12). The activating receptors recognize cell surface molecules typically expressed on cells infected with viruses and intracellular bacteria, as well as cells stressed by DNA damage and malignant transformation. Thus, NK cells eliminate cells infected with intracellular microbes as well as irreparably injured cells and tumor cells. One of the well-defined activating receptors of NK cells is called NKG2D; it recognizes molecules that resemble class I major histocompatibility complex (MHC) proteins and is expressed in

response to many types of cellular stress. Another activating receptor, called CD16, is specific for immunoglobulin G (IgG) antibodies bound to cells. The recognition of antibody-coated cells results in killing of these cells, a phenomenon called **antibody-dependent cellular cytotoxicity** (ADCC). NK cells are the principal mediators of ADCC. The role of this reaction in antibody-mediated immunity is described in Chapter 8. Activating receptors on NK cells have signaling subunits that contain immunoreceptor tyrosine-based activation motifs (ITAMs) in their cytoplasmic tails. ITAMs, which also are present in subunits of lymphocyte antigen receptor–associated signaling molecules, become phosphorylated on tyrosine residues when the receptors recognize their activating ligands. The phosphorylated ITAMs bind and promote the activation of cytoplasmic protein tyrosine kinases, and these enzymes phosphorylate, and thereby activate, other substrates in several different downstream signal transduction pathways, eventually leading to cytotoxic granule exocytosis and production of IFN-γ.

The inhibitory receptors of NK cells, which block signaling by activating

receptors, are specific for self class I MHC molecules, which are expressed on all healthy nucleated cells. Therefore, class I MHC expression protects healthy cells from destruction by NK cells. (In Chapter 3 we describe the important function of MHC molecules in displaying peptide antigens to T lymphocytes.) Two major families of NK cell inhibitory receptors are the killer cell immunoglobulin-like receptors (KIRs), so called because they share structural homology with Ig molecules (see Chapter 4), and receptors consisting of a protein called CD94 and a lectin subunit called NKG2. Both families of inhibitory receptors contain in their cytoplasmic domains structural motifs called immunoreceptor tyrosine-based inhibitory motifs (ITIMs), which become phosphorylated on tyrosine residues when the receptors bind class I MHC molecules. The phosphorylated ITIMs bind and promote the activation of cytoplasmic protein tyrosine phosphatases. These phosphatases remove phosphate groups from the tyrosine residues of various signaling molecules, thereby counteracting the function of the ITAMs and blocking the activation of NK cells through activating receptors. Therefore, when the inhibitory receptors of NK cells encounter self MHC molecules on normal host cells, the NK cells are shut off (see Fig. 2–12). Many viruses have developed mechanisms to block expression of class I molecules in infected cells, which allows them to evade killing by virus-specific CD8$^+$ CTLs. When this happens, the NK cell inhibitory receptors are not engaged, and if the virus induces expression of activating ligands at the same time, the NK cells become activated and eliminate the virus-infected cells.

The role of NK cells and CTLs in defense illustrates how hosts and microbes are engaged in a constant struggle for survival. The host uses CTLs to recognize MHC-displayed viral antigens, viruses inhibit MHC expression to evade killing of the infected cells by CTLs, and NK cells can compensate for the defective CTL response because the NK cells are more effective in the absence of MHC molecules. The winner of this struggle, the host or the microbe, determines the outcome of the infection. The same principles may apply to the functions of NK cells in eradication of tumors, many of which also attempt to escape from CTL-mediated killing by reducing expression of class I MHC molecules.

Other Classes of Lymphocytes

Several types of lymphocytes that have some features of T and B lymphocytes also function in the early defense against microbes and may be considered as part of the innate immune system. A unifying characteristic of these lymphocytes is that they express somatically rearranged antigen receptors (as do classical T and B cells), but the receptors have limited diversity. As mentioned earlier, γδ T cells are present in epithelia. **NK-T cells,** some of which express surface molecules typically found on NK cells, are present in epithelia and lymphoid organs. They recognize microbial lipids bound to a class I MHC–related molecule called CD1. **B-1 cells** are a population of B lymphocytes that are found mostly in the peritoneal cavity and mucosal tissues, where they produce antibodies in response to microbes and microbial toxins that pass through the walls of the intestine. Most of the circulating IgM antibodies found in the blood of normal individuals, called **natural antibodies,** are the products of B-1 cells, and many of these antibodies are specific for carbohydrates that are present in the cell walls of many bacteria. Another type of B lymphocyte, **marginal-zone B cells,** is present at the edges of lymphoid follicles in the spleen and other organs and also is involved in rapid antibody responses to blood-borne polysaccharide-rich microbes.

Thus, these populations of lymphocytes make responses that are characteristic of adaptive immunity (e.g., antibody production) but have features of innate immunity (rapid responses, limited diversity of antigen recognition).

Complement System

The complement system is a collection of circulating and membrane-associated proteins that are important in defense against microbes. Many complement proteins are proteolytic enzymes, and complement activation involves the sequential activation of these enzymes, sometimes called an enzymatic cascade. The complement cascade may be activated by any of three pathways (Fig. 2–13). The **alternative pathway** is triggered when some complement proteins are activated on microbial surfaces and cannot be controlled, because complement regulatory proteins are not present on microbes (but are present on host cells). The alternative pathway is a

FIGURE 2–13 Pathways of complement activation. The activation of the complement system may be initiated by three distinct pathways, all of which lead to the production of C3b (the early steps). C3b initiates the late steps of complement activation, culminating in the formation of a multi-protein complex called the membrane attack complex (MAC), which includes C5b, C6, C7, C8 and C9, and causes lysis of thin-walled microbes. Peptide by-products released during complement activation are the inflammation-inducing C3a and C5a. The principal functions of proteins produced at different steps are shown. The activation, functions, and regulation of the complement system are discussed in more detail in Chapter 8.

component of innate immunity. The **classical pathway** is most often triggered after antibodies bind to microbes or other antigens and is thus a component of the humoral arm of adaptive immunity. The **lectin pathway** is activated when a carbohydrate-binding plasma protein, mannose-binding lectin (MBL), binds to terminal mannose residues on the surface glycoproteins of microbes. This lectin activates proteins of the classical pathway, but because it is initiated by a microbial product in the absence of antibody, it is a component of innate immunity. Activated complement proteins function as proteolytic enzymes to cleave other complement proteins, in an enzymatic cascade that can be rapidly amplified. The central component of complement is a plasma protein called C3, which is cleaved by enzymes generated in the early steps. The major proteolytic fragment of C3, called C3b, becomes covalently attached to microbes and is able to activate downstream complement proteins on the microbial surface. The three pathways of complement activation differ in how they are initiated, but they share the late steps and perform the same effector functions.

The complement system serves three functions in host defense. First, C3b coats microbes and promotes the binding of these microbes to phagocytes, by virtue of receptors for C3b that are expressed on the phagocytes. Thus, microbes that are coated with complement proteins are rapidly ingested and destroyed by phagocytes. This process of coating a microbe with molecules that are recognized by receptors on phagocytes is called **opsonization.** Second, some proteolytic fragments of complement proteins, especially C5a and C3a, are chemoattractants for leukocytes (mainly neutrophils and monocytes), so they promote leukocyte recruitment (inflammation) at the site of complement activation. Third, complement activation culminates in the formation of a polymeric protein complex that inserts into the microbial cell membrane, disturbing the permeability barrier and causing either osmotic lysis or apoptosis of the microbe. A more detailed discussion of the activation and functions of complement is presented in Chapter 8, where we consider the effector mechanisms of humoral immunity.

Other Plasma Proteins of Innate Immunity

Several circulating proteins in addition to complement proteins are involved in defense against infections. Plasma MBL recognizes microbial carbohydrates and can coat microbes for phagocytosis or activate the complement cascade by the lectin pathway, as discussed earlier. MBL belongs to a family of proteins called the collectins, because they are structurally similar to collagen and contain a carbohydrate-binding (lectin) domain. Surfactant proteins in the lung also belong to the collectin family and protect the airways from infection. C-reactive protein (CRP) is a pentraxin (five-headed molecule) that binds to phosphorylcholine on microbes and opsonizes the microbes for phagocytosis by macrophages, which express a receptor for CRP. CRP can also activate proteins of the classical complement pathway.

The circulating levels of many of these plasma proteins increase rapidly after infection. This protective response is called the **acute-phase response** to infection.

Cytokines of Innate Immunity

In response to microbes, dendritic cells, macrophages, and other cells secrete cytokines that mediate many of the cellular reactions of innate immunity (Fig. 2–14). As mentioned earlier, cytokines are soluble proteins that mediate immune and

---

FIGURE 2–14 Cytokines of innate immunity. A, Dendritic cells and macrophages responding to microbes produce cytokines that stimulate inflammation (leukocyte recruitment) and activate natural killer (NK) cells to produce the macrophage-activating cytokine interferon-γ (IFN-γ). **B,** Some important characteristics of the major cytokines of innate immunity are listed. Note that IFN-γ and transforming growth factor beta (TGF-β) are cytokines of both innate and adaptive immunity (see Chapter 5). The name tumor necrosis factor (TNF) arose from an experiment showing that a cytokine induced by lipopolysaccharide killed tumors in mice. We now know that this effect is the result of TNF-induced thrombosis of tumor blood vessels, which is an exaggerated form of a reaction seen in inflammation. The name interferon arose from the ability of these cytokines to interfere with viral infection. IFN-γ is a weak antiviral cytokine compared with the type I IFNs. More information about these cytokines and their receptors is provided in Appendix II. MHC, Major histocompatibility complex.

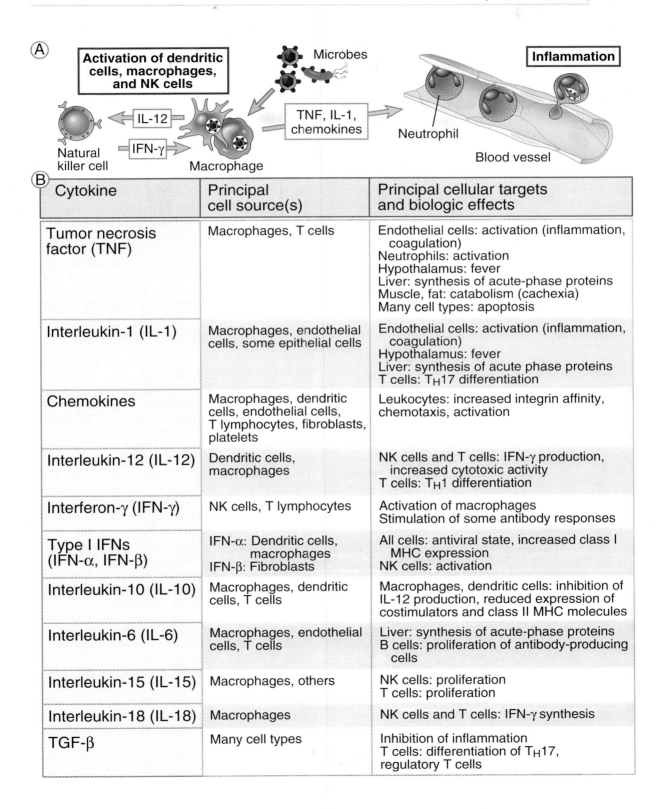

Ⓐ

Activation of dendritic cells, macrophages, and NK cells

Microbes

Inflammation

IL-12

IFN-γ

TNF, IL-1, chemokines

Natural killer cell

Macrophage

Neutrophil

Blood vessel

Ⓑ

Cytokine	Principal cell source(s)	Principal cellular targets and biologic effects
Tumor necrosis factor (TNF)	Macrophages, T cells	Endothelial cells: activation (inflammation, coagulation) Neutrophils: activation Hypothalamus: fever Liver: synthesis of acute-phase proteins Muscle, fat: catabolism (cachexia) Many cell types: apoptosis
Interleukin-1 (IL-1)	Macrophages, endothelial cells, some epithelial cells	Endothelial cells: activation (inflammation, coagulation) Hypothalamus: fever Liver: synthesis of acute phase proteins T cells: T_H17 differentiation
Chemokines	Macrophages, dendritic cells, endothelial cells, T lymphocytes, fibroblasts, platelets	Leukocytes: increased integrin affinity, chemotaxis, activation
Interleukin-12 (IL-12)	Dendritic cells, macrophages	NK cells and T cells: IFN-γ production, increased cytotoxic activity T cells: T_H1 differentiation
Interferon-γ (IFN-γ)	NK cells, T lymphocytes	Activation of macrophages Stimulation of some antibody responses
Type I IFNs (IFN-α, IFN-β)	IFN-α: Dendritic cells, macrophages IFN-β: Fibroblasts	All cells: antiviral state, increased class I MHC expression NK cells: activation
Interleukin-10 (IL-10)	Macrophages, dendritic cells, T cells	Macrophages, dendritic cells: inhibition of IL-12 production, reduced expression of costimulators and class II MHC molecules
Interleukin-6 (IL-6)	Macrophages, endothelial cells, T cells	Liver: synthesis of acute-phase proteins B cells: proliferation of antibody-producing cells
Interleukin-15 (IL-15)	Macrophages, others	NK cells: proliferation T cells: proliferation
Interleukin-18 (IL-18)	Macrophages	NK cells and T cells: IFN-γ synthesis
TGF-β	Many cell types	Inhibition of inflammation T cells: differentiation of T_H17, regulatory T cells

inflammatory reactions and are responsible for communications between leukocytes and between leukocytes and other cells. Most of the molecularly defined cytokines are called **interleukins,** by convention, implying that these molecules are produced by leukocytes and act on leukocytes. (In reality, this is too limited a definition, because many cytokines are produced by or act on cells other than leukocytes, and many cytokines that do mediate communications between leukocytes are given other names for historical reasons.) In innate immunity, the principal sources of cytokines are dendritic cells and macrophages activated by recognition of microbes, although epithelial cells and other cell types may also secrete cytokines. Recognition of bacterial components such as LPS or of viral molecules such as dsRNA by TLRs and other microbial sensors is powerful stimuli for cytokine secretion by dendritic cells and macrophages. In adaptive immunity, a major source of cytokines is helper T lymphocytes (see Chapter 5).

Cytokines are secreted in small amounts in response to an external stimulus and bind to high-affinity receptors on target cells. Most cytokines act on the cells that produce them (autocrine actions) or on adjacent cells (paracrine actions). In innate immune reactions against infections, enough dendritic cells and macrophages may be activated that large amounts of cytokines are produced, and they may be active distant from their site of secretion (endocrine actions).

The cytokines of innate immunity serve various functions in host defense. Tumor necrosis factor (TNF), interleukin-1 (IL-1), and chemokines (chemoattractant cytokines) are the principal cytokines involved in recruiting blood neutrophils and monocytes to sites of infection (described later). TNF and IL-1 also have systemic affects, including inducing fever by acting on the hypothalmus, and these as well as IL-6 stimulate liver cells to produce various proteins called acute phase reactants, such as C reactive protein, and fibrinogen, which contributes to microbial killing. At high concentrations, TNF promotes thrombus formation on the endothelium and reduces blood pressure by a combination of reduced myocardial contractility and vascular dilation and leakiness. Severe, disseminated bacterial infections sometimes lead to a potentially lethal clinical syndrome called **septic shock,** which is characterized by low blood pressure (the defining feature of shock), disseminated intravascular coagulation, and metabolic disturbances. The early clinical and pathologic manifestations of septic shock are caused by high levels of TNF, which is produced in response to the bacteria. Dendritic cells and macrophages also produce IL-12 in response to LPS and other microbial molecules. The role of IL-12 in activating NK cells, ultimately leading to macrophage activation, was mentioned previously. NK cells produce IFN-γ, whose function as a macrophage-activating cytokine was also described earlier. Because IFN-γ is produced by T cells as well, it is considered a cytokine of both innate immunity and adaptive immunity. In viral infections, a subset of dendritic cells, and, to a lesser extent, other infected cells, produce type I IFNs, which inhibit viral replication and prevent spread of the infection to uninfected cells.

INNATE IMMUNE REACTIONS

The principal reactions of the innate immune system that function to eliminate microbes are the acute inflammatory response and antiviral defense mechanisms. Now that we have covered how the innate immune system recognizes microbes and the properties and functions of the major cellular and protein components of innate immunity, we discuss in more detail these innate immune responses. Different types of reactions may occur with different microbes, with each type being particularly effective in eliminating the type of microbe that stimulates the reaction. The major protective innate immune responses to different types of microbes are the following:

- Extracellular bacteria and fungi are combated mainly by the acute inflammatory response, in which neutrophils and monocytes are recruited to the site of infection, and by the complement system.
- Defense against phagocytosed and intracellular bacteria is mediated by macrophages, which are activated by Toll-like receptors and other sensors as well as by cytokines.
- Defense against viruses is provided by type I interferons and natural killer cells.

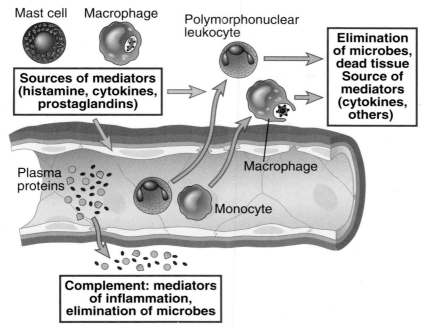

FIGURE 2–15 Acute inflammatory response. Cytokines and other mediators are produced by macrophages, dendritic cells (not shown), mast cells, and other cells in tissues in response to microbial products and damaged host cells. These mediators increase the permeability of blood vessels, leading to the entry of plasma proteins (e.g., complement proteins) into the tissues and promote the movement of leukocytes from the blood into the tissues, where the leukocytes destroy microbes, clear damaged cells, and promote more inflammation and repair.

Inflammation

Inflammation is a tissue reaction that rapidly delivers mediators of host defense—circulating cells and proteins—to the locations where they are needed, the sites of infection and tissue damage (Fig. 2–15). The process of inflammation consists of multiple steps, including recruitment of cells and leakage of plasma proteins through blood vessels, engulfment of microbes and dead material by phagocytes, and destruction of these potentially harmful substances.

Recruitment of Phagocytes to Sites of Infection and Tissue Damage

Neutrophils and monocytes migrate to extravascular sites of infection or tissue damage by binding to venular endothelial adhesion molecules and in response to chemoattractants produced by tissue cells in response to PAMPs and DAMPs. Leukocyte migration from the blood into tissues is a multistep process that consists of initial weak adhesive interactions of the leukocytes to endothelial cells, followed by firm adhesion and then transmigration through the endothelium (Fig. 2–16).

If an infectious microbe breaches an epithelium and enters the subepithelial tissue, resident macrophages and other cells recognize the microbe and respond by producing cytokines. Two of these cytokines, TNF and IL-1, act on the endothelium of venules near the site of infection. These cytokines stimulate the endothelial cells to rapidly express two adhesion molecules of the **selectin** family called E-selectin and P-selectin (selectin refers to the carbohydrate-binding, or lectin, property of these molecules). Circulating neutrophils and monocytes express surface carbohydrates that bind weakly to the selectins. The neutrophils become tethered to the endothelium, flowing blood disrupts this binding, the bonds re-form downstream, and so on, resulting in the rolling of the leukocytes along the endothelial surface.

Leukocytes express another set of adhesion molecules called **integrins,** because they

FIGURE 2–16 Sequence of events in migration of blood leukocytes to sites of infection. At sites of infection, macrophages, dendritic cells, and other cells that have encountered microbes produce cytokines such as tumor necrosis factor (TNF) and interleukin-1 (IL-1) that activate the endothelial cells of nearby venules to express selectins and ligands for integrins, and to secrete chemokines. Selectins mediate weak tethering and rolling of blood neutrophils on the endothelium, integrins mediate firm adhesion of neutrophils, and chemokines activate the neutrophils and stimulate their migration through the endothelium to the site of infection. Blood monocytes and activated T lymphocytes use the same mechanisms to migrate to sites of infection.

integrate extrinsic signals into cytoskeletal alterations. Integrins are present in a low-affinity state on unactivated leukocytes. Within a site of infection, tissue macrophages and endothelial cells produce **chemokines**, which bind to glycoproteins on the luminal surface of endothelial cells and are thus displayed at a high concentration to the leukocytes that are rolling on the endothelium. These chemokines stimulate a rapid increase in the affinity of the leukocyte integrins for their ligands on the endothelium. Concurrently, TNF and IL-1 act on the endothelium to stimulate expression of ligands for integrins. The firm binding of integrins to their ligands arrests the rolling leukocytes on the endothelium. The cytoskeleton of the leukocytes is reorganized, and the cells spread out on the endothelial surface. Chemokines also stimulate the motility of leukocytes, as do bacterial

products and products of complement activation. As a result, the leukocytes begin to migrate between endothelial cells, through the vessel wall, and along the concentration gradient of these chemoattractants to the site of infection.

The sequence of selectin-mediated rolling, chemokine-dependent integrin-mediated firm adhesion, and chemokine-mediated motility leads to the migration of blood leukocytes to an extravascular site of infection within minutes after the infection. (As discussed in Chapter 6, the same sequence of events is responsible for the migration of activated T lymphocytes into infected tissues.) Inherited deficiencies in integrins and selectin ligands lead to defective leukocyte recruitment to sites of infection and increased susceptibility to infections. These disorders are called **leukocyte adhesion deficiencies** (LADs).

FIGURE 2–17 Phagocytosis and intracellular killing of microbes. Macrophages and neutrophils express many surface receptors that may bind microbes for subsequent phagocytosis; select examples of such receptors are shown. Microbes are ingested into phagosomes, which fuse with lysosomes, and the microbes are killed by enzymes and several toxic substances produced in the phagolysosomes. The same substances may be released from the phagocytes and may kill extracellular microbes (not shown). iNOS, Inducible nitric oxide synthase; NO, nitric oxide; ROS, reactive oxygen species.

Microbial products and inflammatory cytokines such as TNF cause capillaries to become leaky, allowing circulating proteins, including complement proteins and antibodies, to exit the blood vessels and enter the tissue site of infection. These proteins work together with phagocytes to destroy the offending agents. In some infections, blood leukocytes other than neutrophils and macrophages, such as eosinophils, may be recruited to sites of infection and provide defense against the pathogens.

Phagocytosis and Destruction of Microbes
Neutrophils and macrophages ingest (phagocytose) microbes and destroy the ingested microbes in intracellular vesicles (Fig. 2–17). **Phagocytosis** is a process of ingestion of particles larger than 0.5 μm in diameter. It begins with membrane receptors binding to the microbe. The principal phagocytic receptors are some pattern recognition receptors, such as mannose receptors and other lectins, and receptors for antibodies and complement. Microbes opsonized with antibodies and complement

fragments are able to bind avidly to specific receptors on phagocytes, resulting in greatly enhanced internalization (see Chapter 8). Binding of the microbe to the cell is followed by extension of the phagocyte plasma membrane around the particle. The membrane then closes up and pinches off, and the microbe is internalized in a membrane-bound vesicle, called a phagosome. The phagosomes fuse with lysosomes to form phagolysosomes. At the same time as the microbe is being bound by the phagocyte's receptors and ingested, the phagocyte receives signals from various receptors that activate several enzymes in the phagolysosomes. One of these enzymes, called phagocyte oxidase, rapidly converts molecular oxygen into superoxide anion and free radicals, a process called the oxidative burst (or respiratory burst). These free radicals are called **reactive oxygen species** (ROS) and are toxic to the ingested microbes. A second enzyme, called inducible nitric oxide synthase (iNOS), catalyzes the conversion of arginine to **nitric oxide** (NO), also a microbicidal substance. The third set of enzymes, the lysosomal proteases, breaks down microbial proteins. All these microbicidal substances are produced mainly within lysosomes and phagolysosomes, where they act on the ingested microbes but do not damage the phagocytes.

In addition to intracellular killing, neutrophils use additional mechanisms to destroy microbes. They can release microbicidal granule contents into the extracellular environment. In response to pathogens and inflammatory mediators, neutrophils die, and during this process they extrude their nuclear contents to form networks of histones (powerful antimicrobial proteins) and other components, which are called Neutrophil Extracellular Traps (NETs). These NETs trap bacteria and fungi and kill the organisms. In some cases, the enzymes and ROS that are liberated into the extracellular space may injure host tissues. This is the reason why inflammation, normally a protective host response to infections, may cause tissue injury as well.

Inherited deficiency of the phagocyte oxidase enzyme is the cause of an immunodeficiency disorder called **chronic granulomatous disease** (CGD). In CGD, phagocytes are unable to eradicate intracellular microbes, and the host tries to contain the infection by calling in more macrophages and lymphocytes, resulting in collections of cells around the microbes called granulomas.

Antiviral Defense

Defense against viruses is a special type of host response that involves interferons, NK cells, and other mechanisms.

Type I interferons induce resistance to viral infection and replication, called an antiviral state. Type I IFNs, which include several forms of IFN-α and one IFN-β, are secreted by many cell types infected by viruses. A major source of these cytokines is a type of dendritic cell called the plasmacytoid dendritic cell (see Chapter 3). When type I IFNs secreted from dendritic cells or other infected cells bind to the IFN receptor on adjacent uninfected cells, signaling pathways are activated that inhibit viral replication and destroy viral genomes (Fig. 2–18). This action is the basis for the use of IFN-α to treat some forms of chronic viral hepatitis.

Virus-infected cells may be destroyed by NK cells, as described earlier. Type I IFNs enhance the ability of NK cells to kill infected cells. In addition, part of the innate response to viral infections includes enhanced apoptosis of infected cells. Death of the infected cells eliminates the reservoir of infection.

Regulation of Innate Immune Responses

Innate immune responses are regulated by a variety of mechanisms that are designed to prevent excessive damage to tissues. These regulatory mechanisms include the production of antiinflammatory cytokines by macrophages and dendritic cells, including interleukin-10 (IL-10), which inhibits the microbicidal and proinflammatory functions of macrophages (classical pathway of macrophage activation), and IL-1 receptor antagonist, which blocks the actions of IL-1. There are also many feedback mechanisms in which signals that induce proinflammatory cytokine production also induce expression of inhibitors of cytokine signaling. For example, TLR signaling stimulates expression of proteins called suppressors of cytokine signaling (SOCS), which block the responses of cells to various cytokines, including IFNs.

MICROBIAL EVASION OF INNATE IMMUNITY

Pathogenic microbes have evolved to resist the mechanisms of innate immunity and are thus

Production of Type I IFN

IFNs induce expression of enzymes that block viral replication

Type I IFN

IFN receptor

Virus-infected cell

Uninfected cell

Phosphorylation of translation initiation factor

RNAase

Inhibition of protein synthesis

Degradation of viral RNA

Inhibition of viral gene expression and virion assembly

Antiviral state: inhibition of viral replication

FIGURE 2–18 Antiviral actions of type I interferons. Type I interferons (IFN-α, IFN-β) are produced by virus-infected cells in response to intracellular TLR signaling and other sensors of viral RNA. Type I interferons bind to receptors on neighboring uninfected cells and activate signaling pathways that induce expression of various enzymes that interfere with viral replication at different steps, including inhibition of viral protein translation, increasing viral RNA degradation, and inhibition of viral gene expression and virion assembly. Type I IFNs also bind to receptors on infected cells and induce expression of genes whose products enhance the cell's susceptibility to CTL-mediated killing (not shown).

able to enter and colonize their hosts (Fig. 2–19). Some intracellular bacteria resist destruction inside phagocytes. *Listeria monocytogenes* produces a protein that enables it to escape from phagocytic vesicles and enter the cytoplasm of infected cells, where it is no longer susceptible to ROS or NO (which are produced mainly in phagolysosomes). The cell walls of mycobacteria contain a lipid that inhibits fusion of vesicles containing ingested bacteria with lysosomes. Other microbes have cell walls that are resistant to the actions of complement proteins. As discussed in Chapters 6 and 8, these mechanisms also enable microbes to resist the effector mechanisms of cell-mediated and humoral immunity, the two arms of adaptive immunity.

ROLE OF INNATE IMMUNITY IN STIMULATING ADAPTIVE IMMUNE RESPONSES

So far we have focused on how the innate immune system recognizes microbes and functions to combat infections. We mentioned at the beginning of this chapter that, in addition to its defense functions, the innate immune response to microbes serves an important warning function by alerting the adaptive immune system that an effective immune response is needed. In this final section, we summarize some of the mechanisms by which innate immune responses stimulate adaptive immune responses.

Innate immune responses generate molecules that provide signals, in addition to antigens, that are required to activate naive T and B lymphocytes. In Chapter 1 we introduced the concept that full activation of antigen-specific lymphocytes requires two signals. Antigen may be referred to as signal 1, and innate immune responses to microbes and to host cells damaged by microbes may provide signal 2 (Fig. 2–20). The stimuli that warn the adaptive immune system that it needs to respond have also been called danger signals. This requirement for microbe-dependent second signals ensures that lymphocytes respond to infectious agents and not to harmless, noninfectious substances. In experimental situations or for vaccination, adaptive immune responses may be induced by antigens without microbes. In all such instances, the antigens need to be administered with substances called **adjuvants** that elicit the same innate immune reactions as microbes do. In fact, many potent adjuvants are the products of microbes. The nature and mechanisms of action of second signals are described in the discussion of the activation of T and B lymphocytes in Chapters 5 and 7, respectively. Here we describe two illustrative examples of second

Mechanism of immune evasion	Organism (example)	Mechanism
Resistance to phagocytosis	Pneumococci	Capsular polysaccharide inhibits phagocytosis
Resistance to reactive oxygen intermediates in phagocytes	Staphylococci	Production of catalase, which breaks down reactive oxygen intermediates
Resistance to complement activation (alternative pathway)	*Neisseria meningitidis*	Sialic acid expression inhibits C3 and C5 convertases
	Streptococci	M protein blocks C3 binding to organism and C3b binding to complement receptors
Resistance to antimicrobial peptide antibiotics	*Pseudomonas*	Synthesis of modified LPS that resists action of peptide antibiotics

FIGURE 2–19 Evasion of innate immunity by microbes. This table provides select examples by which microbes may evade or resist innate immunity. LPS, Lipopolysaccharide.

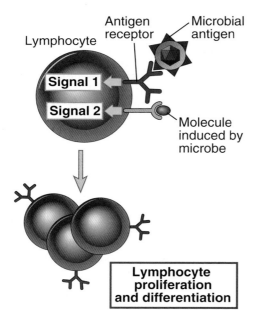

FIGURE 2–20 Two-signal requirement for lymphocyte activation. Antigen recognition by lymphocytes provides signal 1 for activation of the lymphocytes, and substances produced during innate immune responses to microbes (or components of microbes) provide signal 2. In this illustration, the lymphocytes could be T cells or B cells. By convention, the major second signals for T cells are called costimulators because they function together with antigens to stimulate the cells. The nature of second signals for T and B lymphocytes is described further in later chapters.

signals that are generated during innate immune reactions.

Microbes (or IFN-γ produced by NK cells in response to microbes) stimulate dendritic cells and macrophages to produce two types of second signals that can activate T lymphocytes. First, dendritic cells increase their expression of surface molecules called **costimulators,** which bind to receptors on naive T cells and function together with antigen recognition to activate the T cells. Second, the dendritic cells and macrophages secrete cytokines such as IL-12, IL-1, and IL-6, which stimulate the differentiation of naive T cells into effector cells of cell-mediated adaptive immunity.

Blood-borne microbes activate the complement system by the alternative pathway. One of the proteins produced during complement activation, called C3d, becomes covalently attached to the microbe. At the same time as B lymphocytes recognize microbial antigens by their antigen receptors, the B cells recognize the C3d bound to the microbe by a receptor for C3d. The combination of antigen recognition and C3d recognition initiates the process of B cell differentiation into antibody-secreting cells. Thus, a complement product serves as the second signal for humoral immune responses.

These examples illustrate an important feature of second signals: these signals not only stimulate adaptive immunity, but also guide the nature of the adaptive immune response. Intracellular and phagocytosed microbes need to be eliminated by cell-mediated immunity, the adaptive response mediated by T lymphocytes. Microbes that are encountered and ingested by dendritic cells or macrophages induce the second signals—that is, costimulators and IL-12—that stimulate T cell responses. By contrast, blood-borne microbes need to be combated by antibodies, which are produced by B lymphocytes during humoral immune responses. Blood-borne microbes activate the plasma complement system, which in turn stimulates B cell activation and antibody production. Thus, different types of microbes induce different innate immune responses, which then stimulate the types of adaptive immunity that are best able to combat different infectious pathogens.

SUMMARY

- All multicellular organisms contain intrinsic mechanisms of defense against infections, which constitute innate immunity.
- The mechanisms of innate immunity respond to microbes and not to nonmicrobial substances, are specific for structures present on various classes of microbes, are mediated by receptors encoded in the germline, and are not enhanced by repeat exposures to microbes.
- Toll-like receptors (TLRs), expressed on plasma membranes and in endosomes of many cell types, are a major class of innate immune system receptors that recognize different microbial products, including bacterial cell wall constituents and viral nucleic acids. Some receptors of the NLR family recognize microbes, products of damaged cells, and other substances, and these receptors signal through a cytosolic multiprotein complex, the inflammasome, to induce secretion of the proinflammatory cytokine interleukin-1.
- The principal components of innate immunity are epithelia, phagocytes, dendritic cells, natural killer cells, cytokines, and plasma proteins, including the proteins of the complement system.

- Epithelia provide physical barriers against microbes, produce antibiotics, and contain lymphocytes that may prevent infections.
- The principal phagocytes—neutrophils and monocytes/macrophages—are blood cells that are recruited to sites of infection, where they are activated by engagement of different receptors. Activated macrophages destroy microbes and dead cells and initiate tissue repair; these functions may be carried out by different populations of macrophages.
- Natural killer (NK) cells kill host cells infected by intracellular microbes and produce the cytokine interferon-γ, which activates macrophages to kill phagocytosed microbes.
- The complement system is a family of proteins that are activated sequentially on encounter with some microbes and by antibodies (in humoral arm of adaptive immunity). Complement proteins coat (opsonize) microbes for phagocytosis, stimulate inflammation, and lyse microbes.
- Cytokines of innate immunity function to stimulate inflammation (TNF, IL-1, chemokines), activate NK cells (IL-12), activate macrophages (IFN-γ), and prevent viral infections (type I IFNs).
- Inflammation consists of recruiting phagocytes to sites of infection and tissue damage, a process mediated by binding to endothelial adhesion molecules that are induced by the cytokines TNF and IL-1, and responding to soluble chemoattractants, including chemokines, complement fragments, and bacterial peptides. This is followed by ingestion and destruction of microbes and damaged cells.
- Antiviral defense is mediated by type I interferons, which inhibit viral replication, and NK cells, which kill infected cells.
- In addition to providing early defense against infections, innate immune responses provide signals that work together with antigens to activate B and T lymphocytes. The requirement for these second signals ensures that adaptive immunity is elicited by microbes (the inducers of innate immune reactions) and not by nonmicrobial substances.

REVIEW QUESTIONS

1. How does the specificity of innate immunity differ from that of adaptive immunity?
2. What are examples of microbial substances recognized by the innate immune system, and what are the receptors for these substances?
3. What is the inflammasome, and how is it stimulated?
4. What are the mechanisms by which the epithelium of the skin prevents the entry of microbes?
5. How do phagocytes ingest and kill microbes?
6. What is the role of MHC molecules in the recognition of infected cells by NK cells, and what is the physiologic significance of this recognition?
7. What are the roles of the cytokines TNF, IL-12, and type I interferons in defense against infections?
8. How do innate immune responses enhance adaptive immunity?

Answers to and discussion of the Review Questions are available at studentconsult.com.

Antigen Capture and Presentation to Lymphocytes
What Lymphocytes See

Adaptive immune responses are initiated by the recognition of antigens by antigen receptors of lymphocytes. B and T lymphocytes differ in the types of antigens they recognize. The antigen receptors of B lymphocytes—namely, membrane-bound antibodies—can recognize a variety of macromolecules (proteins, polysaccharides, lipids, nucleic acids), in soluble form or cell surface–associated form, as well as small chemicals. Therefore, B cell–mediated humoral immune responses may be generated against many types of microbial cell wall and soluble antigens. The antigen receptors of most T lymphocytes, on the other hand, can see only peptide fragments of protein antigens, and only when these peptides are presented by specialized peptide display molecules on host cells. Therefore, T cell–mediated immune responses may be generated only against protein antigens that are either produced in or taken up by host cells. This chapter focuses on the nature of the antigens that are recognized by lymphocytes. Chapter 4 describes the receptors used by lymphocytes to detect these antigens.

The induction of immune responses by antigens is a remarkable process that must overcome many seemingly insurmountable barriers. The first is the low frequency of naive lymphocytes specific for any one antigen, which may be less than 1 in 10^5 lymphocytes. This small fraction of the body's lymphocytes needs to locate and react rapidly to the antigen, wherever it is introduced. Second, different types of adaptive immune responses are required to defend against different types of microbes. In fact, the immune system has to react in different ways even to the same microbe at different stages of its life. For example, defense against a microbe (e.g., a virus) that has entered the circulation and is free in the blood depends on antibodies that bind the microbe, prevent it from infecting host cells, and help to eliminate it. After it has infected host cells, however, the microbe is safe from antibodies, which cannot enter the cells. As a result, activation of cytotoxic T lymphocytes (CTLs) may be necessary to kill the infected cells and eliminate the reservoir of infection. Thus, we are faced with two important questions:

- How do the rare lymphocytes specific for any microbial antigen find that microbe, especially considering that microbes may enter anywhere in the body?
- How does the immune system produce the effector cells and molecules best able to eradicate a particular type of infection, such as antibodies that bind to extracellular microbes and CTLs that kill infected cells harboring microbes in their cytoplasm?

The answer to both questions is that the immune system has developed a highly specialized system for capturing and displaying antigens to lymphocytes. Research by immunologists, cell biologists, and biochemists has led to a sophisticated understanding of how protein antigens are captured, broken down, and displayed for recognition by T lymphocytes. This is the major topic of discussion in this chapter. We know less about how protein and nonprotein antigens are captured and presented for recognition by B lymphocytes, as summarized in the final section.

ANTIGENS RECOGNIZED BY T LYMPHOCYTES

The majority of T lymphocytes recognize peptide antigens that are bound to and displayed by major histocompatibility complex (MHC) molecules of antigen-presenting cells. The MHC is a genetic locus whose principal protein products function as the peptide display molecules of the immune system. In every individual, different clones of CD4+ and CD8+ T cells can see peptides only when these peptides are

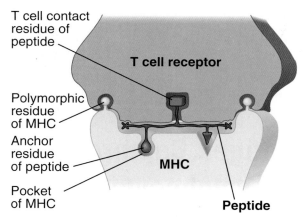

FIGURE 3–1 This model shows how a T cell receptor recognizes a complex of peptide antigen displayed by a MHC molecule. Major histocompatibility complex (MHC) molecules are expressed on antigen-presenting cells and function to display peptides derived from protein antigens. Peptides bind to the MHC molecules by anchor residues, which attach the peptides to pockets in the MHC molecules. The receptor of every T cell recognizes some residues of the peptide and some (polymorphic) residues of the MHC molecule.

displayed by that individual's MHC molecules. This property of T cells is called **MHC restriction.** The T cell receptor (TCR) recognizes some residues of peptide antigen and simultaneously also recognizes residues of the MHC molecule that is displaying that peptide (Fig. 3–1). The properties of MHC molecules and the significance of MHC restriction are described later in this chapter. How T cells learn to recognize peptides presented only by self MHC molecules is described in Chapter 4. Also, some small populations of T cells recognize lipid and other nonpeptide antigens presented by nonpolymorphic class I MHC–like molecules or without any apparent requirement for a specialized antigen display system.

The cells that capture microbial antigens and display them for recognition by T lymphocytes are called **antigen-presenting cells** (APCs). Naive T lymphocytes need to see protein antigens presented by dendritic cells, the most effective and specialized, or professional, APCs to initiate clonal expansion and differentiation of the T cells into effector and memory cells. Differentiated effector T cells again need to see antigens, which may be presented by various APCs, to activate the effector functions of the T cells in both humoral and cell-mediated immune

Skin   Gastrointestinal tract   Respiratory tract

Microbe   Epithelium

Dendritic cell–associated antigen

Cell-free antigen

Antigen that enters blood-stream

Lymphatic vessel

Venule

Connective tissue

To lymph node

To circulation and spleen

Lymph node

Spleen

Lymph node collects antigen from epithelium and connective tissue

Blood-borne antigens are captured by antigen-presenting cells in the spleen

FIGURE 3–2 Capture and display of microbial antigens. Microbes enter through an epithelium and are captured by antigen-presenting cells resident in the tissue, or microbes enter lymphatic vessels or blood vessels. The microbes and their antigens are transported to peripheral lymphoid organs, the lymph nodes, and the spleen, where protein antigens are displayed for recognition by T lymphocytes.

responses. We first describe the way in which APCs present antigens to trigger immune responses and then examine the role of MHC molecules in these processes.

CAPTURE OF PROTEIN ANTIGENS BY ANTIGEN-PRESENTING CELLS

Protein antigens of microbes that enter the body are captured mainly by dendritic cells

and concentrated in the peripheral lymphoid organs, where immune responses are initiated (Fig. 3–2). Microbes usually enter the body through the skin (by contact), the gastrointestinal tract (by ingestion), and the respiratory tract (by inhalation). Some insect-borne microbes may be injected into the bloodstream as a result of insect bites, and some infections are acquired through the genitourinary tract. Microbial antigens can also be produced in any infected tissue. It would be impossible for lymphocytes to patrol

FIGURE 3–3 Dendritic cells. A, Immature dendritic cells reside in tissues including epithelia, such as the skin, and form a network of cells with interdigitating processes, seen as blue cells on the section of skin stained with an antibody that recognizes dendritic cells. **B,** Mature dendritic cells reside in the T cell–rich areas of lymph nodes (and spleen, not shown) and are seen in the section of a lymph node stained with fluorochrome-conjugated antibodies against dendritic cells (red) and B cells in follicles (green). Note that the dendritic cells are in the same regions of the lymph node as T cells (see Fig. 1–15, *B*). (*A, Micrograph of skin courtesy Dr. Y-J. Liu, MD, Anderson Cancer Center, Houston; B, courtesy of Drs. Kathryn Pape and Jennifer Walter, University of Minnesota Medical School, Minneapolis.*)

all these sites searching for foreign invaders; instead, antigens are taken to the lymphoid organs through which lymphocytes recirculate.

All the interfaces between the body and the external environment are lined by continuous epithelia, whose principal function is to provide a barrier to infection. The epithelia and subepithelial tissues contain a network of **dendritic cells;** the same cells are present in the T cell–rich areas of peripheral lymphoid organs and, in smaller numbers, in most other organs (Fig. 3–3). There are two major populations of dendritic cells, called conventional and plasmacytoid, which differ in their locations and responses (Fig. 3–4). The majority of dendritic cells in tissues and lymphoid organs belong to the conventional subset. In the skin, the epidermal dendritic cells are called Langerhans cells. Plasmacytoid dendritic cells are named because of their morphologic resemblance to plasma

cells; they are present in the blood and tissues. Plasmacytoid dendritic cells are also the major source of type I interferons in innate immune responses to viral infections (see Chapter 2).

Dendritic cells use various membrane receptors to bind microbes, such as lectin receptors for carbohydrate structures typical of microbial but not mammalian glycoproteins. These captured microbes or their antigens typically enter the dendritic cells by receptor-mediated endocytosis; some soluble antigens may enter by pinocytosis. At the same time as the dendritic cells are capturing antigens, products of the microbes stimulate innate immune reactions by binding to Toll-like receptors (TLRs) and other sensors of microbes in the dendritic cells, as well as in parenchymal cells and resident macrophages in the tissue (see Chapter 2). This results in production of inflammatory cytokines such as tumor necrosis factor (TNF) and

Feature	Conventional dendritic cells	Plasmacytoid dendritic cells
Surface markers	CD11c high CD11b high	CD11c low CD11b negative B220 high
Major location	Tissues	Blood and tissue
Expression of Toll-like receptors	TLRs 4, 5, 8 high	TLRs 7, 9 high
Major cytokines produced	TNF, IL-6, IL-12	Type I interferons
Postulated major functions	Induction of T cell responses against most antigens	Antiviral innate immunity and induction of T cell responses against viruses

FIGURE 3–4 Populations of dendritic cells. This table lists the properties of two major classes of dendritic cell, conventional and plasmacytoid. Many subsets of conventional dendritic cells have been described (not shown), which may perform specialized functions in different tissues. IL, Interleukin; TNF, tumor necrosis factor.

interleukin-1 (IL-1). The combination of TLR signaling and cytokines activates the dendritic cells, resulting in several changes in phenotype, migration, and function.

When conventional dendritic cells that encounter microbes at epithelial barriers are activated, they lose their adhesiveness for epithelia and begin to express the chemokine receptor CCR7, which is specific for chemoattracting cytokines (chemokines) produced by lymphatic endothelium and by stromal cells in the T cell zones of lymph nodes. These chemokines direct the dendritic cells to exit the epithelium and migrate through lymphatic vessels to the lymph nodes draining that epithelium (Fig. 3–5). During the process of migration, the dendritic cells mature from cells designed to capture antigens into APCs capable of stimulating T lymphocytes. This maturation is reflected by increased synthesis and stable expression of MHC molecules, which display antigen to T cells, and of other molecules, called costimulators, that are required for full T cell responses (discussed later). Soluble antigens in the lymph are picked up by dendritic cells that reside in the lymph nodes, and bloodborne antigens are handled in essentially the same way by dendritic cells in the spleen.

The net result of this sequence of events is that the protein antigens of microbes that enter the body are transported to and concentrated in the regions of lymph nodes where the antigens are most likely to encounter T lymphocytes. Recall that naive T lymphocytes continuously recirculate through lymph nodes and also express CCR7, which promotes their entry into the T cell zones of lymph nodes (see Chapter 1). Therefore, dendritic cells bearing captured antigen and naive T cells poised to recognize antigens come together in lymph nodes. This process is remarkably efficient; it is estimated that if microbial antigens are introduced at any site in the body, a T cell response to these antigens begins in the lymph nodes draining that site within 12 to 18 hours.

Different types of APC serve distinct functions in T cell–dependent immune responses (Fig. 3–6). Dendritic cells are the principal inducers of such responses, because these cells are the most potent APCs for activating naive T lymphocytes. Another important type of APC is the macrophage, which is abundant in all tissues. In cell-mediated immune reactions, macrophages phagocytose microbes and display the antigens of these microbes to effector T cells, which activate the macrophages to kill the microbes (see Chapter 6). B lymphocytes ingest protein antigens and display them to helper T cells within lymphoid tissues; this process is important for the development of humoral immune responses (Chapter 7). As

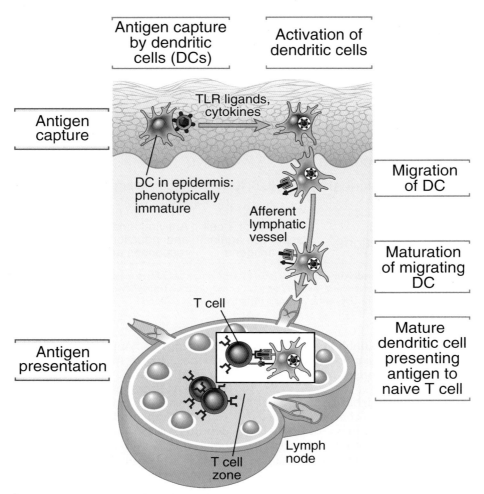

FIGURE 3–5 Capture and presentation of protein antigens by dendritic cells. Immature dendritic cells in the epithelium (skin, as shown here, where the dendritic cells are called Langerhans cells) capture microbial antigens, are activated, and leave the epithelium. The dendritic cells migrate to draining lymph nodes, being attracted there by chemokines produced in the lymphatics and nodes. In response to signals induced by the microbe, such as Toll-like receptor (TLR) signals and cytokines, the dendritic cells mature and acquire the ability to present antigens to naive T lymphocytes in the lymph nodes. Dendritic cells at different stages of their maturation may express different membrane proteins. Immature dendritic cells express surface receptors that capture microbial antigens, whereas mature dendritic cells express high levels of major histocompatibility complex (MHC) molecules and costimulators, which function to stimulate T cells.

discussed later in this chapter, all nucleated cells can present antigens derived from microbes in the cytoplasm to CD8+ CTLs.

Now that we know how protein antigens are captured, transported to, and concentrated in peripheral lymphoid organs, we next ask, how are these antigens displayed to T lymphocytes? To answer this question, we first need

to understand what MHC molecules are and how they function in immune responses.

STRUCTURE AND FUNCTION OF MAJOR HISTOCOMPATIBILITY COMPLEX MOLECULES

MHC molecules are membrane proteins on APCs that display peptide antigens for

Cell type	Expression of		Principal function
	Class II MHC	Costimulators	
Dendritic cells	Constitutive; increases with maturation; increased by IFN-γ	Constitutive; increases with maturation; inducible by TLR ligands, IFN-γ, and T cells (CD40-CD40L interactions)	Initiation of T cell responses to protein antigens
Macrophages	Low or negative; inducible by IFN-γ	Low, inducible by TLR ligands, IFN-γ, and T cells (CD40-CD40L interactions)	Effector phase of cell-mediated immune responses
B lymphocytes	Constitutive; increased by IL-4	Induced by T cells (CD40-CD40L interactions), antigen receptor cross-linking	Antigen presentation to CD4$^+$ helper T cells in humoral immune responses (cognate T cell–B cell interactions)

FIGURE 3–6 Major antigen-presenting cells (APCs). This table lists the properties of the principal class II MHC–expressing APCs, which present antigens to CD4$^+$ helper T cells. Other cell types, such as vascular endothelial cells, also express class II MHC, but their roles in immune responses are not established. In the thymus, epithelial cells express class II MHC molecules and play a role in the maturation and selection of T cells. All nucleated cells can present class I MHC–associated peptides to CD8$^+$ T cells. IFN-γ, interferon-γ; IL-4, interleukin-4; TLR, Toll-like receptor.

recognition by T lymphocytes. The MHC was discovered as the genetic locus that is the principal determinant of acceptance or rejection of tissue grafts exchanged between individuals (tissue, or *histo*, compatibility). In other words, individuals who are identical at their MHC locus (inbred animals and identical twins) will accept grafts from one another, and individuals who differ at their MHC loci will reject such grafts. Because graft rejection is not a natural biologic phenomenon, MHC genes and the molecules they encode must have evolved to perform other functions. We now know that the physiologic role of MHC molecules is to display peptides derived from microbial protein antigens to antigen-specific T lymphocytes as a first step in protective T cell–mediated immune responses to microbes. This function of MHC molecules is the explanation for the phenomenon of MHC restriction of T cells, as mentioned earlier.

The collection of genes that make up the MHC locus is found in all mammals (Fig. 3–7) and includes genes that encode MHC and other proteins. Human MHC proteins are called **human leukocyte antigens** (HLAs) because they were discovered as antigens of leukocytes that could be identified with specific antibodies. In all species, the MHC locus contains two sets of highly polymorphic genes, called the class I and class II MHC genes. These genes encode the class I and class II MHC molecules that display peptides to T cells. In addition to the polymorphic genes, the MHC locus contains many nonpolymorphic genes, some of which code for proteins involved in antigen presentation.

Structure of MHC Molecules

Class I and class II MHC molecules are membrane proteins that each contains a peptide-binding cleft at the amino-terminal end. Although the two classes of molecules differ in subunit composition, they are very similar in overall structure (Fig. 3–8).

Each **class I MHC molecule** consists of an α chain noncovalently associated with a protein called β_2-microglobulin that is encoded by a gene outside the MHC. The amino-terminal $\alpha 1$ and $\alpha 2$ domains of the class I MHC molecule form a peptide-binding cleft, or groove, that is large enough to accommodate peptides of 8 to 11 amino acids. The floor of the peptide-binding cleft is the region that binds peptides for display to T lymphocytes, and the sides and tops of the cleft are the regions that are contacted by the T cell receptor (which also contacts part of

FIGURE 3–7 Genes of the major histocompatibility complex (MHC) locus. Schematic maps show the human MHC, called the human leukocyte antigen (HLA) complex, and the mouse MHC, called the H-2 complex, illustrating the major genes that code for molecules involved in immune responses. Sizes of genes and intervening DNA segments are not shown to scale. Class II loci are shown as single blocks, but each consists of at least two genes. The products of some of the genes (DM, proteasome components, TAP) are involved in antigen processing. "Class III" MHC locus refers to genes that encode molecules other than peptide display molecules; this term is not typically used. There are also multiple class I–like genes and pseudogenes (not shown). LT, Lymphotoxin; TAP, transporter associated with antigen processing; TNF, tumor necrosis factor.

displayed peptide; see Fig. 3–1). The polymorphic residues of class I molecules, that is, the amino acids that differ among different individuals' MHC molecules, are located in the α1 and α2 domains of the α chain. Some of these polymorphic residues contribute to variations in the floor of the peptide-binding cleft and thus in the ability of different MHC molecules to bind peptides. Other polymorphic residues contribute to variations in the tops of the clefts and thus influence recognition by T cells. The α3 domain is invariant and contains the binding site for the T cell coreceptor CD8 but not CD4. As discussed in Chapter 5, T cell activation requires recognition of MHC-associated peptide antigen by the TCR and simultaneous recognition of the MHC molecule by the coreceptor. Therefore, CD8+ T cells can only respond to peptides displayed by class I MHC molecules, the MHC molecules to which the CD8 coreceptor binds.

Each **class II MHC molecule** consists of two chains, called α and β. The amino-terminal regions of both chains, called the α1 and β1 domains, contain polymorphic residues and

form a cleft that is large enough to accommodate peptides of 10 to 30 residues. The nonpolymorphic β2 domain contains the binding site for the T cell coreceptor CD4. Because CD4 binds to class II MHC molecules but not to class I, CD4+ T cells can only respond to peptides presented by class II MHC molecules.

Properties of MHC Genes and Proteins

Several features of MHC genes and molecules are important for the normal function of these molecules (Fig. 3–9).

MHC genes are codominantly expressed, meaning that the alleles inherited from both parents are expressed equally. Because there are three polymorphic class I genes, called HLA-A, HLA-B, and HLA-C in humans, and each person inherits one set of these genes from each parent, any cell can express six different class I molecules. In the class II locus, every individual inherits one pair of HLA-DP genes (called DPA1 and DPB1, encoding the α and β chains), one pair of HLA-DQ genes (DQA1 and DQB1,

Class I MHC

Class II MHC

FIGURE 3–8 Structure of class I and class II MHC molecules. Schematic diagrams (at left) and models of the crystal structures (at right) of class I MHC and class II MHC molecules illustrate the domains of the molecules and the fundamental similarities between them. Both types of MHC molecules contain peptide-binding clefts and invariant portions that bind CD8 (the α3 domain of class I) or CD4 (the β2 domain of class II). β2m, β2-microglobulin; Ig, immunoglobulin. *(Crystal structures courtesy of Dr. P. Bjorkman, California Institute of Technology, Pasadena.)*

can inherit six to eight class II MHC alleles, three or four from each parent (one set each of DP and DQ, and one or two of DR, β alleles). Because of the extra DRβ genes, and because some DQα molecules encoded on one chromosome can associate with DQβ molecules encoded from the other chromosome, the total number of expressed class II molecules may be considerably more than six.

The set of MHC alleles present on each chromosome is called an **MHC haplotype.** In humans, each HLA allele is given a numeric designation. For example, an HLA haplotype of an individual could be HLA-A2, HLA-B5, HLA-DR3, and so on. All heterozygous individuals have two HLA haplotypes, one from each chromosome.

MHC genes are highly polymorphic, meaning that many different alleles are present among the different individuals in the population. The total number of HLA alleles in the population is estimated to be more than 5000, with about 2500 for the HLA-B locus alone, making MHC genes the most polymorphic of all genes in mammals. The polymorphism of MHC genes is so great that any two individuals in an outbred population are extremely unlikely to have exactly the same MHC genes and molecules. These different polymorphic variants are inherited and not generated de novo in individuals by somatic gene recombination, as are antigen receptor genes (see Chapter 4). Because the polymorphic residues determine which peptides are presented by which MHC molecules, the existence of multiple alleles ensures that there are always some members of the population who will be able to present any particular microbial protein antigen. MHC polymorphism may have evolved because it ensures that a population will be able to deal with the diversity of microbes and at least some individuals will be able to mount effective immune responses to the peptide antigens of these microbes. Thus, everyone will not succumb to a newly encountered or mutated microbe.

Class I molecules are expressed on all nucleated cells, but class II molecules are expressed mainly on dendritic cells, macrophages, and B lymphocytes. The physiologic significance of this strikingly different expression pattern is described later. Class II molecules also are expressed on thymic epithelial cells and endothelial cells and can be induced on other cell types by the cytokine interferon-γ.

encoding the α and β chains), one HLA-DRα gene from each parent (DRA1), and one or two HLA-DRβ genes from each parent (DRB1 and DRB 3, 4, or 5). The polymorphism resides in the β chains. Thus, a heterozygous individual

Feature	Significance	
Co-dominant expression: Both parental alleles of each MHC gene are expressed	Increases number of different MHC molecules that can present peptides to T cells	
Polymorphic genes: Many different alleles are present in the population	Ensures that different individuals are able to present and respond to different microbial peptides	
MHC-expressing cell types: Class II: Dendritic cells, macrophages, B cells	CD4+ helper T lymphocytes interact with dendritic cells, macrophages, B lymphocytes	
Class I: All nucleated cells	CD8+ CTLs can kill any virus-infected cell	

FIGURE 3–9 Properties of MHC molecules and genes. This table lists some of the important features of MHC molecules, and their significance for immune responses. CTLs, Cytotoxic T lymphocytes.

Peptide Binding to MHC Molecules

The peptide-binding clefts of MHC molecules bind peptides derived from protein antigens and display these peptides for recognition by T cells (Fig. 3–10). There are pockets in the floors of the peptide-binding clefts of most MHC molecules. Some of the amino acids in the peptide antigens fit into these MHC pockets and anchor the peptides in the cleft of the MHC molecule; these amino acids are called anchor residues. Other residues of the bound peptide project upward and are recognized by the antigen receptors of T cells. Several features of the interaction of peptide antigens with MHC molecules are important for understanding the peptide display function of MHC molecules (Fig. 3–11).

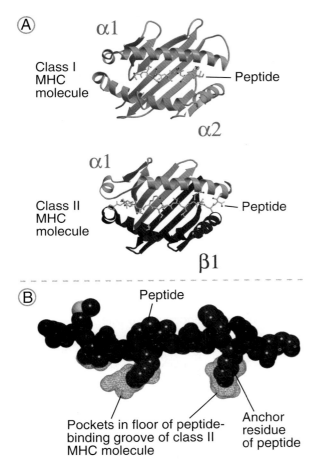

FIGURE 3–10 Binding of peptides to MHC molecules. **A,** These views of the crystal structures of MHC molecules show how peptides (in yellow) lie on the floors of the peptide-binding clefts and are available for recognition by T cells. **B,** The side view of a cutout of a peptide bound to a class II MHC molecule shows how anchor residues of the peptide hold it in the pockets in the cleft of the MHC molecule. (*A,* courtesy of Dr. P. Bjorkman, California Institute of Technology, Pasadena, California; *B* from Scott CA, Peterson PA, Teyton L, Wilson IA: Crystal structures of two I-Ad-peptide complexes reveal that high affinity can be achieved without large anchor residues. Immunity 8:319-329, 1998. © Cell Press; with permission.)

Each MHC molecule can present only one peptide at a time, because there is only one binding cleft, but each MHC molecule is capable of presenting many different peptides. As long as the pockets of the MHC molecule can accommodate the anchor residues of the peptide, that peptide can be displayed by the MHC molecule. Therefore, only one or two residues in a peptide determine if that peptide will bind in the cleft of a particular MHC molecule. Thus, MHC molecules are said to have a broad specificity for peptide binding; each MHC molecule can bind many but not all possible peptides. This feature is essential for the antigen display function of MHC molecules, because each individual has only a few different MHC molecules that must be able to present a vast number and variety of antigens.

MHC molecules bind only peptides and not other types of antigens. Among various classes of molecules, only peptides have the structural and charge characteristics that permit binding to the clefts of MHC molecules. This is why MHC-restricted CD4+ T cells and CD8+ T cells can recognize and respond only to protein antigens, the natural source of peptides.

MHC molecules acquire their peptide cargo during their biosynthesis, assembly, and transport inside cells. Therefore, MHC molecules display peptides derived from protein antigens that are inside host cells (produced inside cells or ingested from the extracellular environment). This explains why MHC-restricted T cells recognize cell-associated microbes. Importantly, class I MHC molecules acquire peptides from cytosolic proteins and class II molecules from proteins that are taken up into intracellular vesicles. The mechanisms and significance of these processes are discussed later.

Only peptide-loaded MHC molecules are stably expressed on cell surfaces. The reason for this is that MHC molecules must assemble both their chains and bound peptides to achieve a stable structure, and empty molecules are degraded inside cells. This requirement for peptide binding ensures that only useful MHC molecules, that is, those displaying peptides, are expressed on cell surfaces for recognition by T cells. Once peptides bind to MHC molecules, they stay bound for a long time, even up to days. The slow off-rate ensures that after an MHC molecule has acquired a peptide, it will display the peptide long enough to maximize the chance that a particular T cell will find the peptide it can recognize and initiate a response.

In each individual, the MHC molecules can display peptides derived from the individual's own proteins, as well as peptides from foreign (i.e., microbial) proteins. This inability of MHC molecules to discriminate between self antigens and foreign antigens raises two questions. First, at any time, the quantity of

Feature	Significance	
Broad specificity	Many different peptides can bind to the same MHC molecule	
Each MHC molecule displays one peptide at a time	Each T cell responds to a single peptide bound to an MHC molecule	
MHC molecules bind only peptides	MHC-restricted T cells respond only to protein antigens, and not to other chemicals	
Peptides are acquired during intracellular assembly	Class I and class II MHC molecules display peptides from different cellular compartments	
Stable surface expression of MHC molecule requires bound peptide	Only peptide-loaded MHC molecules are expressed on the cell surface for recognition by T cells	
Very slow off-rate	MHC molecule displays bound peptide for long enough to be located by T cell	

FIGURE 3–11 Features of peptide binding to MHC molecules. This table lists some of the important features of peptide binding to MHC molecules, with their significance for immune responses. ER, Endoplasmic reticulum; I$_i$, invariant chain.

self proteins is certain to be much greater than that of any microbial antigens. Why, then, are the available MHC molecules not constantly occupied by self peptides and unable to present foreign antigens? The likely answer is that new MHC molecules are constantly being synthesized, ready to accept peptides, and they are adept at capturing any peptides that are present in cells. Also, a single T cell may need to see a peptide displayed by only as few as 0.1% to 1% of the approximately 10^5 MHC molecules on the surface of an APC, so that even rare MHC molecules displaying a peptide are enough to initiate an immune response. The second problem is that if MHC molecules are constantly displaying self peptides, why do we not develop immune responses to self antigens, so-called autoimmune responses? The answer is that T cells specific for self antigens are either killed or inactivated (see Chapter 9). Thus, T cells are constantly patrolling the body looking at MHC-associated peptides, and if there is an infection, only those T cells that recognize microbial peptides will respond, while self peptide–specific T cells will either be absent or will have been previously inactivated.

MHC molecules are capable of displaying peptides, but not intact microbial protein antigens. Therefore, mechanisms must exist for converting naturally occurring proteins into peptides able to bind to MHC molecules. This conversion, called **antigen processing,** is described next.

PROCESSING AND PRESENTATION OF PROTEIN ANTIGENS

Extracellular proteins that are internalized by specialized APCs (dendritic cells, macrophages, B cells) are processed in endocytic vesicles and displayed by class II MHC molecules, whereas proteins in the cytosol of any nucleated cell are processed by cytoplasmic organelles and displayed by class I MHC molecules (Fig. 3–12). These two

FIGURE 3–12 Pathways of intracellular processing of protein antigens. The class II MHC pathway converts protein antigens that are endocytosed into vesicles of antigen-presenting cells into peptides that bind to class II MHC molecules for recognition by CD4+ T cells. The class I MHC pathway converts proteins in the cytoplasm into peptides that bind to class I MHC molecules for recognition by CD8+ T cells. CTL, Cytotoxic T lymphocyte; ER, endoplasmic reticulum; TAP, transporter associated with antigen processing.

Feature	Class II MHC Pathway	Class I MHC pathway
Composition of stable peptide-MHC complex	Polymorphic α and β chains of MHC, peptide	Polymorphic α chain of MHC, β2-microglobulin, peptide
Cells that express MHC	Dendritic cells, mononuclear phagocytes, B lymphocytes; endothelial cells, thymic epithelium	All nucleated cells
Responsive T cells	CD4+ T cells	CD8+ T cells
Source of protein antigens	Endosomal/lysosomal proteins (mostly internalized from extracellular environment)	Cytosolic proteins (mostly synthesized in the cell; may enter cytosol from phagosomes)
Enzymes responsible for peptide generation	Endosomal and lysosomal proteases (e.g., cathepsins)	Cytoplasmic proteasome
Site of peptide loading of MHC	Specialized vesicles	Endoplasmic reticulum
Molecules involved in transport of peptides and loading of MHC molecules	Invariant chain, DM	TAP

FIGURE 3–13 Features of the pathways of antigen processing. MHC, Major histocompatibility complex; TAP, transporter associated with antigen processing.

pathways of antigen processing involve different cellular organelles and proteins (Fig. 3–13). They are designed to sample all the proteins present in the extracellular and intracellular environments. The segregation of antigen-processing pathways also ensures that different classes of T lymphocytes recognize antigens from different compartments (discussed later).

Processing of Internalized Antigens for Display by Class II MHC Molecules

The main steps in the presentation of peptides by class II MHC molecules include ingestion of the antigen, proteolysis in endocytic vesicles, and association of peptides with class II molecules (Fig. 3–14).

Dendritic cells and macrophages may internalize extracellular microbes or microbial proteins by several mechanisms, including phagocytosis, receptor-mediated endocytosis, and pinocytosis. Microbes may bind to surface receptors specific for microbial products or to receptors that recognize antibodies or products of complement activation (opsonins) attached to the microbes. B lymphocytes internalize proteins that specifically bind to the cells' antigen receptors (see Chapter 7). These APCs may also pinocytose proteins without any specific recognition event. After internalization into APCs

Uptake of extracellular proteins into vesicular compartments of APC	Processing of internalized proteins in endosomal/lysosomal vesicles	Biosynthesis and transport of class II MHC molecules to endosomes	Association of processed peptides with class II MHC molecules in vesicles	Expression of peptide-MHC complexes on cell surface

FIGURE 3–14 Class II major histocompatibility complex pathway of processing of internalized vesicular antigens. Protein antigens are ingested by antigen-presenting cells (APCs) into vesicles, where they are degraded into peptides. Class II MHC molecules enter the same vesicles, where the class II invariant chain peptide (CLIP) that occupies the cleft of newly synthesized class II molecules is removed. These class II molecules are then able to bind peptides derived from the endocytosed protein. The DM molecule facilitates the removal of CLIP and subsequent binding of the antigenic peptide. The peptide–class II MHC complexes are transported to the cell surface and are recognized by CD4+ T cells. ER, Endoplasmic reticulum; I_i, invariant chain.

by any of these pathways, the microbial proteins enter acidic intracellular vesicles, called endosomes or phagosomes, which may fuse with lysosomes. In these vesicles the proteins are broken down by proteolytic enzymes, generating many peptides of varying lengths and sequences.

Class II MHC–expressing APCs constantly synthesize these MHC molecules in the endoplasmic reticulum (ER). Each newly synthesized class II molecule carries with it an attached protein called the **invariant chain** (I_i), which contains a sequence called the class II invariant chain peptide (CLIP) that binds tightly to the peptide-binding cleft of the class II molecule. Thus, the cleft of the newly synthesized class II molecule is occupied and prevented from accepting peptides in the ER that are destined to bind to MHC

Class I molecules (see below). This class II molecule with its associated I_i is targeted to the late endosomal/lysosomal vesicles that contain peptides derived from ingested extracellular proteins. Late endosomes/lysosomes also contain a class II MHC–like protein called DM, whose function is to exchange CLIP in the class II MHC molecule with higher-affinity peptides that may be available in this compartment. Once the class II MHC molecule binds tightly to one of the peptides generated from the ingested proteins, this peptide-MHC complex becomes stable and is delivered to the cell surface. If the MHC molecule does not find a peptide it can bind, the empty molecule is unstable and is degraded by proteases in the vesicles. One protein antigen may give rise to many peptides, only a few of which (perhaps only one or two) may bind to the MHC molecules present in the individual and stimulate immune responses in that individual.

Processing of Cytosolic Antigens for Display by Class I MHC Molecules

The main steps in antigen presentation by class I MHC molecules include generation of antigens in the cytoplasm or nucleus, proteolysis by a specialized organelle and transport into the ER, and binding of peptides to newly synthesized class I molecules (Fig. 3–15).

Antigenic proteins may be produced in the cytoplasm from viruses that are living inside infected cells, from some phagocytosed microbes that may leak from or be transported out of phagosomes into the cytoplasm, and from mutated or altered host genes that encode cytosolic or nuclear proteins, as in tumors. All these proteins, as well as the cell's own misfolded cytoplasmic and nuclear proteins, are targeted for destruction by proteolysis by the ubiquitin-proteasome pathway. These proteins are unfolded, covalently tagged with multiple copies of a peptide called ubiquitin, and threaded through an organelle called the **proteasome,** where the unfolded proteins are degraded by proteolytic enzymes. In cells that have been exposed to inflammatory cytokines (as in an infection), the proteasomes become very efficient at cleaving cytosolic and nuclear proteins into peptides with the size and sequence properties that enable the peptides to bind well to class I MHC molecules.

However, the cell faces another challenge: The peptides are in the cytosol, while the MHC molecules are being synthesized in the ER, and the two need to come together. This problem is overcome by a specialized transport molecule, called the **transporter associated with**

| Production of proteins in the cytosol | Proteolytic degradation of proteins | Transport of peptides from cytosol to ER | Assembly of peptide-class I complexes in ER | Surface expression of peptide-class I complexes |

FIGURE 3–15 Class I major histocompatibility complex pathway of processing of cytosolic antigens. Proteins enter the cytoplasm of cells either from phagocytosed microbes or from endogenous synthesis by microbes, such as viruses, that reside in the cytoplasm of infected cells. Cytoplasmic proteins are unfolded, ubiquitinated, and degraded in proteasomes (Ub, ubiquitin). The peptides that are produced are transported by the transporter associated with antigen processing (TAP) into the endoplasmic reticulum (ER), where the peptides may be further trimmed. Newly synthesized class I MHC molecules are attached to TAP by a linker protein called tapasin, so the MHC molecules are strategically located to receive peptides that are transported into the ER by TAP. The peptide–class I MHC complexes are transported to the cell surface and are recognized by CD8+ T cells. β2m, β2-microglobulin.

antigen processing (TAP), located in the ER membrane. TAP binds proteasome-generated peptides on the cytosolic side of the ER membrane, then actively pumps them into the interior of the ER. Newly synthesized class I MHC molecules, which do not contain bound peptides, associate with a bridging protein called tapasin that links them to TAP molecules in the ER membrane. Thus, as peptides enter the ER, they can easily be captured by the empty class I molecules. (Recall that in the ER, the class II MHC molecules are not able to bind peptides because of the invariant chain.) If a class I molecule finds a peptide with the right fit, the complex is stabilized, released from association with TAP, and transported to the cell surface.

The evolutionary struggle between microbes and their hosts is well illustrated by the numerous strategies that viruses have developed to block the class I MHC pathway of antigen presentation. These strategies include removing newly synthesized MHC molecules from the ER, inhibiting the transcription of MHC genes, and blocking peptide transport by TAP. By inhibiting the class I MHC pathway, viruses reduce presentation of their own antigens to CD8+ T cells and are thus able to evade the adaptive immune system. These viral evasion strategies are partly counterbalanced by the ability of natural killer cells of the innate immune system to recognize and kill virally infected cells that have lost class I MHC expression (see Chapter 2). The mechanisms of immune evasion by viruses are discussed in Chapter 6.

Cross-Presentation of Internalized Antigens to CD8+ T Cells

Dendritic cells are capable of ingesting virus-infected cells and displaying viral antigens bound to class I MHC molecules to CD8+ T lymphocytes. This pathway of antigen presentation seems to violate the rule that internalized proteins are displayed by class II MHC molecules to CD4+ T cells. In order to respond, naive CD8+ T cells, as with CD4+ cells, need to recognize antigens presented by mature dendritic cells. However, some viruses may infect only particular cell types and not dendritic cells, and these infected cells may not produce all the signals needed to initiate T cell activation. How, then, are naive CD8+ T lymphocytes able to respond to the intracellular antigens of infected cells?

Some dendritic cells have the ability to ingest infected cells, process the antigens from these ingested cells, transport the antigens into the cytosol, from where they enter the ER and bind to class I molecules, and display the antigens from the infected cells for recognition by CD8+ T lymphocytes (Fig. 3–16). This process

| Antigen capture | Cross-presentation | T cell response |

FIGURE 3–16 Cross-presentation of microbial antigens from infected cells by dendritic cells (APCs). Cells infected with intracellular microbes (e.g., viruses) are ingested by dendritic cells, and the antigens of the infectious microbes are broken down and presented in association with the major histocompatibility complex (MHC) molecules of the antigen-presenting cells (APCs). T cells recognize the microbial antigens and costimulators expressed on the APCs, and the T cells are activated. In most cases, the term cross-presentation (or cross-priming) is applied to CD8+ T cells (cytotoxic T lymphocytes, CTLs) recognizing class I MHC–associated antigens (as shown); the same cross-presenting APC may display class II MHC–associated antigens from the microbe for recognition by CD4+ helper T cells.

is called **cross-presentation** (or cross-priming), to indicate that one type of cell, dendritic cells, can present the antigens of other, infected, cells, and prime (or activate) naive T lymphocytes specific for these antigens. The dendritic cells that ingest infected cells may also simultaneously present microbial antigens to CD4$^+$ helper T lymphocytes. Thus, both classes of T lymphocytes, CD4$^+$ and CD8$^+$ cells, specific for the same microbe may be activated close to one another. As discussed in Chapter 6, this process may be important for the antigen-stimulated differentiation of naive CD8$^+$ T cells to effector CTLs and memory cells, which often requires help from CD4$^+$ cells. Once the CD8$^+$ T cells have differentiated into CTLs, they kill infected host cells without the need for dendritic cells or signals other than recognition of antigen (see Chapter 6).

Physiologic Significance of MHC-Associated Antigen Presentation

Many fundamental features of T cell–mediated immunity are closely linked to the peptide display function of MHC molecules.

The restriction of T cell recognition to MHC-associated peptides ensures that T cells see and respond only to cell-associated antigens. This is because MHC molecules are cell membrane proteins, and because peptide loading and subsequent expression of MHC molecules depend on intracellular biosynthetic and assembly steps. In other words, MHC molecules can be loaded with peptides only inside cells, where intracellular and ingested antigens are present. Therefore, T lymphocytes can recognize the antigens of intracellular microbes, which require T cell–mediated effector mechanisms, as well as antigens ingested from the extracellular environment, such as those against which antibody responses are generated.

By segregating the class I and class II pathways of antigen processing, the immune system is able to respond to extracellular and intracellular microbes in different ways best able to defend against these microbes (Fig 3–17). Extracellular microbes are captured and ingested by APCs, including B lymphocytes and macrophages, and are presented by class II molecules, which are expressed mainly on these APCs (and on dendritic cells). Because of the specificity of CD4 for class II, class

II–associated peptides are recognized by CD4$^+$ T lymphocytes, which function as helper cells. These helper T cells help B lymphocytes to produce antibodies, and they help phagocytes to destroy ingested microbes, thereby activating the two effector mechanisms best able to eliminate microbes that are internalized from the extracellular environment. Neither of these mechanisms is effective against viruses and other pathogens that survive and replicate in the cytoplasm of host cells. Cytosolic antigens are processed and displayed by class I MHC molecules, which are expressed on all nucleated cells—again, as expected, because all nucleated cells can be infected with some viruses. Class I–associated peptides are recognized by CD8$^+$ T lymphocytes, which differentiate into CTLs. The CTLs kill the infected cells and eradicate the infection, this being the most effective mechanism for eliminating cytoplasmic microbes.

Thus, the nature of the protective immune response to different microbes is optimized by linking several features of antigen presentation and T cell recognition: the pathways of processing of vesicular and cytosolic antigens, the cellular expression of class II and class I MHC molecules, the specificity of CD4 and CD8 coreceptors for class II and class I molecules, and the functions of CD4$^+$ cells as helper cells and of CD8$^+$ cells as CTLs. This function of MHC-associated antigen-processing pathways is important because the antigen receptors of T cells cannot distinguish between extracellular and intracellular microbes. In fact, as previously mentioned, the same virus can be extracellular early after infection and becomes intracellular once the infection is established. During its extracellular life, the virus is fought by antibodies and phagocytes activated by helper T cells, but once the virus has found a haven in the cytoplasm of cells, it can be eradicated only by CTL-mediated killing of the infected cells. The segregation of class I and class II antigen presentation pathways ensures the correct, specialized immune response against microbes in different locations.

The structural constraints on peptide binding to different MHC molecules, including length and anchor residues, account for the immunodominance of some peptides derived from complex protein antigens, and for the inability of some individuals to respond to certain protein antigens. When any protein is proteolytically degraded in APCs,

| Antigen uptake or synthesis | Antigen presentation | T cell effector functions |

Ⓐ **Class II MHC–associated presentation of extracellular antigen to helper T cells**

Macrophage

Antigen in endosome

Extracellular antigen

$CD4^+$ helper T lymphocyte

Cytokines

Macrophage activation: destruction of phagocytosed antigen

Antigen-specific B cell

Extracellular antigen

B cell antibody secretion: antibody binding to antigen

Ⓑ **Class I MHC–associated presentation of cytosolic antigen to cytotoxic T lymphocytes**

Cytosolic antigen

$CD8^+$ cytotoxic T lymphocyte

Killing of antigen-expressing target cell

FIGURE 3–17 Role of MHC-associated antigen presentation in recognition of microbial antigens by CD4$^+$ and CD8$^+$ T cells. A, Protein antigens of microbes that are endocytosed from the extracellular environment by macrophages and B lymphocytes enter the class II MHC pathway of antigen processing. As a result, these proteins are recognized by CD4$^+$ helper T lymphocytes, whose functions are to activate macrophages to destroy phagocytosed microbes and activate B cells to produce antibodies against extracellular microbes and toxins. **B,** Protein antigens of microbes that live in the cytoplasm of infected cells enter the class I MHC pathway of antigen processing. As a result, these proteins are recognized by CD8$^+$ cytotoxic T lymphocytes, whose function is to kill infected cells.

many peptides may be generated, but only those peptides able to bind to the MHC molecules in that individual can be presented for recognition by T cells. These MHC-binding peptides are the **immunodominant** peptides of the antigen. Even microbes with complex protein antigens express a limited number of immunodominant peptides. Many attempts have been made to identify these peptides in order to develop vaccines, but it is difficult to select a small number of peptides from any microbe that would be immunogenic in a large number of people, because of the enormous polymorphism (variability) of MHC molecules in the population. The polymorphism of the MHC also means that some

individuals may not express MHC molecules capable of binding any peptide derived from a particular antigen. These individuals would be nonresponders to that antigen. One of the earliest observations that established the physiologic importance of the MHC was the discovery that some inbred animals did not respond to simple protein antigens and responsiveness (or lack of) mapped to genes called immune response (Ir) genes, later shown to be genes in the MHC locus.

This chapter began with two questions: how do rare antigen-specific lymphocytes find antigens, and how are the appropriate immune responses generated against extracellular and intracellular microbes? Understanding the biology of APCs and the role of MHC molecules in displaying the peptides of protein antigens has provided satisfying answers to both questions, specifically for T cell–mediated immune responses.

Functions of Antigen-Presenting Cells in Addition to Antigen Display

Antigen-presenting cells not only display peptides for recognition by T cells, but in response to microbes, also express additional signals for T cell activation. The two-signal hypothesis of lymphocyte activation was introduced in Chapters 1 and 2 (see Fig. 2–20), and we return to this concept when we discuss the responses of T and B cells in Chapters 5 and 7. Recall that antigen is the necessary signal 1, and signal 2 is provided by APCs reacting to microbes. The expression of molecules in APCs that serve as second signals for lymphocyte activation is part of the innate immune response to different microbial products. For example, many bacteria produce a substance called lipopolysaccharide (LPS, endotoxin). When the bacteria are captured by APCs for presentation of their protein antigens, LPS acts on the same APCs, through a TLR, and stimulates the expression of costimulators and the secretion of cytokines. The costimulators and cytokines act in concert with antigen recognition by the T cell to stimulate the proliferation of the T cells and their differentiation into effector and memory cells.

ANTIGENS RECOGNIZED BY B CELLS AND OTHER LYMPHOCYTES

B lymphocytes use membrane-bound antibodies to recognize a wide variety of antigens, including proteins, polysaccharides, lipids, and small chemicals. These antigens may be expressed on microbial surfaces (e.g., capsular or envelope antigens) or may be in soluble form (e.g., secreted toxins). B cells differentiate in response to antigen and other signals into cells that secrete antibodies (see Chapter 7). The secreted antibodies enter the circulation and mucosal fluids and bind to the antigens, leading to their neutralization and elimination. The antigen receptors of B cells and the antibodies that are secreted usually recognize antigens in the native

conformation, with no requirement for antigen processing or display by a specialized system. Macrophages in lymphatic sinuses and dendritic cells adjacent to follicles may capture antigens that enter lymph nodes and present the antigens, in intact (unprocessed) form, to B lymphocytes in the follicles. However, it is not known if there is a requirement for a specialized population of APCs to present antigens to naive B cells in order to initiate humoral immune responses.

The B cell–rich lymphoid follicles of the lymph nodes and spleen contain a population of cells called **follicular dendritic cells** (FDCs), whose function is to display antigens to activated B cells. The antigens that FDCs display are coated with antibodies or by complement byproducts such as C3b and C3d. FDCs use receptors called Fc receptors, specific for one end of antibody molecules, to bind the antigen-antibody complexes, and receptors for complement proteins, to bind antigens with these proteins attached. These antigens are seen by specific B lymphocytes during humoral immune responses, and they function to select B cells that bind the antigens with high affinity. This process is discussed in Chapter 7.

Although this chapter has focused on peptide recognition by MHC-restricted CD4+ and CD8+ T cells, there are other, smaller populations of T cells that recognize different types of antigens. Natural killer T cells (called NK-T cells), which are distinct from natural killer (NK) cells described in Chapter 2, are specific for lipids displayed by class I–like CD1 molecules, and γδ T cells recognize a wide variety of molecules, some displayed by class I–like molecules and others apparently requiring no specific processing or display. The functions of these cells and the significance of their unusual specificities are poorly understood.

SUMMARY

* The induction of immune responses to the protein antigens of microbes depends on a specialized system for capturing and displaying these antigens for recognition by the rare naive T cells specific for any antigen. Microbes and microbial antigens that enter the body through epithelia are

captured by dendritic cells located in the epithelia and transported to regional lymph nodes, or by dendritic cells in lymph nodes and spleen. The protein antigens of the microbes are displayed by the antigen-presenting cells (APCs) to naive T lymphocytes that recirculate through the lymphoid organs.

* Molecules encoded in the major histocompatibility complex (MHC) perform the function of displaying peptides derived from protein antigens.

* MHC genes are highly polymorphic. Their major products are class I and class II MHC molecules, which contain peptide-binding clefts, where the polymorphic residues are concentrated, and invariant regions, which bind the co-receptors CD8 and CD4, respectively.

* Proteins that are ingested by APCs from the extracellular environment are proteolytically degraded within the vesicles of the APCs, and the peptides generated bind to the clefts of newly synthesized class II MHC molecules. CD4 binds to an invariant part of class II MHC, because of which $CD4^+$ helper T can only be activated by class II MHC–associated peptides derived mainly from extracellular proteins.

* Proteins that are produced in the cytoplasm of infected cells, or that enter the cytoplasm from phagosomes, are degraded by proteasomes, transported into the endoplasmic reticulum by TAP, and bind to the clefts of newly synthesized class I MHC molecules. CD8 binds class I MHC molecules, so $CD8^+$ cytotoxic T lymphocytes can be activated only by class I MHC–associated peptides derived from cytosolic proteins.

* The role of MHC molecules in antigen display ensures that T cells only recognize cell-associated protein antigens, and that the correct type of T cell (helper or cytotoxic) responds to the type of microbe the T cell is best able to combat.

* Microbes activate APCs to express membrane proteins (costimulators) and to secrete cytokines that provide signals functioning in concert with antigens to stimulate specific T cells. The requirement for these second signals ensures that T cells respond to microbial antigens and not to harmless, nonmicrobial substances.

* B lymphocytes recognize proteins as well as nonprotein antigens, even in their native conformations. Follicular dendritic cells display antigens to germinal center B cells and select high-affinity B cells during humoral immune responses.

REVIEW QUESTIONS

1. When antigens enter through the skin, in what organs are they concentrated? What cell type(s) play important roles in this process of antigen capture?

2. What are MHC molecules? What are human MHC molecules called? How were MHC molecules discovered, and what is their function?

3. What are the differences between the antigens that are displayed by class I and class II MHC molecules?

4. Describe the sequence of events by which class I and class II MHC molecules acquire antigens for display.

5. Which subsets of T cells recognize antigens presented by class I and class II MHC molecules? What molecules on T cells contribute to their specificity for either class I or class II MHC–associated peptide antigens?

Answers to and discussion of the Review Questions are available at studentconsult.com.

Antigen Recognition in the Adaptive Immune System

Structure of Lymphocyte Antigen Receptors and Development of Immune Repertoires

Antigen receptors serve critical roles in the maturation of lymphocytes from progenitors and in all adaptive immune responses. In adaptive immunity, naive lymphocytes recognize antigens to initiate responses, and effector T cells and antibodies recognize antigens to perform their functions. **B and T lymphocytes express different receptors that recognize antigens: membrane-bound antibodies on B cells and T cell receptors (TCRs) on T lymphocytes.**

The principal function of cellular receptors in the immune system, as in other biologic systems, is to detect external stimuli (antigens, for the antigen receptors of the adaptive immune system) and trigger responses of the cells on which the receptors are expressed. To recognize a large variety of different antigens, the antigen receptors of lymphocytes must be able to bind to and distinguish between many, often closely related, chemical structures. Antigen receptors are clonally distributed, meaning that each lymphocyte clone is specific for a distinct antigen and has a unique receptor, different from the receptors of all other clones. (Recall that a clone consists of a parent cell and its progeny.) The total number of distinct lymphocyte clones is very large, and this entire collection makes up the immune **repertoire**. Although each clone of B lymphocytes or T lymphocytes recognizes a different antigen, the antigen receptors transmit biochemical signals that are fundamentally the same in all lymphocytes and are unrelated to specificity. These features of lymphocyte recognition and antigen receptors raise the following questions:

- How do the antigen receptors of lymphocytes recognize extremely diverse antigens and transmit activating signals to the cells?
- What are the differences in the recognition properties of antigen receptors on B cells and T cells?
- How is the vast diversity of receptor structures in the lymphocyte repertoire generated? The diversity of antigen recognition implies the existence of many structurally different antigen receptor proteins, more than can reasonably be encoded in the inherited genome

(germline). Therefore, special mechanisms must exist for generating this diversity.

In this chapter, we describe the structures of the antigen receptors of B and T lymphocytes and how these receptors recognize antigens. We also discuss how the diversity of antigen receptors is generated during the process of lymphocyte development, thus giving rise to the repertoire of mature lymphocytes. The process of antigen-induced lymphocyte activation is described in later chapters.

ANTIGEN RECEPTORS OF LYMPHOCYTES

The antigen receptors of B and T lymphocytes have several features that are important for the functions of these receptors in adaptive immunity (Fig. 4–1). Although these receptors have many similarities in terms of structure and mechanisms of signaling, there are fundamental differences related to the types of antigenic structures that B cells and T cells recognize. **The plasma membrane antibodies that function as antigen receptors of B lymphocytes can recognize a much broader range of chemical structures than the antigen receptors of T cells.** B lymphocyte antigen receptors and the antibodies that B cells secrete are able to recognize the shapes, or conformations, of native macromolecules, including proteins, lipids, carbohydrates, and nucleic acids, as well as simple, small chemical groups. This broad specificity of B cells for structurally different types of molecules enables antibodies to recognize diverse microbes and toxins in their native form. In striking contrast, most T cells see only peptides, and only when these peptides are displayed on antigen-presenting cells (APCs) bound to membrane proteins encoded in the major histocompatibility complex (MHC) genetic locus. Thus, T cells are able to detect cell-associated microbes (see Chapter 3). **Antigen receptor molecules consist of regions (domains) involved in antigen recognition—and therefore varying between clones of lymphocytes—and other regions required for structural integrity and effector functions—and thus relatively conserved among all clones.** The antigen-recognizing domains of the receptors are called **variable (V) regions,** and the conserved

portions are the **constant (C) regions.** Even within each V region, most of the sequence variability is concentrated within short stretches, which are called hypervariable regions, or complementarity-determining regions (CDRs), because they form the parts of the receptor that bind antigens (i.e., they are complementary to the shapes of antigens). By concentrating sequence variation in small regions of the receptor, it is possible to maximize the variability of the antigen-binding part while retaining the basic structure of the receptors. As discussed later, special mechanisms exist in developing lymphocytes to create genes that encode different variable regions of antigen receptor proteins in individual clones.

Antigen receptor chains are associated with invariant membrane proteins whose function is to deliver intracellular signals that are triggered by antigen recognition (see Fig. 4–1). These signals, which are transmitted to the cytosol and the nucleus, may cause a lymphocyte to divide, to differentiate, or in certain circumstances to die. Thus, the two functions of lymphocyte receptors for antigen—specific antigen recognition and signal transduction—are mediated by different polypeptides. This again allows variability to be segregated in one set of molecules—the receptors themselves—while leaving the conserved function of signal transduction in other, invariant proteins. The associated set of plasma membrane antigen receptor and signaling molecules in B lymphocytes is called the **B cell receptor (BCR) complex,** and in T lymphocytes, it is called the **T cell receptor (TCR) complex.** When antigen molecules bind to antigen receptors of lymphocytes, the associated signaling proteins of the receptor complexes are brought into proximity. As a result, enzymes attached to the cytoplasmic portions of the signaling proteins catalyze the phosphorylation of other proteins. Phosphorylation triggers complex signaling cascades that culminate in the transcriptional activation of many genes and the production of numerous proteins that mediate the responses of the lymphocytes. We return to the processes of T and B lymphocyte activation in Chapters 5 and 7, respectively.

Antibodies exist in two forms—as membrane-bound antigen receptors on B cells or as secreted proteins—but TCRs exist only as membrane receptors on T cells. Secreted antibodies are present in the blood and

Feature or function	Antibody (Immunoglobulin)	T cell receptor (TCR)
Forms of antigens recognized	Macromolecules (proteins, polysaccharides, lipids, nucleic acids), small chemicals Conformational and linear epitopes	Peptides displayed by MHC molecules on APCs Linear epitopes
Diversity	Each clone has a unique specificity; potential for >10^9 distinct specificities	Each clone has a unique specificity; potential for >10^{11} distinct specificities
Antigen recognition is mediated by:	Variable (V) regions of heavy and light chains of membrane Ig	Variable (V) regions of α and β chains
Signaling functions are mediated by:	Proteins (Igα and Igβ) associated with membrane Ig	Proteins (CD3 and ζ) associated with TCR
Effector functions are mediated by:	Constant (C) regions of secreted Ig	TCR does not perform effector functions

FIGURE 4–1 Properties of antibodies and T cell antigen receptors (TCRs). Antibodies (also called immunoglobulins) may be expressed as membrane receptors or secreted proteins; TCRs only function as membrane receptors. When immunoglobulin (Ig) or TCR molecules recognize antigens, signals are delivered to the lymphocytes by proteins associated with the antigen receptors. The antigen receptors and attached signaling proteins form the B cell receptor (BCR) and TCR complexes. Note that single antigen receptors are shown recognizing antigens, but signaling typically requires the binding of two or more receptors to adjacent antigen molecules. The important characteristics of these antigen-recognizing molecules are summarized. APCs, Antigen-presenting cells; MHC, major histocompatibility complex.

mucosal secretions, where they function to neutralize and eliminate microbes and toxins (i.e., they are the effector molecules of humoral immunity). Antibodies are also called **immunoglobulins** (Igs), referring to immunity-conferring proteins with the characteristic slow electrophoretic mobility of globulins. Secreted antibodies recognize microbial antigens and toxins by their variable domains, the same as the membrane-bound antigen receptors of B lymphocytes. The constant regions of some secreted antibodies have the ability to bind to other molecules that participate in the elimination of antigens: these molecules include receptors on phagocytes and proteins of the complement system. Thus, antibodies serve different functions at different stages of humoral immune responses: membrane-bound antibodies on B cells recognize antigens to initiate the responses, and secreted antibodies neutralize and eliminate microbes and their toxins in the effector phase of humoral immunity. In cell-mediated immunity, the effector function of microbe elimination is performed by T lymphocytes themselves and by other leukocytes responding to the T cells. The antigen receptors of T cells are involved only in antigen recognition and T cell activation, and these proteins are not secreted and do not mediate effector functions.

With this introduction, we describe next the antigen receptors of lymphocytes, first antibodies and then T cell receptors.

Antibodies

An antibody molecule is composed of four polypeptide chains, including two identical heavy (H) chains and two identical light (L) chains, with each chain containing a variable region and a constant region (Fig. 4–2). The four chains are assembled to form a Y-shaped molecule. Each light chain is attached to one heavy chain, and the two heavy chains are attached to each other, all by disulfide bonds. A light chain is made up of one V and one C domain, and a heavy chain has one V and three or four C domains. Each domain folds into a characteristic three-dimensional shape, called the immunoglobulin domain (Fig. 4–2, D). An Ig domain consists of two layers of β-pleated sheet held together by a disulfide bridge. The adjacent strands of each β-sheet are connected by short, protruding loops; in Ig molecules, these loops

make up the three CDRs responsible for antigen recognition. Ig domains are present in many other proteins in the immune system, as well as outside the immune system, and most of these proteins are involved in responding to stimuli from the environment and from other cells. All these proteins are said to be members of the immunoglobulin superfamily, and they may have evolved from a common ancestral gene.

The antigen-binding site of an antibody is composed of the V regions of both the heavy chain and the light chain, and the core antibody structure contains two identical antigen binding sites (see Fig. 4–2). Each variable region of the heavy chain (called V_H) or of the light chain (called V_L) contains three hypervariable regions, or CDRs. Of these three, the greatest variability is in CDR3, which is located at the junction of the V and C regions. As may be predicted from this variability, CDR3 is also the portion of the Ig molecule that contributes most to antigen binding. Functionally distinct portions of antibody molecules were first identified based on fragments generated by proteolysis. The fragment of an antibody that contains a whole light chain (with its single V and C domains) attached to the V and first C domains of a heavy chain contains the portion of the antibody required for antigen recognition and is therefore called **Fab** (fragment, antigen-binding). The remaining heavy-chain C domains make up the **Fc** (fragment, crystalline) region; this fragment tends to crystallize in solution. In each Ig molecule, there are two identical Fab regions that bind antigen and one Fc region that is responsible for most of the biologic activity and effector functions of the antibodies. (As discussed later, some antibodies exist as multimers of two or five antibody molecules attached to one another.) Between the Fab and Fc regions of most antibody molecules is a flexible portion called the hinge region. The hinge allows the two antigen-binding Fab regions of each antibody molecule to move independent of each other, enabling them to simultaneously bind antigen epitopes that are separated from one another by varying distances. The C-terminal end of the heavy chain may be anchored in the plasma membrane, as seen in B cell receptors, or it may terminate in a tail piece that lacks the membrane anchor so that the antibody is produced as a secreted protein. Light chains are not attached to cell membranes.

FIGURE 4–2 Structure of antibodies. Schematic diagrams of **A,** a secreted immunoglobulin G (IgG) molecule, and **B,** a molecule of a membrane-bound form of IgM, illustrating the domains of the heavy and light chains and the regions of the proteins that participate in antigen recognition and effector functions. N and C refer to the amino-terminal and carboxy-terminal ends of the polypeptide chains, respectively. **C,** The crystal structure of a secreted IgG molecule illustrates the domains and their spatial orientation; the heavy chains are colored blue and red, the light chains are green, and carbohydrates are gray. **D,** The ribbon diagram of the Ig V domain shows the basic β-pleated sheet structure and the projecting loops that form the three CDRs. CDR, Complementarity determining region. *(**C** courtesy of Dr. Alex McPherson, University of California, Irvine.)*

The two types of light chains, called κ and λ, differ in their C regions. Each B cell expresses either κ or λ, but not both. There are five types of heavy chains, called μ, δ, γ, ε, and α, which differ in their C regions. Each type of light chain may complex with any type of heavy chain in an antibody molecule. Antibodies that contain different heavy chains belong to different **classes,** or **isotypes,** and are named according to their heavy chains (IgM, IgD, IgG, IgE, and IgA), regardless of the light-chain class. Each isotype has distinct physical and biologic properties and effector functions (Fig. 4–3). The antigen receptors of naive B lymphocytes, which are mature B cells that have not encountered antigen, are membrane-bound IgM and IgD. After stimulation by antigen and helper T lymphocytes, the antigen-specific B lymphocyte clone may expand and differentiate into progeny that secrete antibodies. Some of the progeny of IgM and IgD expressing B cells may secrete IgM, and other progeny of the same B cells may produce antibodies of other heavy-chain classes. This change in Ig isotype production is called **heavy-chain class** (or **isotype**) **switching;** its mechanism and importance are discussed in Chapter 7. Although heavy-chain C regions may switch during humoral immune responses, each clone of B cells maintains its specificity, because the V regions do not change. The light-chain class (κ or λ) also remains fixed throughout the life of each B cell clone.

Antibodies are capable of binding a wide variety of antigens, including macromolecules and small chemicals. The reason for this is that the antigen-binding CDR loops of antibody molecules can come together either to form clefts capable of accommodating small molecules or to form flat surfaces capable of accommodating many larger molecules, including portions of proteins (Fig. 4–4). Antibodies bind to antigens by reversible, noncovalent interactions, including hydrogen bonds, hydrophobic interactions, and charge-based interactions. The parts of antigens that are recognized by antibodies are called **epitopes,** or **determinants.** Different epitopes of protein antigens may be recognized based on the sequence of a stretch of amino acids (linear epitopes) or on the shape (conformational epitopes). Some of these epitopes are hidden within antigen molecules and are exposed as a result of a physicochemical change.

The strength with which one antigen-binding surface of an antibody binds to one epitope of an antigen is called the **affinity** of the interaction. Affinity often is expressed as the dissociation constant (K_d), which is the molar concentration of an antigen required to occupy half the available antibody molecules in a solution; the lower the K_d, the higher the affinity. Most antibodies produced in a primary immune response have a K_d in the range of 10^{-6} to 10^{-9} M, but with repeated stimulation (e.g., in a secondary immune response), the affinity increases to a K_d of 10^{-8} to 10^{-11} M. This increase in antigen-binding strength is called **affinity maturation** (see Chapter 7). Each IgG, IgD, and IgE antibody molecule has two antigen-binding sites. Secreted IgA is a dimer and therefore has four antigen-binding sites, and secreted IgM is a pentamer, with 10 antigen-binding sites. Therefore, each antibody molecule can bind 2 to 10 epitopes of an antigen, or epitopes on two or more neighboring antigens. The total strength of binding is much greater than the affinity of a single antigen-antibody bond and is called the **avidity** of the interaction. Antibodies produced against one antigen may bind other, structurally similar antigens. Such binding to similar epitopes is called a **cross-reaction.**

In B lymphocytes, membrane-bound Ig molecules are noncovalently associated with two other proteins, called Igα and Igβ, and the three proteins make up the BCR complex. When the B cell receptor recognizes antigen, Igα and Igβ transmit signals to the interior of the B cell that initiate the process of B cell activation. These and other signals in humoral immune responses are discussed in Chapter 7.

The realization that one clone of B cells makes an antibody of only one specificity has been exploited to produce **monoclonal antibodies,** one of the most important technical advances in immunology, with far-reaching implications for clinical medicine and research. To produce monoclonal antibodies, B cells, which have a short lifespan in vitro, are obtained from an animal immunized with an antigen, and fused with myeloma cells (tumors of plasma cells), which can be propagated indefinitely in tissue culture (Fig. 4–5). The myeloma cell line used lacks a specific enzyme, as a result of which these cells cannot grow in the presence of a certain toxic drug; fused cells, containing both myeloma and normal B cell nuclei, however, do grow in

Isotype of antibody	Subtypes	H chain	Plasma concentr. (mg/mL)	Plasma half-life (days)	Secreted form	Functions
IgA	IgA1,2	α (1 or 2)	3.5	6	Monomer, dimer **IgA (dimer)**	Mucosal immunity
IgD	None	δ	Trace		None	Naive B cell antigen receptor
IgE	None	ε	0.05	2	Monomer **IgE**	Mast cell activation (immediate hypersensitivity) Defense against helminthic parasites
IgG	IgG1-4	γ (1,2,3 or 4)	13.5	23	Monomer **IgG**	Opsonization, complement activation, antibody-dependent cell-mediated cytotoxicity, neonatal immunity, feedback inhibition of B cells
IgM	None	μ	1.5	5	Pentamer **IgM**	Naive B cell antigen receptor, complement activation

FIGURE 4–3 Features of the major isotypes (classes) of antibodies. This table summarizes some important features of the major antibody isotypes of humans. Isotypes are classified on the basis of their heavy (H) chains; each isotype may contain either κ or λ light chain. The schematic diagrams illustrate the distinct shapes of the secreted forms of these antibodies. Note that IgA consists of two subclasses, called IgA1 and IgA2, and IgG consists of four subclasses, called IgG1, IgG2, IgG3, and IgG4. (IgG subclasses are given different names in other species, for historical reasons; in mice, they are called IgG1, IgG2a, IgG2b, IgG2c, and IgG3.) The plasma concentrations are average values in normal individuals.

FIGURE 4–4 Binding of an antigen by an antibody. This model of a protein antigen bound to an antibody molecule shows how the antigen-binding site can accommodate soluble macromolecules in their native (folded) conformation. The heavy chains of the antibody are red, the light chains are yellow, and the antigens are blue. *(Courtesy of Dr. Dan Vaughn, Cold Spring Harbor Laboratory, Cold Spring Harbor, NY.)*

the presence of this drug because the normal B cells provide the missing enzyme. Thus, by fusing the two cell populations and culturing them with the drug, it is possible to grow out fused cells derived from the B cells and the myeloma, which are called **hybridomas.** From a population of hybridomas, one can select and expand the continuously growing cells that secrete the antibody of desired specificity; such antibodies, derived from a single B cell clone, are monoclonal antibodies. By this means, monoclonal antibodies against virtually any antigen can be produced.

Most monoclonal antibodies are made by fusing cells from immunized mice with mouse myelomas. Such mouse monoclonal antibodies cannot be injected repeatedly into human subjects, because the human immune system sees the mouse Ig as foreign and mounts an immune response against the injected antibodies. This problem has been overcome by genetic engineering approaches that retain the antigen-binding V regions of the mouse monoclonal antibody and replace the rest of the Ig with human Ig; such humanized antibodies are suitable for administration to people (although with prolonged use, even some humanized monoclonal antibodies may elicit anti-Ig antibody responses in treated individuals). More recently, monoclonal antibodies have been generated by using recombinant DNA technology to clone the DNA encoding human antibodies of desired specificity. Another approach is to replace the Ig genes of mice with human antibody genes and then immunize these mice with an antigen to produce specific human antibodies. Monoclonal antibodies are now in widespread use as therapeutic and diagnostic reagents for many diseases in humans.

T Cell Receptors for Antigens

The TCR, which recognizes peptide antigens displayed by MHC molecules, is a membrane-bound heterodimer composed of an α chain and a β chain, each chain containing one variable (V) region and one constant (C) region (Fig. 4–6). The V and C regions are homologous to immunoglobulin V and C regions. In the V region of each TCR chain, there are three hypervariable, or complementarity-determining, regions, each corresponding to a loop in the V domain. As in antibodies, CDR3 is the most variable among different TCRs.

Both the α chain and the β chain of the TCR participate in specific recognition of MHC molecules and bound peptides (Fig. 4–7). One of the remarkable features of T cell antigen recognition that has emerged from x-ray crystallographic analyses of TCRs bound to MHC-peptide complexes is that each TCR recognizes as few as one to three residues of the MHC-associated peptide. We also know that only a few peptides of even complex microbes, the immunodominant epitopes, are actually recognized by the immune system. This means that T cells can distinguish complex microbes on the basis of few amino acid differences between the immunodominant epitopes of the microbes.

From 5% to 10% of T cells in the body express receptors composed of gamma (γ) and delta (δ) chains, which are structurally similar to the αβ TCR but have very different specificities. The γδ TCR may recognize a variety of protein and nonprotein antigens, usually not displayed by classical MHC molecules. T cells expressing γδ TCRs are abundant in epithelia. This observation suggests that γδ T cells recognize microbes usually encountered at epithelial surfaces, but neither the specificity nor the function of these T cells is well established. Another subpopulation of T cells, comprising less than 5% of all T cells, express markers of natural killer cells and are called natural killer T cells (NK-T cells). NK-T cells express αβ TCRs with limited diversity, and they recognize lipid antigens displayed by nonpolymorphic class I MHC–like molecules. The functions of NK-T cells also are not well understood.

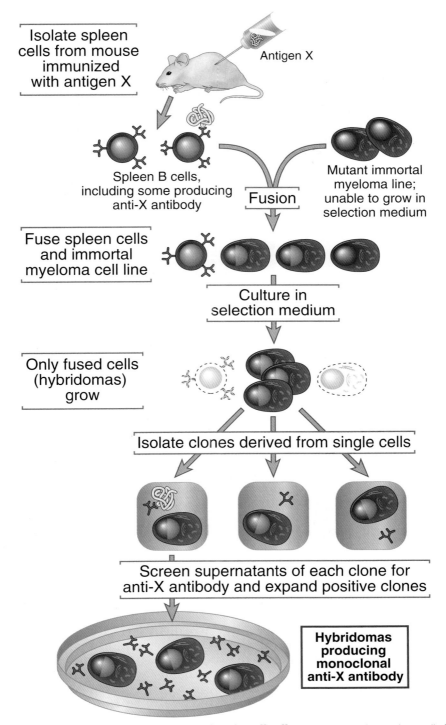

FIGURE 4–5 Generation of hybridomas and monoclonal antibodies. In this procedure, spleen cells from a mouse that has been immunized with a known antigen are fused with an enzyme-deficient myeloma cell line that does not secrete its own immunoglobulins. The fused cells are then placed in a selection medium that permits the survival of only immortalized hybrids—the normal B cells provide the enzyme that the myeloma lacks, and unfused B cells cannot survive indefinitely. These hybrid cells are then grown as single-cell clones and tested for the secretion of antibody of the desired specificty. The clone producing this antibody is expanded and becomes a source of the monoclonal antibody.

FIGURE 4–6 Structure of the T cell antigen receptor (TCR). The schematic diagram of the αβ TCR (left) shows the domains of a typical TCR specific for a peptide-MHC complex. The antigen-binding portion of the TCR is formed by the Vα and Vβ domains. N and C refer to the amino-terminal and carboxy-terminal ends of the polypeptides. The ribbon diagram (right) shows the structure of the extracellular portion of a TCR as revealed by x-ray crystallography. *(From Bjorkman PJ. MHC restriction in three dimensions: a view of T cell receptor/ligand interactions. Cell 89.167–170, 1997. © Cell Press; with permission.)*

The TCR recognizes antigen, but as with membrane Ig on B cells, it is incapable of transmitting signals to the T cell on its own. Associated with the TCR is a complex of proteins, called the CD3 and ζ proteins, which make up the TCR complex (see Fig. 4–1). The CD3 and ζ chains transmit some of the signals that are initiated when the TCR recognizes antigen. In addition, T cell activation requires engagement of the coreceptor molecule CD4 or CD8, which recognize nonpolymorphic portions of MHC molecules and also transmit activating signals. The functions of these TCR-associated proteins and coreceptors are discussed in Chapter 5.

Antigen recognition is similar for B and T lymphocyte receptors but also differs in important ways (Fig. 4–8). Antibodies can bind many different types of chemical structures, often with high affinities, which is why antibodies can bind to and neutralize many different microbes and toxins that may be present at low concentrations in the circulation. TCRs only recognize peptide-MHC complexes and bind these with relatively low affinity, which may be why the binding of T cells to APCs has to be strengthened by additional cell surface adhesion molecules (see Chapter 5). The three-dimensional structure of

the TCR is similar to that of the Fab region of an Ig molecule. Unlike in antibodies, both TCR chains are anchored in the plasma membrane; TCRs are not produced in a secreted form and do not undergo class switching or affinity maturation during the life of a T cell.

DEVELOPMENT OF IMMUNE REPERTOIRES

Now that we have discussed the structure of antigen receptors of B and T lymphocytes and how these receptors recognize antigens, the next question is how the enormous diversity of these receptors is produced. As the clonal selection hypothesis predicted, there are many clones of lymphocytes with distinct specificities, perhaps as many as 10^9, and these clones arise before encounter with antigen. There are not enough genes in the human genome for every possible receptor to be encoded by a different gene. In fact, the immune system has developed mechanisms for generating extremely diverse antigen receptors from a limited number of inherited genes, and the generation of diverse receptors is intimately linked to the process of B and T lymphocyte maturation.

FIGURE 4–7 Recognition of peptide-MHC complex by T cell antigen receptor. This ribbon diagram is drawn from the crystal structure of the extracellular portion of a peptide-MHC complex bound to a TCR that is specific for the peptide displayed by the MHC molecule. The peptide can be seen attached to the cleft at the top of the MHC molecule, and one residue of the peptide contacts the V region of a TCR. The structure of MHC molecules and their function as peptide display proteins are described in Chapter 3. β_2m, β_2-Microglobulin; MHC, major histocompatibility complex; TCR, T cell receptor. *(From Bjorkman PJ: MHC restriction in three dimensions: a view of T cell receptor/ligand interactions. Cell 89:167–170, 1997. © Cell Press; with permission.)*

Early Lymphocyte Development

The development of lymphocytes from bone marrow stem cells involves commitment of hematopoietic progenitors to the B or T cell lineage, the proliferation of these progenitors, the rearrangement and expression of antigen receptor genes, and selection events to identify and expand cells that express potentially useful antigen receptors (Fig. 4–9). These events are common to B and T lymphocytes, even though B lymphocytes mature in the bone marrow and T lymphocytes mature in the thymus. Each of the processes that occur during lymphocyte maturation plays a special role in the generation of the lymphocyte repertoire.

Commitment to the B cell or T cell lineages is associated with changes in common lymphoid progenitors in the bone marrow. These changes include the activation of several lineage-specific transcription factors and increased accessibility of Ig and TCR genes to the gene recombination machinery, described later.

Immature lymphocytes undergo proliferation at several stages during their maturation. Proliferation of developing lymphocytes is necessary to ensure that an adequate number of cells will be available to express useful antigen receptors and mature into functionally competent lymphocytes. Survival and proliferation of the earliest lymphocyte precursors are stimulated mainly by the growth factor interleukin-7 (IL-7), which is produced by stromal cells in the bone marrow and the thymus. IL-7 maintains and expands the number of lymphocyte progenitors (mainly T cell progenitors in humans, and both B and T cell precursors in mice) before they express antigen receptors, thus generating a large pool of cells in which diverse antigen receptors may be produced. Even greater proliferative expansion of the B and T cell lineages occurs after the developing lymphocytes have completed rearrangement of the first antigen receptor genes and the assembly of a preantigen receptor. This step is a quality control checkpoint in lymphocyte development that ensures preservation of cells with functional receptors.

Antigen receptors are encoded by several gene segments that are separate from one another in the germline and that recombine during lymphocyte maturation. Diversity is generated during this recombination process mainly by varying the nucleotide sequences at the sites of recombination. The expression of diverse antigen receptors is the central event in lymphocyte maturation and is described in the next section.

Lymphocytes are selected at multiple steps during their maturation to preserve the useful specificities. Selection is based on the expression of intact antigen receptor components and what they recognize. As discussed later, many attempts to generate antigen receptors fail because of errors during the gene recombination process. Therefore, checkpoints are needed at which only cells with intact, functional antigen receptors are selected to survive and proliferate. Prelymphocytes and immature lymphocytes that fail to express antigen receptors die by apoptosis (see Fig. 4–9). Immature T cells are also selected to recognize self MHC molecules in the

Feature	Antigen-binding molecule	
	Immunoglobulin (Ig)	T cell receptor (TCR)
	Antigen — Ig	CD4 — Peptide — TCR
Antigen binding	Made up of three CDRs in V_H and three CDRs in V_L	Made up of three CDRs in $V\alpha$ and three CDRs in $V\beta$
Changes in constant regions	Heavy-chain class switching and change from membrane to secretory Ig	None
Affinity of antigen binding	K_d 10^{-7}-10^{-11} M; average affinity of Igs increases during immune response	K_d 10^{-5}-10^{-7} M; no change during immune responses
On-rate and off-rate	Rapid on-rate, variable off-rate	Slow on-rate, slow off-rate

FIGURE 4–8 Features of antigen recognition by immunoglobulins and T cell antigen receptors. This table summarizes the important similarities and differences of Ig and TCR molecules, the antigen receptors of B and T lymphocytes, respectively.

thymus. This process, called **positive selection,** ensures the cells that complete maturation will be capable of recognizing antigens displayed by the same MHC molecules on APCs (which are the only MHC molecules these cells can normally encounter). Strongly self-reactive B or T cells are eliminated to prevent the development of autoimmune responses; this process is called **negative selection.**

The processes of B and T lymphocyte maturation and selection share some important features but also differ in many respects. We start with the central event that is common to both lineages: the recombination and expression of antigen receptor genes.

Production of Diverse Antigen Receptors

The formation of functional genes that encode B and T lymphocyte antigen receptors is initiated by somatic recombination of gene segments that code for the variable regions of the receptors, and diversity is generated during this process. Hematopoietic stem cells in the bone marrow as well as early lymphoid progenitors contain Ig and TCR genes in their inherited, or germline, configuration. In this configuration, Ig heavy-chain and light-chain loci and the TCR α-chain and β-chain loci each contain multiple variable region (V) gene segments, numbering about 100, and one or a few constant region (C) genes (Fig. 4–10). Between the V and C genes are groups of several short coding sequences called diversity (D) and joining (J) gene segments. (All antigen receptor gene loci contain V, J, and C genes, but only the Ig heavy-chain and TCR β-chain loci also contain D gene segments.) The commitment of a lymphocyte progenitor to become a B lymphocyte is associated with the recombination of randomly selected gene segments in the Ig heavy chain locus—first one D gene segment with one J

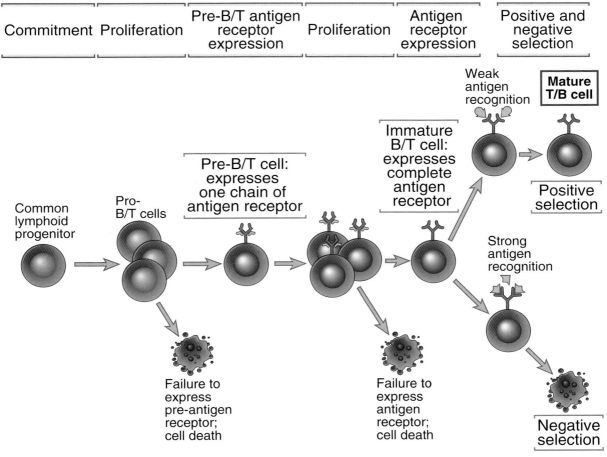

FIGURE 4–9 Steps in maturation of lymphocytes. During their maturation, B and T lymphocytes go through cycles of proliferation and expression of antigen receptor proteins by gene recombination. Cells that fail to express intact, functional receptors die by apoptosis, because they do not receive necessary survival signals. At the end of the process, the cells undergo positive and negative selection. The lymphocytes shown may be B or T cells.

segment, followed by the rearrangement of a V segment to the fused D-J element (Fig. 4–11). Thus, the committed but still-developing B cell now has a recombined V-D-J exon in the heavy-chain locus. This gene is transcribed, and in the primary transcript, the VDJ exon is spliced to the C-region exons of the μ chain, the most 5′ C region, to form a complete μ messenger RNA (mRNA). The μ mRNA is translated to produce the μ heavy chain, which is the first Ig protein synthesized during B cell maturation. Essentially, the same sequence of DNA recombination and RNA splicing leads to production of a light chain in B cells, except that the light-chain loci lack D segments, so a V region exon recombines directly

with a J segment. The rearrangement of TCR α-chain and β-chain genes in T lymphocytes is similar to that of Ig L and H chains, respectively.

The somatic recombination of V and J, or of V, D, and J, gene segments is mediated by a lymphoid-specific enzyme, VDJ recombinase, and additional enzymes, most of which are not lymphocyte specific and are involved in repair of double-stranded DNA breaks. The VDJ recombinase is composed of the recombinase-activating gene 1 and 2 (RAG-1 and RAG-2) proteins. It recognizes DNA sequences that flank all antigen receptor V, D, and J gene segments. As a result of this recognition, the recombinase brings two Ig or TCR gene segments close together and

FIGURE 4–10 Germline organization of antigen receptor gene loci. In the germline, inherited antigen receptor gene loci contain coding segments (exons, shown as colored blocks of various sizes) that are separated by segments that are not expressed (introns, shown as gray sections). Each immunoglobulin heavy-chain constant (C) region and T cell receptor (TCR) C region consists of multiple exons that encode the domains of the C regions; the organization of the Cμ exons in the Ig heavy-chain locus is shown as an example. The diagrams illustrate the antigen receptor gene loci in humans; the basic organization is the same in all species, although the precise order and number of gene segments may vary. The sizes of the segments and the distances between them are not drawn to scale. D, Diversity; J, joining; L, leader sequence (a small stretch of nucleotides that encodes a peptide that guides proteins through the endoplasmic reticulum and is cleaved from the mature proteins); V, variable.

cleaves the DNA at specific sites. The DNA breaks are then repaired by ligases, producing a full-length recombined V-J or V-D-J exon without the intervening DNA segments (see Fig. 4–11). The VDJ recombinase is expressed only in immature B and T lymphocytes. Although the same enzyme can mediate recombination of all Ig and TCR genes, intact Ig heavy-chain and light-chain genes are rearranged and expressed only in B cells, and TCR α and β genes are rearranged and expressed only in T cells. The lineage specificity of receptor gene rearrangement appears to be linked to the expression of lineage-specific transcription factors.

Diversity of antigen receptors is produced by the use of different combinations of V, D, and J gene segments in different clones of lymphocytes (called combinatorial diversity) and even more by changes in nucleotide sequences introduced at the

FIGURE 4–11 Recombination and expression of immunoglobulin (Ig) genes. The expression of an Ig heavy chain involves two gene recombination events (D-J joining, followed by joining of a V region to the DJ complex, with deletion and loss of intervening gene segments). The recombined gene is transcribed, and the VDJ segment is spliced onto the first heavy-chain RNA (which is μ), to give rise to the μ mRNA. The mRNA is translated to produce the μ heavy-chain protein. The recombination of other antigen receptor genes, that is, the Ig light chain and the T cell receptor (TCR) α and β chains, follows essentially the same sequence, except that in loci lacking D segments (Ig light chains and TCR α), a V gene recombines directly with a J gene segment.

junctions of the recombining V, D, and J gene segments (called **junctional diversity**) (Fig. 4–12). Combinatorial diversity is limited by the number of available V, D, and J gene segments, but junctional diversity is almost unlimited. Junctional diversity is produced by

three types of sequence changes, each of which generates more sequences than are present in the germline genes. First, exonucleases may remove nucleotides from V, D, and J gene segments at the sites of recombination. Second, a lymphocyte-specific enzyme called terminal

	Immunoglobulin		T cell receptor	
	Heavy chain	κ	α	β
Number of V gene segments	~100	35	54	67
Number of diversity (D) gene segments	27	0	0	2
Number of joining (J) gene segments	6	5	61	4

Mechanism

Combinatorial diversity:	
Number of possible V-(D)-J combinations	Ig: ~10^6 TCR: ~3×10^6
Junctional diversity:	

V1 D1 J1 C

D1 J1 C   V1   V1 D1 J1 C

Removal of nucleotides   Addition of nucleotides (N-region or P-nucleotides)

Total potential repertoire with junctional diversity	Ig: ~10^{11} TCR: ~10^{16}

FIGURE 4–12 Mechanisms of diversity in antigen receptors. Diversity in immunoglobulins and T cell receptors is produced by random combinations of V, D, and J gene segments, which is limited by the numbers of these segments and by removal and addition of nucleotides at the V-J or V-D-J junctions, which is almost unlimited. Junctional diversity maximizes the variations in the CDR3 regions of the antigen receptor proteins, because CDR3 is the site of V-J and V-D-J recombination. The estimated contributions of these mechanisms to the potential size of the mature B and T cell repertoires are shown. Also, diversity is increased by the ability of different Ig heavy and light chains, or different TCR α and β chains, to associate in different cells, forming different receptors (not shown). Although the upper limit on the number of immunoglobulin (Ig) and T cell receptor (TCR) proteins that may be expressed is extremely large, each individual contains on the order of only 10^7 clones of B cells and T cells with distinct specificities and receptors; in other words, only a fraction of the potential repertoire may actually be expressed. *(Modified from Davis MM, Bjorkman PJ: T-cell antigen receptor genes and T-cell recognition. Nature 334:395–402, 1988.)*

	Stem cell	Pro-B	Pre-B	Immature B	Mature B
Ig DNA, RNA	Germline DNA	Germline DNA	Recombined H chain gene (VDJ); μ mRNA	Recombined H chain gene, κ or λ genes; μ and κ or λ mRNA	Alternative splicing of primary transcript to form Cμ and Cδ mRNA
Ig expression	None	None	Cytoplasmic μ and pre-B receptor–associated μ	Membrane IgM (μ+κ or λ light chain)	Membrane IgM and IgD

FIGURE 4–13 Steps in maturation and selection of B lymphocytes. The maturation of B lymphocytes proceeds through sequential steps, each of which is characterized by particular changes in immunoglobulin (Ig) gene expression and in the patterns of Ig protein expression. At the pro-B cell and pre-B cell stages, failure to express functional antigen receptors (Ig heavy chain and Ig light chain, respectively) results in death of the cells by a default pathway of apoptosis. The pre-BCR consists of a membrane-associated Ig μ protein attached to two other proteins called surrogate light chains because they take the place of the light chain in a complete Ig molecule. BCR, B cell receptor.

deoxyribonucleotidyl transferase (TdT) catalyzes the random addition of nucleotides that are not part of germline genes to the junctions between V and D segments and D and J segments, forming so-called N regions. Third, during an intermediate stage in the process of V(D)J recombination, before breaks in the DNA are repaired, overhanging DNA sequences may be generated that are then filled in, forming P-nucleotides, introducing even more variability at the sites of recombination.

As a result of these mechanisms, the nucleotide sequence at the site of V(D)J recombination in antibody or TCR molecules made by one clone of lymphocytes differs from the sequence at the V(D)J site of antibody or TCR molecules made by every other clone. These junctional sequences and the D and J segments encode the amino acids of the CDR3 loop, mentioned earlier as the most variable of the CDRs and the most important for antigen recognition. Thus, junctional diversity maximizes the variability in the antigen-binding regions of antibodies and TCRs. In the process of creating junctional diversity, many genes may be produced with sequences that cannot code for proteins and are therefore useless. This is a price the immune system pays for generating

tremendous diversity. The risk of producing nonfunctional genes also is why the process of lymphocyte maturation contains checkpoints at which only cells with useful receptors are selected to survive.

Maturation and Selection of B Lymphocytes

The maturation of B lymphocytes occurs mainly in the bone marrow (Fig. 4–13). Progenitors committed to the B cell lineage proliferate, giving rise to a large number of precursors of B cells, called **pro-B cells.** These cells begin to rearrange Ig genes, initially in the heavy-chain locus. Cells that make productive VDJ rearrangements at the Ig heavy-chain locus develop into **pre-B cells**, defined by the presence of the Ig μ heavy-chain protein, mainly in the cytoplasm. Some of the μ protein is expressed on the cell surface in association with two other, invariant proteins, called the surrogate light chains because they resemble light chains and associate with a heavy chain. The μ chain and surrogate light chains associate with the Igα and Igβ signaling molecules to form the pre-B cell receptor (pre-BCR) complex. The assembled pre-BCR delivers signals that promote the survival and proliferation of B lineage cells that have made a productive rearrangement at the Ig H-chain locus. This is the first checkpoint in B cell development, and it selects and expands the pre-B cells that express a functional μ heavy chain (an essential component of the pre-BCR and BCR). Pre-B cells that make out-of-frame (nonproductive) rearrangements at the heavy-chain locus fail to make the μ protein, cannot express a pre-BCR or receive pre-BCR signals, and die by programmed cell death (apoptosis).

The pre-BCR complex also signals to shut off recombination of Ig heavy chain genes on the second chromosome, because of which each B cell can express an Ig heavy chain from only one of the two inherited parental alleles. This process is called **allelic exclusion,** and it helps ensure that each cell can only express a receptor of a single specificity. The pre-BCR also triggers recombination at the Ig κ light-chain locus; the λ light chain is produced only if the recombined κ chain locus fails to express a functional protein or if the κ chain generates a potentially harmful self-reactive receptor and has to be eliminated, by the process called receptor editing (see Chapter 9). Whichever functional light chain is produced associates with the μ chain to form the complete membrane-associated IgM antigen receptor. This receptor again delivers signals that promote survival, thus preserving cells that express complete antigen receptors, the second checkpoint during maturation. Signals from the antigen receptor also shut off production of the recombinase enzyme and further recombination at unrecombined light chain loci. As a result, each B cell produces either one κ or one λ light chain from one of the inherited parental alleles. The presence of two sets of light-chain genes simply increases the chance of completing successful gene recombination and receptor expression.

The IgM-expressing B lymphocyte is the **immature B cell.** Its further maturation may occur in the bone marrow or after it leaves the bone marrow and enters the spleen. The final maturation step involves coexpression of IgD with IgM, which occurs because in any given B cell, the recombined VDJ heavy-chain gene exon may be spliced onto the Cμ exons or the Cδ exons, giving rise to a μ or δ mRNA, respectively. We know that the ability of B cells to respond to antigens develops together with the coexpression of IgM and IgD, but why both classes of receptor are needed is not known. The IgM⁺IgD⁺ cell is the **mature B cell,** able to respond to antigen in peripheral lymphoid tissues.

The B cell repertoire is further shaped by negative selection. In this process, if an immature B cell binds a multivalent antigen in the bone marrow with high affinity, it may reactivate the VDJ recombinase enzyme, undergo additional light-chain V-J recombination, generate a different light chain, and thus change the specificity of the antigen receptor, a process called receptor editing. The antigens most often found in the bone marrow are self antigens that are abundantly expressed throughout the body (i.e., are ubiquitous), such as blood proteins, and membrane molecules common to all cells. Negative selection may also involve deletion of self-reactive B cells. Negative selection therefore eliminates potentially dangerous cells that can recognize and react against ubiquitous self antigens.

The process of Ig gene recombination is random and cannot be inherently biased toward recognition of microbes. However, the receptors produced are able to recognize the antigens of many, varied microbes that the immune system must defend against. The repertoire of B lymphocytes is likely generated randomly, selected positively for expression of intact receptors, and selected negatively against strong recognition of self antigens. What is left after these selection processes is a large collection of mature B cells, which by chance include some that are able to recognize almost any microbial antigen that may be encountered.

Most mature B cells are called follicular B cells because they are found within lymph node and spleen follicles. Marginal-zone B cells, which are found at the margins of splenic follicles, develop from the same progenitors (pro-B cells) as do follicular B cells. B-1 lymphocytes, a distinct population found in lymphoid organs and the peritoneal cavity, may develop earlier and from different precursors. The role of these B cell subsets in humoral immunity is described in Chapter 7.

Maturation and Selection of T Lymphocytes

The process of T lymphocyte maturation has some unique features, primarily related to the specificity of different subsets of T cells for peptides displayed by different classes of MHC molecules. T cell progenitors migrate from the bone

FIGURE 4–14 Steps in the maturation and selection of major histocompatibility complex (MHC)–restricted T lymphocytes. The maturation of T lymphocytes in the thymus proceeds through sequential steps often defined by the expression of the CD4 and CD8 coreceptors. The TCR β chain is first expressed at the double-negative pre-T cell stage, and the complete T cell receptor is expressed in double-positive cells. The pre-TCR consists of the TCR β chain associated with a protein called pre-Tα. Maturation culminates in the development of CD4+ and CD8+ single-positive T cells. As with B cells, failure to express antigen receptors at any stage leads to death of the cells by apoptosis.

marrow to the thymus, where the entire process of maturation occurs (Fig. 4–14). The most immature progenitors are called **pro-T cells** or **double-negative T cells** (or double-negative thymocytes) because they do not express CD4 or CD8. These cells expand in number mainly under the influence of IL-7 produced in the thymus. TCR β gene recombination, mediated by the VDJ recombinase, occurs in some of these double-negative cells. (The γδ T cells undergo similar recombination involving TCR γ and δ loci, but they belong to a distinct lineage and are not discussed further.) If VDJ recombination is successful in one of the two inherited loci and a TCR β-chain protein is synthesized, it is expressed on

the surface in association with an invariant protein called pre-Tα, to form the pre-TCR complex of **pre-T cells.** If the recombination in one of the two inherited loci is not successful, recombination will take place on the other locus. If a complete TCR β chain is not produced in a pro-T cell, that cell dies. The pre-TCR complex delivers intracellular signals once it is assembled, similar to the signals from the pre-BCR complex in developing B cells. These signals promote survival, proliferation, and TCR α gene recombination and inhibit VDJ recombination at the second TCR β-chain locus (allelic exclusion). Failure to express the α chain and the complete TCR again results in death of the cell. The surviving cells express the complete αβ TCR and both the CD4 and CD8 coreceptors; these cells are called **double-positive T cells** (or double-positive thymocytes).

Different clones of double-positive T cells express different αβ TCRs. If the TCR of a T cell recognizes an MHC molecule in the thymus, which must be a self MHC molecule displaying a self peptide, and if the interaction is of low or moderate affinity, this T cell is selected to survive. T cells that do not recognize an MHC molecule in the thymus die by apoptosis; these T cells would not be useful because they would be incapable of seeing MHC-displayed cell-associated antigens in that individual. This preservation of self MHC–restricted (i.e., useful) T cells is the process of **positive selection.** During this process, T cells whose TCRs recognize class I MHC–peptide complexes preserve the expression of CD8, the coreceptor that binds to class I MHC, and lose expression of CD4, the coreceptor specific for class II MHC molecules. Conversely, if a T cell recognizes class II MHC–peptide complexes, this cell maintains expression of CD4 and loses expression of CD8. Thus, what emerges are **single-positive T cells** (or single-positive thymocytes), which are either CD8+ class I MHC restricted or CD4+ class II MHC restricted. During positive selection, the T cells also become functionally segregated: the CD8+ T cells are capable of becoming CTLs on activation, and the CD4+ cells are helper cells.

Immature, double-positive T cells whose receptors strongly recognize MHC-peptide complexes in the thymus undergo apoptosis. This is the process of **negative selection,** and it serves to eliminate T lymphocytes that could react in a harmful way against self proteins that are expressed in the thymus. Some of these self proteins are present throughout the body, and others are tissue proteins that are expressed in thymic epithelial cells by special mechanisms, as discussed in Chapter 9 in the context of self-tolerance. It may seem surprising that both positive selection and negative selection are mediated by recognition of the same set of self MHC–self peptide complexes in the thymus. (Note that the thymus can contain only self MHC molecules and self peptides; microbial peptides are concentrated in peripheral lymphoid tissues and tend not to enter the thymus.) The likely explanation for these distinct outcomes is that if the antigen receptor of a T cell recognizes a self MHC–self peptide complex with low avidity, the result is positive selection, whereas high-avidity recognition leads to negative selection. High-avidity recognition occurs if the T cell expresses a TCR that has a high affinity for that self peptide, and if the self peptide is present in the thymus at a higher concentration than positively selecting peptides. If such a T cell were allowed to mature, antigen recognition could lead to harmful immune responses against the self antigen, so the T cell must be eliminated.

As with B cells, the ability of T cells to recognize foreign antigens relies on the generation of a very diverse repertoire of clonal antigen receptors. T cells that weakly recognize self antigens in the thymus may strongly recognize and respond to foreign microbial antigens in the periphery.

SUMMARY

* In the adaptive immune system, the molecules responsible for specific recognition of antigens are antibodies and T cell antigen receptors.
* Antibodies (also called immunoglobulins) may be produced as membrane receptors of B lymphocytes and as proteins secreted by antigen-stimulated B cells that have differentiated into antibody-secreting plasma cells. Secreted antibodies are the effector molecules of humoral immunity, capable of neutralizing microbes and microbial toxins and eliminating them by activating various effector mechanisms.
* T cell receptors (TCRs) are membrane receptors and are not secreted.
* The core structure of antibodies consists of two identical heavy chains and two identical light chains forming a disulfide-linked complex. Each chain consists of a variable (V) region, which is the portion that recognizes antigen, and a constant (C) region, which provides structural stability and, in heavy chains, performs the effector functions of antibodies. The V region of one heavy chain and of one light chain together form the antigen-binding site, and thus the core structure has two identical antigen-binding sites.
* T cell receptors consist of an α chain and a β chain. Each chain contains one V

region and one C region, and both chains participate in the recognition of antigens, which for most T cells are peptides displayed by MHC molecules.

- The V regions of immunoglobulin (Ig) and TCR molecules contain hypervariable segments, also called complementarity-determining regions (CDRs), which are the regions of contact with antigens.

- The genes that encode antigen receptors consist of multiple segments separate in the germline and brought together during maturation of lymphocytes. In B cells, the Ig gene segments undergo recombination as the cells mature in the bone marrow, and in T cells the TCR gene segments undergo recombination during maturation in the thymus.

- Receptors of different specificities are generated in part by different combinations of V, D, and J gene segments. The process of recombination introduces variability in the nucleotide sequences at the sites of recombination by adding or removing nucleotides from the junctions. The result of this introduced variability is the development of a diverse repertoire of lymphocytes, in which clones of cells with different antigen specificities express receptors that differ in sequence and recognition, and most of the differences are concentrated at the regions of gene recombination.

- During their maturation, lymphocytes are selected to survive at several checkpoints; only cells with complete functional antigen receptors are preserved and expanded. In addition, T lymphocytes are positively selected to recognize peptide antigens displayed by self MHC molecules and to ensure that the recognition of the appropriate type of MHC molecule matches the co-receptor preserved.

- Immature lymphocytes that strongly recognize self antigens are negatively selected and prevented from completing their maturation, thus eliminating cells with the potential of reacting in harmful ways against self tissues.

REVIEW QUESTIONS

1. What are the functionally distinct domains (regions) of antibody and TCR molecules? What features of the amino acid sequences in these regions are important for their functions?
2. What are the differences in the types of antigens recognized by antibodies and TCRs?
3. What mechanisms contribute to the diversity of antibody and TCR molecules? Which of these mechanisms contributes the most to the diversity?
4. What are some of the checkpoints during lymphocyte maturation that ensure survival of the useful cells?
5. What is the phenomenon of negative selection, and what is its importance?

Answers to and discussion of the Review Questions are available at studentconsult.com.

T Cell–Mediated Immunity
Activation of T Lymphocytes by Cell-Associated Antigens

T lymphocytes perform multiple functions in defending against infections by various kinds of microbes. A major role for T lymphocytes is in **cell-mediated immunity (CMI),** which provides defense against infections by intracellular microbes. Two types of infections may lead to microbes finding a haven inside cells, from where they must be eliminated by cell-mediated immune responses (Fig. 5–1). First, microbes are ingested by phagocytes as part of the early defense mechanisms of innate immunity, but some of these microbes have evolved to resist the microbicidal activities of phagocytes. Many pathogenic intracellular bacteria and protozoa are able to survive, and even replicate, in the vesicles of phagocytes. Some of these phagocytosed microbes may enter the cytosol of infected cells and multiply in this compartment, using the nutrients of the infected cells. Cytosolic microbes are protected from the microbicidal mechanisms of phagocytes, because these mechanisms are confined to vesicular compartments, where they cannot damage the host cells. Second, viruses may bind to receptors on a wide variety of cells and are able to infect and replicate in the cytoplasm of these cells. These cells often do not possess intrinsic mechanisms for destroying the viruses.

In addition to CMI, T lymphocytes also play important roles in defense against microbes that do not reproduce inside cells nor survive in phagocytes, including several types of bacteria, fungi, and helminthic parasites. T cells that mediate defense against these organisms include subsets of CD4+ helper T lymphocytes that were not known to exist when the classic role of T cells in CMI was first defined. A major role of some of these subsets is to help B cells to produce antibodies, as part of humoral immune responses (see Chapter 7). Another role of some of these helper T cell subsets is to promote inflammatory responses rich in activated leukocytes that are particularly efficient at killing extracellular microbes. We will discuss these T cell subsets and

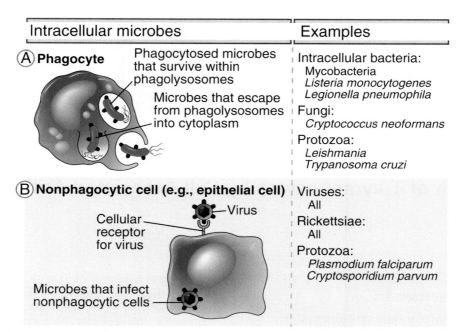

Intracellular microbes		Examples
(A) **Phagocyte**	Phagocytosed microbes that survive within phagolysosomes Microbes that escape from phagolysosomes into cytoplasm	Intracellular bacteria: Mycobacteria *Listeria monocytogenes* *Legionella pneumophila* Fungi: *Cryptococcus neoformans* Protozoa: *Leishmania* *Trypanosoma cruzi*
(B) **Nonphagocytic cell (e.g., epithelial cell)** Cellular receptor for virus —Virus Microbes that infect nonphagocytic cells		Viruses: All Rickettsiae: All Protozoa: *Plasmodium falciparum* *Cryptosporidium parvum*

FIGURE 5–1 Types of intracellular microbes combated by T cell–mediated immunity. A, Microbes may be ingested by phagocytes and may survive within vesicles (phagolysosomes) or escape into the cytoplasm, where they are not susceptible to the microbicidal mechanisms of the phagocytes. **B,** Viruses may bind to receptors on many cell types, including nonphagocytic cells, and may replicate in the cytoplasm of the infected cells. Some viruses establish latent infections, in which viral proteins are produced in infected cells (not shown).

their functions later in this chapter and in Chapter 6.

The major functions of T lymphocytes—activation of phagocytes, killing of infected cells, and help for B cells—require that the T lymphocytes interact with other cells, which may be phagocytes, infected host cells, or B lymphocytes. Recall that the specificity of T cells for peptides displayed by major histocompatibility complex (MHC) molecules ensures that the T cells can see and respond only to antigens associated with other cells (see Chapters 3 and 4). This chapter discusses the way in which T lymphocytes are activated by recognition of cell-associated antigens and other stimuli. We address the following questions:

- What signals are needed to activate T lymphocytes, and what cellular receptors are used to sense and respond to these signals?
- How are the few naive T cells specific for any microbe converted into the large number of effector T cells that have specialized

functions and the ability to eliminate diverse microbes?
- What molecules are produced by T lymphocytes that mediate their communications with other cells, such as macrophages, B lymphocytes, and other leukocytes?

After describing here how T cells recognize and respond to the antigens of cell-associated microbes, in Chapter 6 we discuss how these T cells function to eliminate the microbes.

PHASES OF T CELL RESPONSES

Naive T lymphocytes recognize antigens in the peripheral lymphoid organs, which stimulates their proliferation and differentiation into effector and memory cells, and the effector cells are activated by the same antigens in peripheral tissues or lymphoid organs (Fig. 5–2). Naive T cells express antigen

Induction of response

Antigen recognition in lymphoid organs

CD4+ T cells

CD8+ T cells

CD4+ effector T cells

CD8+ T cells (CTLs)

T cell expansion and differentiation

Differentiated effector T cells enter circulation

Migration of effector T cells and other leukocytes to site of infection

Effector T cells encounter antigens in peripheral tissues

Cells with intracellular microbes

Cytokines

Activation of effector T cells

T cell effector functions

Leukocyte activation (inflammation); phagocytosis and killing of microbes

CTL killing of infected cell

FIGURE 5–2 Induction and effector phases of cell-mediated immunity. (1) Induction of response: Naive CD4+ T cells and CD8+ T cells recognize peptides that are derived from protein antigens and presented by antigen-presenting cells in peripheral lymphoid organs. The T lymphocytes are stimulated to proliferate and differentiate into effector cells, many of which enter the circulation. (2) Migration of effector T cells and other leukocytes to site of antigen: Effector T cells and other leukocytes migrate through blood vessels in peripheral tissues by binding to endothelial cells that have been activated by cytokines produced in response to infection in these tissues. (3) T cell effector functions: CD4+ T cells recruit and activate phagocytes to destroy microbes, and CD8+ cytotoxic T lymphocytes (CTLs) kill infected cells.

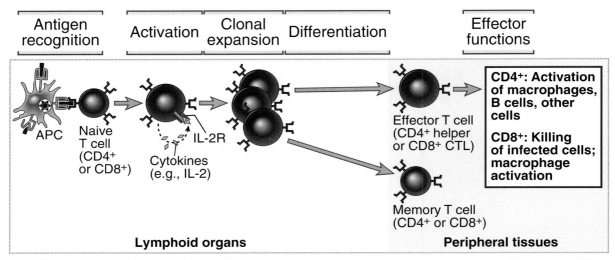

FIGURE 5–3 Steps in the activation of T lymphocytes. Naive T cells recognize major histocompatibility complex (MHC)–associated peptide antigens displayed on antigen-presenting cells and other signals (not shown). The T cells respond by producing cytokines, such as interleukin-2 (IL-2), and expressing receptors for these cytokines, leading to an autocrine pathway of cell proliferation. The result is clonal expansion of the T cells. Some of the progeny differentiate into effector cells, which serve various functions in CMI, and memory cells, which survive for long periods. APC, Antigen-presenting cell; CTL, cytotoxic T lymphocyte; IL-2R, interleukin-2 receptor.

receptors and coreceptors that function in recognizing cells harboring microbes, but these cells are incapable of performing the effector functions required for eliminating the microbes. Differentiated effector cells are capable of performing these functions, which they do in lymphoid organs and in peripheral, nonlymphoid tissues. In this chapter we focus on the responses of naive T cells to antigens, as well as the generation of effector cells. The functions of effector T lymphocytes in CMI are described in Chapter 6 and the roles of helper T cells in antibody responses in Chapter 7.

The responses of naive T lymphocytes to cell-associated microbial antigens consist of a series of sequential steps that result in an increase in the number of antigen-specific T cells and the conversion of naive T cells to effector and memory cells (Fig. 5–3). One of the earliest responses is the secretion of **cytokines,** whose multiple functions in CMI are described later in this chapter. Some cytokines stimulate the proliferation of the antigen-activated T cells, resulting in a rapid increase in the number of antigen-specific lymphocytes, a process called **clonal expansion.** Some of these activated lymphocytes undergo the process of **differentiation,** which results

in the conversion of naive T cells into a population of effector T cells, which function to eliminate microbes. Many of the effector T cells leave the lymphoid organs, enter the circulation, and migrate to any site of infection, where they can eradicate the infection. Some effector T cells may remain in the lymph node, where they function to eradicate infected cells at that site or provide signals to B cells that promote antibody responses against the microbes. Some of the progeny of the T cells that have proliferated in response to antigen develop into **memory T cells,** which are long-lived and functionally inactive, circulate for months or years, and are ready to respond rapidly to repeated exposure to the same microbe. As effector T cells eliminate the infectious agent, the stimuli that triggered T cell expansion and differentiation also are eliminated. As a result, most of the cells in the greatly expanded clone of antigen-specific lymphocytes die, returning the system to a resting state, with memory cells being the cells remaining from the immune response. This sequence of events is common to CD4+ T lymphocytes and CD8+ T lymphocytes, although there are important differences in the properties and effector functions of CD4+ and CD8+ cells, as discussed later.

Central to the function of T cells is their regulated migration through various tissues. As discussed in previous chapters, naive T lymphocytes constantly recirculate through peripheral lymphoid organs searching for foreign protein antigens. The antigens of microbes are transported from the portals of entry of the microbes to the same regions of peripheral lymphoid organs through which naive T cells recirculate. In these organs, the antigens are processed and displayed by MHC molecules on dendritic cells, the antigen-presenting cells (APCs) that are the most efficient stimulators of naive T cells (see Chapter 3). When a T cell recognizes antigen, it is transiently arrested on the dendritic cell and it initiates an activation program. Following activation, the cells may leave the lymphoid organ and migrate preferentially to the inflamed tissue, the original source of the antigen. The control of this directed migration is discussed in Chapter 6.

With this overview, we proceed to a description of the stimuli required for T cell activation and regulation. Three types of stimuli are critical for full T cell activation: antigen recognition initiates the process, costimulation maximizes the response, and cytokines amplify the response and direct it along various specialized differentiation pathways. We then describe the biochemical signals that are generated by antigen recognition and translated into the biologic responses of the lymphocytes.

ANTIGEN RECOGNITION AND COSTIMULATION

The initiation of T cell responses requires multiple receptors on the T cells recognizing ligands on APCs. The T cell receptor (TCR) recognizes MHC-associated peptide antigens, CD4 or CD8 coreceptors recognize the MHC molecules, adhesion molecules strengthen the binding of T cells to APCs, and receptors for costimulators recognize second signals provided by the APCs (Fig. 5–4). The roles of these molecules in T cell responses to antigens are described next.

Recognition of MHC-Associated Peptides

The T cell receptor for antigen (the TCR) and the CD4 or CD8 coreceptor together recognize the complex of peptide antigens and MHC molecules on APCs, and this recognition provides the initiating, or first, signal for T cell activation (Fig. 5–5). The TCR expressed on all CD4$^+$ and CD8$^+$ T cells consists of an α chain and a β chain, both of which participate in antigen recognition (see Chapter 4, Fig. 4–6). (A small subset of T cells expresses TCRs composed of γ and δ chains.) The TCR of a T cell specific for a foreign (e.g., microbial) peptide recognizes the displayed peptide and simultaneously recognizes residues of the MHC molecule located around the peptide-binding cleft. Every mature MHC-restricted T cell expresses either CD4 or CD8, both of which are called coreceptors because they function with the TCR to bind MHC molecules. At the time when the TCR is recognizing the peptide-MHC complex, CD4 or CD8 recognizes the class II or class I MHC molecule, respectively, at a site separate from the peptide-binding cleft. As discussed in Chapter 3, when protein antigens are ingested by APCs from the extracellular milieu into vesicles, these antigens are processed into peptides that are displayed by class II MHC molecules. By contrast, protein antigens present in the cytosol are processed into peptides displayed by class I MHC molecules. Thus, CD4$^+$ T cells recognize antigens ingested from extracellular microbes, and CD8$^+$ T cells recognize peptides derived from cytosolic or nuclear antigens. The specificity of CD4 and CD8 for different classes of MHC molecules and the distinct pathways for the processing of vesicular and cytosolic antigens ensure that different classes of T cells respond to and defend against different types of microbes (see Fig. 3–17). The TCR and its coreceptor need to be engaged simultaneously to initiate the T cell response, and multiple TCRs likely need to be triggered for T cell activation to occur. Once these conditions are achieved, the T cell begins its activation program.

The biochemical signals that lead to T cell activation are triggered by a set of proteins linked to the TCR that are part of the TCR complex and by the CD4 or CD8 coreceptor (see Fig. 5–5). In lymphocytes, antigen recognition and subsequent signaling are performed by different sets of molecules. The TCR αβ heterodimer recognizes antigens, but it is not able to transmit biochemical signals to the interior of the cell. The TCR is noncovalently associated with a complex of transmembrane signaling molecules including three CD3 proteins and a protein called the ζ chain. The TCR, CD3, and ζ chain make up

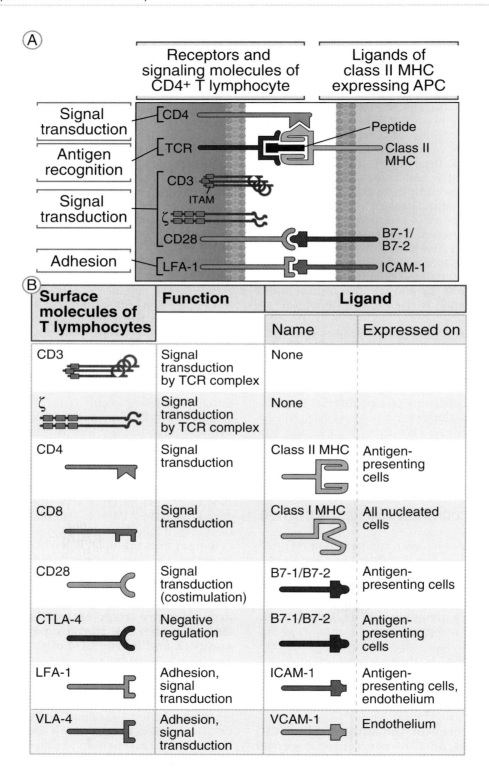

Ⓐ

	Receptors and signaling molecules of CD4+ T lymphocyte	Ligands of class II MHC expressing APC
Signal transduction	CD4	Peptide
Antigen recognition	TCR	Class II MHC
Signal transduction	CD3 — ITAM, ζ, CD28	B7-1/ B7-2
Adhesion	LFA-1	ICAM-1

Ⓑ

Surface molecules of T lymphocytes	Function	Ligand	
		Name	Expressed on
CD3	Signal transduction by TCR complex	None	
ζ	Signal transduction by TCR complex	None	
CD4	Signal transduction	Class II MHC	Antigen-presenting cells
CD8	Signal transduction	Class I MHC	All nucleated cells
CD28	Signal transduction (costimulation)	B7-1/B7-2	Antigen-presenting cells
CTLA-4	Negative regulation	B7-1/B7-2	Antigen-presenting cells
LFA-1	Adhesion, signal transduction	ICAM-1	Antigen-presenting cells, endothelium
VLA-4	Adhesion, signal transduction	VCAM-1	Endothelium

FIGURE 5–4 Molecules involved in T cell activation. A, Major surface molecules of CD4$^+$ T cells involved in the activation of these cells and corresponding ligands on antigen-presenting cells. CD8$^+$ T cells use most of the same molecules, except that the TCR recognizes peptide-class I MHC complexes, and the coreceptor is CD8, which recognizes class I MHC. Immunoreceptor tyrosine-based activation motifs (ITAMs) are the regions of signaling proteins that are phosphorylated on tyrosine residues and become docking sites for other signaling molecules (see Fig. 5–9). CD3 is composed of three polypeptide chains, δ, ε, and γ, arranged in two pairs (δε and γε); we show CD3 as three protein chains. **B,** Important properties of major surface molecules of T cells involved in functional responses. The functions of most of these molecules are described in this chapter; the role of CTLA-4 in shutting off T cell responses is described in Chapter 9. VLA-4, like LFA-1, is an integrin involved in leukocyte binding to endothelium (see Chapter 6). APC, Antigen-presenting cell; ICAM-1, intercellular adhesion molecule 1; LFA-1, leukocyte function–associated antigen 1; MHC, major histocompatibility complex; TCR, T cell receptor; VLA, very late antigen.

the TCR complex. Although the α and β TCRs must vary among T cell clones to recognize diverse antigens, the signaling functions of TCRs are the same in all clones, and therefore the CD3 and ζ proteins are invariant among different T cells. The mechanisms of signal transduction by these proteins of the TCR complex are discussed later in the chapter.

T cells can also be activated experimentally by molecules that bind to the TCRs of many or all clones of T cells, regardless of the peptide-MHC specificity of the TCR. These polyclonal activators of T cells include antibodies specific for the TCR or associated CD3 proteins, polymeric carbohydrate-binding proteins such as phytohemagglutinin (PHA), and certain microbial proteins called superantigens. Polyclonal activators often are used as experimental tools to study T cell responses, and in clinical settings to test for T cell function or to prepare metaphase spreads for chromosomal analyses. Microbial superantigens may cause systemic inflammatory disease by inducing excessive cytokine release from many T cells.

Role of Adhesion Molecules in T Cell Responses

Adhesion molecules on T cells recognize their ligands on APCs and stabilize the binding of the T cells to the APCs. Most TCRs bind the peptide-MHC complexes for which they are specific with low affinity. A possible reason for this weak recognition is that T cells are positively selected during their maturation by weak recognition of self MHC with self peptides, and not by foreign antigens because these antigens are not present in the thymus where T cells are maturing (see Chapter 4). To induce a response, the binding of T cells to APCs must be stabilized for a sufficiently long period that the necessary signaling threshold is achieved. This stabilization function is performed by adhesion molecules on the T cells that bind to ligands expressed on APCs. The most important of these adhesion molecules belong to the family of heterodimeric (two-chain) proteins called **integrins.** The major T cell integrin involved in binding to APCs is leukocyte function–associated antigen 1 (LFA-1), whose ligand on APCs is called intercellular adhesion molecule 1 (ICAM-1).

FIGURE 5–5 Antigen recognition and signal transduction during T cell activation. Different T cell molecules recognize antigen and deliver biochemical signals to the interior of the cell as a result of antigen recognition. The CD3 and ζ proteins are noncovalently attached to the T cell receptor (TCR) α and β chains by interactions between charged amino acids in the transmembrane domains of these proteins (not shown). The figure illustrates a CD4$^+$ T cell; the same interactions are involved in the activation of CD8$^+$ T cells, except that the co-receptor is CD8 and the TCR recognizes a peptide–class I MHC complex. APC, Antigen-presenting cell; MHC, major histocompatibility complex.

FIGURE 5–6 Role of costimulation in T cell activation. Resting antigen-presenting cells (APCs), which have not been exposed to microbes or adjuvants, may present peptide antigens, but they do not express costimulators and are unable to activate naive T cells. T cells that recognize antigen without costimulation may become unresponsive (tolerant) to subsequent exposure to antigen. Microbes, as well as cytokines produced during innate immune responses to microbes, induce the expression of costimulators, such as B7 molecules, on the APCs. The B7 costimulators are recognized by the CD28 receptor on naive T cells, providing signal 2. In conjunction with antigen recognition (signal 1), this recognition initiates T cell responses. Activated APCs also produce cytokines that stimulate the differentiation of naive T cells into effector cells. IL, Interleukin.

On resting naive T cells, which are cells that have not previously recognized and been activated by antigen, the LFA-1 integrin is in a low-affinity state. Antigen recognition by a T cell increases the affinity of that cell's LFA-1. Therefore, once a T cell sees antigen, it increases the strength of its binding to the APC presenting that antigen, providing a positive feedback loop. Thus, integrin-mediated adhesion is critical for the ability of T cells to bind to APCs displaying microbial antigens. Integrins also play an important role in directing the migration of effector T cells and other leukocytes from the circulation to sites of infection. This process is described in Chapters 2 and 6.

Role of Costimulation in T Cell Activation

The full activation of T cells depends on the recognition of costimulators on APCs in addition to antigen (Fig. 5–6). We have previously referred to costimulators as second signals for T cell activation (see Chapters 2 and 3). The name **costimulator** derives from the fact that these molecules provide stimuli to T cells that function together with stimulation by antigen. The best-defined costimulators for T cells are two related proteins called B7-1 (CD80) and B7-2 (CD86), both of which are expressed on APCs and whose expression is increased when the APCs encounter microbes. These B7 proteins are recognized by a receptor called CD28, which is expressed on virtually all T cells. The binding of CD28 on T cells to B7 on the APCs generates signals in the T cells that work together with signals generated by TCR recognition of antigen presented by MHC proteins on the same APCs. CD28-mediated signaling is essential for the responses of naive T cells; in the absence of CD28-B7 interactions, antigen recognition by the TCR is insufficient for T cell activation. The requirement for costimulation ensures that naive T lymphocytes are activated fully by microbial antigens, and not by harmless foreign substances (or by self antigens), because, as stated previously, microbes stimulate the expression of B7 costimulators on APCs.

Another set of molecules that participate in T cell responses are CD40 ligand (CD40L, or CD154) on activated T cells and CD40 on APCs. These molecules do not directly enhance T cell activation. Instead, CD40L expressed on an antigen-stimulated T cell binds to CD40 on APCs and activates the APCs to express more B7 costimulators and to secrete cytokines (e.g., IL-12) that enhance T cell differentiation. Thus, the CD40L-CD40 interaction promotes T cell activation by making APCs better at stimulating T cells.

The role of costimulation in T cell activation explains an observation mentioned in earlier chapters. Protein antigens, such as those used in vaccines, fail to elicit T cell–dependent immune responses unless these antigens are administered with substances that activate APCs, especially dendritic cells. Such substances are called **adjuvants,** and they function mainly by inducing the expression of costimulators on APCs and by stimulating the APCs to secrete cytokines that activate T cells. Most adjuvants are products of microbes (e.g., killed mycobacteria) or substances that mimic microbes, and they bind to pattern recognition receptors of the innate immune system, such as Toll-like receptors (see Chapter 2). Thus, adjuvants trick the immune system into responding to purified protein antigens in a vaccine as if they were parts of infectious microbes.

Understanding the nature and biology of costimulators is an evolving story, and much remains to be learned about the regulation and functions of this family of proteins. These issues are of practical importance because enhancing the expression of costimulators may be useful for stimulating T cell responses (e.g., against tumors), and blocking costimulators may be a strategy for inhibiting unwanted responses. Agents that block B7:CD28 are used in the treatment of rheumatoid arthritis, other inflammatory diseases, and graft rejection, and antibodies to block CD40:CD40L interactions are being tested in inflammatory diseases and in transplant recipients to reduce or prevent graft rejection.

Proteins homologous to CD28 also are critical for limiting and terminating immune responses. Thus, different members of the CD28 family are involved in activating and inhibiting T cells. The prototypes of the inhibitory receptors are CTLA-4, which, like CD28, recognizes B7-1 and B7-2 on APCs, and PD-1, which recognizes different but structurally related ligands on many cell types. Both CTLA-4 and PD-1 are induced in activated T cells, and genetic deletion of these molecules in mice results in excessive lymphocyte expansion and autoimmune disease. CTLA-4 and PD-1 are also involved in inhibiting responses to some tumors, and PD-1 inhibits responses to some chronic viral infections. These discoveries are the basis for the use of antibodies that block CTLA-4 or PD-1 to enhance immune responses to tumors in patients with cancer. The role of these inhibitory receptors in maintaining unresponsiveness to self antigens is discussed in Chapter 9.

Stimuli for Activation of CD8+ T Cells

The activation of CD8+ T cells is stimulated by recognition of class I MHC–associated peptides and requires costimulation and/or helper T cells (Fig. 5–7). The responses of CD8+ T cells may differ in several ways from responses of CD4+ T lymphocytes. One feature unique to CD8+ T cell activation is that its initiation often requires cytoplasmic antigen from one cell (e.g., virus-infected cells) to be cross-presented by dendritic cells (see Fig. 3–16). Another characteristic of CD8+ T cells is that their differentiation into fully active cytotoxic T lymphocytes (CTLs), and into memory cells, may require the concomitant activation of CD4+ helper T cells. When virus-infected cells are ingested by dendritic cells the APC may present antigens from the cytosol in complex with class I MHC molecules and from vesicles in complex with class II MHC molecules. Thus, both CD8+ T cells and CD4+ T cells specific for viral antigens are activated near one another. The CD4+ T cells may produce cytokines or membrane molecules that help to activate the CD8+ T cells. This requirement for helper T cells in CD8+ T cell responses is the likely explanation for the defective CTL responses to many viruses in patients infected with the human immunodeficiency virus (HIV), which kills CD4+ but not CD8+ T cells. CTL responses to some viruses do not appear to require help from CD4+ T cells.

FIGURE 5–7 Activation of CD8⁺ T cells. Antigen-presenting cells (APCs), principally dendritic cells, may ingest infected cells and present microbial antigens to CD8⁺ T cells (cross-presentation) and to CD4⁺ helper T cells. Sometimes, the APC may be infected and can directly present antigens (not shown). The helper T cells then produce cytokines that stimulate the expansion and differentiation of the CD8⁺ T cells. It is also postulated that helper cells may activate APCs to make them potent stimulators of CD8⁺ T cells (not shown) CTLs, Cytotoxic T lymphocytes.

Now that we have described the stimuli required to activate naive T lymphocytes, we next consider the biochemical pathways triggered by antigen recognition and other stimuli.

BIOCHEMICAL PATHWAYS OF T CELL ACTIVATION

On recognition of antigens and costimulators, T cells express proteins that are involved in proliferation, differentiation, and effector functions of the cells (Fig. 5–8). Naive T cells that have not encountered antigen have a low level of protein synthesis. Within minutes of antigen recognition, new gene transcription and protein synthesis are seen in the activated T cells. These newly expressed proteins mediate many of the subsequent responses of the T cells.

The biochemical pathways that link antigen recognition with T cell responses consist of the activation of enzymes, recruitment of adaptor proteins, and production of active transcription factors (Fig. 5–9). These biochemical pathways are initiated when the TCR complexes and the appropriate coreceptor are brought together by binding to MHC-peptide complexes on the surface of APCs.

In addition, there is an orderly redistribution of other proteins in both the APC and T cell membranes at the point of cell-to-cell contact, such that the TCR complex, CD4/CD8 coreceptors, and CD28 coalesce to the center and the integrins move to form a peripheral ring. This redistribution of signaling and adhesion molecules is thought to be responsible for optimal induction of activating signals in the T cell. The region of contact between the APC and T cell, including the redistributed membrane proteins, is called the **immunologic synapse.** Although the synapse was first described as the site of transduction of activating signals, it may serve other functions. Some effector molecules and cytokines may be secreted through this region, ensuring that they do not diffuse away but are targeted to the APC. Enzymes that serve to degrade or inhibit signaling molecules are also recruited to the synapse, so it may be involved in terminating lymphocyte activation.

The CD4 and CD8 coreceptors facilitate signaling through a protein tyrosine kinase called Lck that is noncovalently attached to the cytoplasmic tails of these coreceptors. As discussed in Chapter 4, several transmembrane signaling proteins are associated with the TCR, including the CD3 and ζ chains. CD3 and ζ contain motifs, each with two tyrosine residues, called

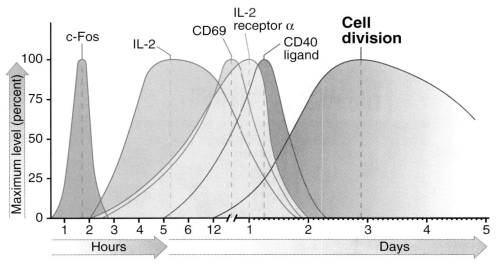

FIGURE 5–8 Proteins produced by antigen-stimulated T cells. Antigen recognition by T cells results in the synthesis and expression of a variety of proteins, examples of which are shown. The kinetics of production of these proteins are approximations and may vary in different T cells and with different types of stimuli. The possible effects of costimulation on the patterns or kinetics of gene expression are not shown. c-Fos is a transcription factor; interleukin-2 (IL-2) is a cytokine that functions as a growth factor for T cells; CD69 is a marker of T cell activation involved in cell migration; CD40 ligand is an effector molecule of T cells.

immunoreceptor tyrosine-based activation motifs (ITAMs), which are critical for signaling. Lck, which is brought near the TCR complex by the CD4 or CD8 molecules, phosphorylates tyrosine residues contained within the ITAMs of the CD3 and ζ proteins. The phosphorylated ITAMs of the ζ chain become docking sites for a tyrosine kinase called ZAP-70 (zeta-associated protein of 70 kD), which also is phosphorylated by Lck and thereby made enzymatically active. The active ZAP-70 then phosphorylates various adaptor proteins and enzymes, which assemble near the TCR complex and mediate additional signaling events. Major signaling pathways linked to ζ-chain phosphorylation and ZAP-70 are the calcium-NFAT pathway, the Ras– and Rac–MAP kinase pathways, the PKCθ–NF-κB pathway, and the PI-3 kinase pathway.

Nuclear factor of activated T cells (NFAT) is a transcription factor present in an inactive phosphorylated form in the cytoplasm of resting T cells. NFAT activation and its nuclear translocation depend on the concentration of calcium (Ca^{2+}) ions in the cell. This signaling pathway is initiated by ZAP-70–mediated phosphorylation and activation of an enzyme called phospholipase Cγ (PLCγ), which catalyzes the hydrolysis of a plasma membrane inositol phospholipid

called phosphatidylinositol 4,5-bisphosphate (PIP_2). One byproduct of PLCγ-mediated PIP_2 breakdown, called inositol 1,4,5-triphosphate (IP_3), binds to IP_3 receptors on the endoplasmic reticulum (ER) membrane and stimulates release of Ca^{2+} from the ER, thereby raising the cytosolic Ca^{2+} concentration. In response to the loss of calcium from intracellular stores, a plasma membrane calcium channel is opened, leading to the influx of extracellular Ca^{2+} into the cell, which sustains the elevated Ca^{2+} concentration for hours. Cytoplasmic Ca^{2+} binds a protein called calmodulin, and the Ca^{2+}-calmodulin complex activates a phosphatase called calcineurin. This enzyme removes phosphates from cytoplasmic NFAT, enabling it to migrate into the nucleus, where it binds to and activates the promoters of several genes, including the genes encoding the T cell growth factor interleukin-2 (IL-2) and components of the IL-2 receptor. A drug called cyclosporine binds to and inhibits the phosphatase activity of calcineurin and thus inhibits the NFAT-dependent production of cytokines by T cells. This agent is widely used as an immunosuppressive drug to prevent graft rejection; its introduction was one of the major factors in the success of organ transplantation (see Chapter 10).

FIGURE 5–9 Signal transduction pathways in T lymphocytes. Antigen recognition by T cells induces early signaling events, which include tyrosine phosphorylation of molecules of the T cell receptor (TCR) complex and the recruitment of adaptor proteins to the site of T cell antigen recognition. These early events lead to the activation of several biochemical intermediates, which in turn activate transcription factors that stimulate transcription of genes whose products mediate the responses of the T cells. The possible effects of costimulation on these signaling pathways are not shown. These signaling pathways are illustrated as independent of one another, for simplicity, but may be interconnected in more complex networks. AP-1, Activating protein 1; APC, antigen-presenting cell; GTP/GDP, guanosine triphosphate/diphosphate; ITAM, immunoreceptor tyrosine-based activation motif; mTOR, mammalian target of rapamycin; NFAT, nuclear factor of activated T cells; PKC, protein kinase C; PLCγ1, γ1 isoform of phosphatidylinositol-specific phospholipase C; PI-3, phosphatidylinositol-3; ZAP-70, zeta-associated protein of 70 kD.

The **Ras/Rac–MAP kinase pathways** include the guanosine triphosphate (GTP)–binding Ras and Rac proteins, several adaptor proteins, and a cascade of enzymes that eventually activate one of a family of mitogen-activated protein (MAP) kinases. These pathways are initiated by ZAP-70–dependent phosphorylation and accumulation of adaptor proteins at the plasma membrane, leading to the recruitment of Ras or Rac, and their activation by exchange of bound guanosine diphosphate (GDP) with GTP. Ras•GTP and Rac•GTP initiate different enzyme cascades, leading to the activation of distinct MAP kinases. The terminal MAP kinases in these pathways, called extracellular signal–regulated kinase (ERK) and c-Jun amino-terminal

(N-terminal) kinase (JNK), respectively induce the expression of a protein called c-Fos and the phosphorylation of another protein called c-Jun. c-Fos and phosphorylated c-Jun combine to form the transcription factor **activating protein 1 (AP-1),** which enhances the transcription of several T cell genes.

Another major pathway involved in TCR signaling consists of activation of the θ isoform of the serine-threonine kinase called protein kinase C (PKCθ) and activation of the transcription factor **nuclear factor κB (NF-κB).** PKC is activated by diacylglycerol, which, like IP$_3$, is generated by PLC-mediated hydrolysis of membrane inositol lipids. PKCθ acts through adaptor proteins recruited to the TCR complex to activate NF-κB. NF-κB exists in the cytoplasm of resting T cells in an inactive form, bound to an inhibitor called IκB. TCR-induced signals, downstream of PKCθ, activate a kinase that phosphorylates IκB and targets it for destruction. As a result, NF-κB is released and moves to the nucleus, where it promotes the transcription of several genes.

T cell receptor signal transduction also involves a lipid kinase called **phosphatidylinositol-3 (PI-3) kinase,** which phosphorylates membrane PIP$_2$ to generate PIP$_3$. The phospholipid PIP$_3$ is required for the activation of a number of crucial targets including a serine-threonine kinase called protein kinase B, or Akt, which has many roles, including stimulating expression of anti-apoptotic proteins and thus promoting survival of antigen-stimulated T cells. The PI-3 kinase/Akt pathway is triggered not only by the TCR but also by CD28 and IL-2 receptors. Closely linked to the Akt pathway is mTOR (mammalian target of rapamycin), a serine-threonine kinase that is involved in stimulating protein translation and in cell survival and growth. A drug that binds to and inactivates mTOR, rapamycin, is used to treat graft rejection.

The various transcription factors, including NFAT, AP-1, and NF-κB, stimulate transcription and subsequent production of cytokines, cytokine receptors, cell cycle inducers, and effector molecules such as CD40L (see Fig. 5–8). All these signals are initiated by antigen recognition, because binding of the TCR and coreceptors to antigen (peptide-MHC complexes) is necessary to initiate signaling in T cells.

As stated earlier, recognition of costimulators, such as B7 molecules, by their receptor (CD28) is essential for full T cell responses. The biochemical signals transduced by CD28 on binding to B7 costimulators are less well defined than are TCR-triggered signals. CD28 engagement likely amplifies some TCR signaling pathways that are triggered by antigen recognition (signal 1) and also initiates a distinct set of signals that complement TCR signals.

Having described the stimuli and biochemical pathways in T cell activation, we now discuss how T cells respond to antigens and differentiate into effector cells capable of combating microbes.

FUNCTIONAL RESPONSES OF T LYMPHOCYTES TO ANTIGEN AND COSTIMULATION

The recognition of antigen and costimulators by T cells initiates an orchestrated set of responses that culminate in the expansion of the antigen-specific clones of lymphocytes and the differentiation of the naive T cells into effector cells and memory cells (see Fig. 5–3). Many of the responses of T cells are mediated by cytokines that are secreted by the T cells and act on the T cells themselves and on many other cells involved in immune defenses. Each component of the biologic responses of T cells is discussed next.

Secretion of Cytokines and Expression of Cytokine Receptors

In response to antigen and costimulators, T lymphocytes, especially CD4$^+$ T cells, rapidly secrete several different cytokines that have diverse activities (Fig. 5–10). Cytokines are a large group of proteins that function as mediators of immunity and inflammation. We have already discussed cytokines in innate immune responses, which are produced mainly by dendritic cells and macrophages (see Chapter 2). In adaptive immunity, cytokines are secreted by T cells, mainly CD4$^+$ cells. These proteins share some important properties (Fig. 5–10, *A*), although different cytokines have distinct activities and play different roles in immune responses (Fig. 5–10, *B*).

The first cytokine to be produced by CD4$^+$ T cells, within 1 to 2 hours after activation, is interleukin-2 (IL-2). Activation also rapidly enhances the ability of T cells to bind and respond to IL-2, by increasing the expression of

A **General properties of T cell cytokines**

Property	Significance
Produced transiently in response to antigen	Provides cytokine when needed
Usually acts on same cell that produces the cytokine (autocrine) or nearby cells (paracrine)	Systemic effects of cytokines usually reflect severe infections or autoimmunity
Pleiotropism: each cytokine has multiple biologic actions	Provides diversity of actions but may limit clinical utility of cytokines because of unwanted effects
Redundancy: multiple cytokines may share the same or similar biologic activities	Blocking any one cytokine may not achieve a desired effect

B **Biologic actions of select T cell cytokines**

Cytokine	Principal action	Cellular source(s)
Interleukin-2 (IL-2)	Survival, proliferation, and differentiation of effector and regulatory T cells	CD4$^+$ and CD8$^+$ T cells
IL-4	B cell switching to IgE	CD4$^+$ T cells, mast cells
IL-5	Activation of eosinophils	CD4$^+$ T cells, mast cells
Interferon-γ (IFN-γ)	Activation of macrophages	CD4$^+$ and CD8$^+$ T cells, natural killer cells
IL-17	Stimulation of acute inflammation	CD4$^+$ T cells; other cells
TGF-β	Inhibition of T cell activation; differentiation of regulatory T cells	CD4$^+$ T cells; many other cell types

FIGURE 5–10 Properties of the major cytokines produced by CD4$^+$ helper T lymphocytes. A, General properties of all cytokines and their importance. **B,** Effector functions of select cytokines involved in T cell–mediated immunity. Transforming growth factor β (TGF-β) functions mainly as an inhibitor of immune responses; its role is discussed in Chapter 9. The cytokines of innate immunity are shown in Figure 2–14. More information about these cytokines and their receptors is provided in Appendix II. IgE, Immunoglobulin E.

the high-affinity IL-2 receptor (Fig. 5–11). The receptor for IL-2 is a three-chain molecule. Naive T cells express two signaling chains but do not express the chain that enables the receptor to bind IL-2 with high affinity. Within hours after activation by antigens and costimulators, the T cells produce the third chain of the receptor, and now the complete IL-2 receptor is able to bind IL-2 strongly. Thus, IL-2 produced by antigen-stimulated T cells preferentially binds to and acts

on the same T cells, an example of autocrine cytokine action. The principal functions of IL-2 are to stimulate the survival and proliferation of T cells, resulting in an increase in the number of the antigen-specific T cells; IL-2 was originally called T cell growth factor. (IL-2 also is essential for the maintenance of regulatory T cells and thus for controlling immune responses, as we discuss in Chapter 9.) Differentiated effector CD4$^+$ T cells produce many other cytokines, and

T cell activation by antigen + costimulator

Secretion of IL-2

Expression of IL-2Rα chain; formation of high-affinity IL-2Rαβγ complex

IL-2–induced T cell proliferation

IL-2Rβγc complex

Resting (naive) T cell

CD28

Costimulator (B7)

IL-2

IL-2Rαβγc complex

IL-2Rβγc

Low-affinity IL-2R ($K_d \sim 10^{-9}$ M)

IL-2Rαβγc

High-affinity IL-2R ($K_d \sim 10^{-11}$ M)

FIGURE 5–11 Role of interleukin-2 and IL-2 receptors in T cell proliferation. Naive T cells express the low-affinity IL-2 receptor (IL-2R) complex, made up of the β and γc chains (γc designates common γ chain, so called because it is component of receptors for several cytokines). On activation by antigen recognition and costimulation, the cells produce IL-2 and express the α chain of the IL-2R, which associates with the β and γc chains to form the high-affinity IL-2 receptor. Binding of IL-2 to its receptor initiates proliferation of the T cells that recognized the antigen. APC, Antigen-presenting cell.

the functions of some of the major cytokines are described later.

CD8+ T lymphocytes that recognize antigen and costimulators do not appear to secrete large amounts of IL-2, but these lymphocytes proliferate prodigiously during immune responses. Antigen recognition and costimulation may be able to drive the proliferation of CD8+ T cells, or IL-2 may be provided by CD4+ helper T cells (see Fig. 5-7).

Clonal Expansion

T lymphocytes activated by antigen and costimulation begin to proliferate within 1 or 2 days, resulting in expansion of antigen-specific clones (Fig. 5–12). This expansion quickly provides a large pool of antigen-specific lymphocytes from which effector cells can be generated to combat infection.

The magnitude of clonal expansion is remarkable, especially for CD8+ T cells. Before infection, the frequency of CD8+ T cells specific for any one

microbial protein antigen is about 1 in 10^5 or 10^6 lymphocytes in the body. At the peak of some viral infections, possibly within a week after the infection, as many as 10% to 20% of all the lymphocytes in the lymphoid organs may be specific for that virus. This means that the antigen-specific clones have increased by more than 10,000-fold, with an estimated doubling time of about 6 hours. Several features of this clonal expansion are surprising. First, this enormous expansion of T cells specific for a microbe is not accompanied by a detectable increase in bystander cells that do not recognize that microbe. Second, even in infections with complex microbes that contain many protein antigens, a majority of the expanded clones are specific for only a few, often less than five, immunodominant peptides of that microbe.

The expansion of CD4+ T cells appears to be much less than that of CD8+ cells, probably 100-fold to 1000-fold. This difference in the magnitude of clonal expansion of CD8+ T cells and CD4+ T cells may reflect differences in their

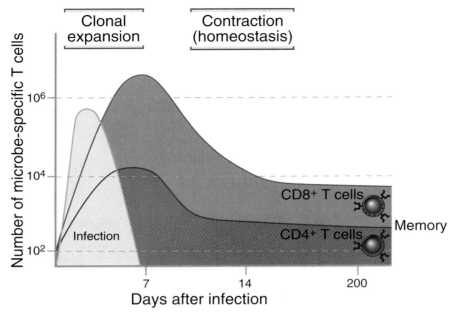

FIGURE 5–12 Expansion and decline of T cell responses. The numbers of CD4⁺ and CD8⁺ T cells specific for various antigens, and the clonal expansion and contraction during immune responses, are illustrated. The numbers are approximations based on studies of model microbial and other antigens in inbred mice; in humans, the numbers of lymphocytes are about 1000-fold greater.

functions. CD8⁺ CTLs are effector cells that kill infected cells by direct contact, and many CTLs may be needed to kill large numbers of infected cells. By contrast, each CD4⁺ effector cell secretes cytokines that activate many other effector cells, so a relatively small number of cytokine producers may be sufficient.

Within a week or two of their activation, some of the expanded T cells have differentiated into effector and memory cells and the majority die as the stimuli that initiated the response are eliminated. The result is contraction of the expanded clones and a return to the baseline steady state. This process is described later.

Differentiation of Naive T Cells into Effector Cells

Some of the progeny of antigen-stimulated, proliferating T cells differentiate into effector cells whose function is eradicate infections. This process of differentiation is the result of changes in gene expression, such as the activation of genes encoding cytokines (in CD4⁺ T cells) or cytotoxic proteins (in CD8⁺ CTLs). It begins in concert with clonal expansion, and differentiated effector cells appear within 3 or 4 days after

exposure to microbes. As mentioned earlier many of these cells leave the peripheral lymphoid organs and migrate to the site of infection. Here the effector cells again encounter the microbial antigens that stimulated their development. On recognition of antigen, the effector cells respond in ways that serve to eradicate the infection. Effector cells of the CD4⁺ and CD8⁺ populations perform different functions and are best described separately. Some differentiated CD4⁺ helper T cells migrate into lymphoid follicles in the lymphoid organs, where they stay to help B cells (see Chapter 7).

Effector cells of the CD4⁺ helper lineage function to activate phagocytes and B lymphocytes by expressing various surface molecules and secreting cytokines (Fig. 5–13). The most important cell surface protein involved in the effector function of CD4⁺ T cells is CD40 ligand, a member of a large family of proteins structurally related to the cytokine tumor necrosis factor (TNF). The *CD40L* gene is transcribed in CD4⁺ T cells in response to antigen recognition and costimulation, and so CD40L is expressed on activated helper T cells. It binds to its receptor, CD40, which is expressed mainly on macrophages, B lymphocytes, and dendritic cells.

CD4+ T cells activate macrophages, B lymphocytes

Effector functions of activated macrophages, B lymphocytes

(A) **Cell-mediated immunity**

Macrophage

CD4+ T lymphocyte

CD40 ligand — CD40

Cytokine — Cytokine receptor

Macrophage activation and killing of phagocytosed microbes

(B) **Humoral immunity**

Antigen-specific B lymphocyte

CD4+ T lymphocyte

CD40 ligand — CD40

Cytokine receptor

Secretion of antibodies with enhanced abilities to neutralize and eliminate antigens

FIGURE 5–13 Molecules involved in effector functions of CD4+ helper T cells. CD4+ T cells that have differentiated into effector cells express CD40L and secrete cytokines. CD40L binds to CD40 on macrophages or B lymphocytes, and cytokines bind to their receptors on the same cells. The combination of signals delivered by CD40 and cytokine receptors (arrows) activates macrophages in CMI **(A)** and activates B cells to produce high-affinity isotype-switched antibodies in humoral immune responses **(B)**.

Engagement of CD40 activates these cells, and thus CD40L is an important participant in the activation of macrophages and B lymphocytes by helper T cells (see Chapters 6 and 7). The interaction of CD40L on T cells with CD40 on dendritic cells stimulates the expression of costimulators on these APCs and the production of T cell–activating cytokines, thus providing a positive feedback (amplification) mechanism for APC-induced T cell activation.

Subsets of CD4+ Helper T Cells Distinguished by Cytokine Profiles

In the 1980s, analysis of cytokine production by helper T cells revealed that functionally distinct subsets of CD4+ T cells exist, distinguished by the cytokines they produce, and more recently, additional subsets have been defined. The existence of these subsets explains how the immune system responds differently to different microbes. For example, intracellular microbes such as mycobacteria are ingested by phagocytes but resist intracellular killing. The adaptive immune response to such microbes results in the activation of the phagocytes to kill the ingested microbes. In contrast, helminthic parasites are too large to be phagocytosed, and the immune response to helminths is dominated by the production of immunoglobulin E (IgE) antibodies and the activation of eosinophils. IgE antibody binds to the helminths, and eosinophils destroy the helminths. Both these types of immune

	Signature cytokines	Immune reactions	Host defense	Role in diseases
T_H1 cell	IFNγ	Macrophage activation; IgG production	Intracellular microbes	Autoimmune diseases; tissue damage associated with chronic infections
T_H2 cell	IL-4 IL-5 IL-13	Mast cell, eosinophil activation; IgE production; alternative macrophage activation	Helminthic parasites	Allergic diseases
T_H17 cell	IL-17A IL-17F IL-22	Neutrophilic, monocytic inflammation	Extracellular bacteria; fungi	Autoimmune and inflammatory diseases

FIGURE 5–14 Characteristics of subsets of CD4+ helper T lymphocytes. A naive CD4+ T cell may differentiate into subsets that produce different cytokines and perform different effector functions. The table summarizes the major differences among T_H1, T_H2, and T_H17 subsets of helper T cells. Note that many helper T cells may not be readily classified into these distinct, polarized subsets. IFN, Interferon; Ig, immunoglobulin; IL, interleukin.

responses depend on CD4+ helper T cells, but for many years it was not clear how the CD4+ helper cells are able to stimulate such distinct immune effector mechanisms. We now know that these responses are mediated by functionally distinct subpopulations of CD4+ effector T cells that produce different cytokines, as described next.

CD4+ helper T cells may differentiate into at least three subsets of effector cells that produce distinct sets of cytokines and perform different functions (Fig. 5–14). The subsets that were defined first are called **T_H1 cells** and **T_H2 cells** (for type 1 helper T cells and type 2 helper T cells); more recently, a third population has been identified and called **T_H17 cells** because its signature cytokine is interleukin-17. (Regulatory T cells, another subset of CD4+ T cells, suppress immune responses and are discussed in Chapter 9 in the context of immunologic tolerance.) The existence of these subpopulations has been an important milestone in understanding immune responses, and provides excellent models for studying the process of cell differentiation. However, it should be noted that many activated CD4+ T cells may produce various mixtures of cytokines and therefore cannot be readily classified into these subsets, and there may be

considerable plasticity in these populations so that one subset may convert into another under some conditions. In addition, the cytokines that are characteristic of these subsets may be produced by cells other than CD4+ T lymphocytes. The contributions of these other cell types to host defense and inflammatory diseases are not fully understood, but are topics of considerable scientific interest.

Functions of CD4+ T Cell Subsets
The T_H1 Subset

T_H1 cells stimulate phagocyte-mediated ingestion and killing of microbes, a key component of cell-mediated immunity (Fig. 5–15). The most important cytokine produced by T_H1 cells is **interferon-γ** (IFN-γ), so called because it was discovered as a cytokine that inhibited (or interfered with) viral infection. IFN-γ is a potent activator of macrophages, especially the ability of macrophages to kill ingested microbes (classical macrophage activation). (The type I IFNs [Chapter 2] are much more potent anti-viral cytokines than is IFN-γ.) IFN-γ also stimulates the production of antibody isotypes that promote the phagocytosis of microbes, because these antibodies bind directly to phagocyte Fc receptors and they activate

FIGURE 5–15 Functions of T$_H$1 cells. T$_H$1 cells produce the cytokine interferon-γ (IFN-γ), which activates phagocytes to kill phagocytosed microbes (classical pathway of macrophage activation) and stimulates the production of antibodies that promote the ingestion of microbes by the phagocytes. The role of T$_H$1 cells in antibody responses is better documented in mice than in humans. APC, Antigen-presenting cell.

complement, generating products that bind to phagocyte complement receptors (see Chapter 8). Because of these actions of IFN-γ, T$_H$1 cells are critical for ingestion and killing of intracellular microbes in phagocytes. Individuals with mutations affecting the generation or function of T$_H$1 cells are extremely susceptible to infections by such organisms, especially atypical mycobacteria, which are common in the environment and usually not pathogenic in healthy people. IFN-γ also stimulates the expression of class II MHC molecules and B7 costimulators on macrophages and dendritic cells, which may serve to amplify T cell responses.

The T$_H$2 subset

T$_H$2 cells stimulate phagocyte-independent, eosinophil-mediated immunity, which is especially effective against helminthic parasites (Fig. 5–16). T$_H$2 cells produce interleukin-4, which stimulates the production of IgE antibodies, and interleukin-5, which activates eosinophils. IgE activates mast cells and binds to eosinophils. These IgE-dependent, mast cell– and eosinophil-mediated reactions are important in killing helminthic parasites. IgE coats the helminths, eosinophils bind to the IgE, eosinophils are activated to release their granule contents, and granule enzymes kill the parasites. In addition, some of the cytokines produced by T$_H$2 cells, such as IL-4 and IL-13, promote the expulsion of parasites from mucosal organs and inhibit the entry of microbes by stimulating mucus secretion. The cytokines of T$_H$2 cells also activate macrophages. Unlike T$_H$1-mediated activation, which enhances the ability of macrophages to kill microbes, T$_H$2-mediated macrophage activation enhances other functions, such as synthesis of extracellular matrix proteins involved in tissue repair. This type of response is called alternative macrophage activation (see Fig. 2-10). Some of the cytokines produced by T$_H$2 cells, such as IL-4, IL-10, and IL-13, inhibit the microbicidal activities of macrophages and thus suppress T$_H$1 cell–mediated immunity. Therefore, the efficacy of cell-mediated immune responses against a microbe may be determined by a balance between the activation of T$_H$1 and T$_H$2 cells in response to that microbe. We return to this concept and its importance in infectious diseases in Chapter 6.

The T$_H$17 Subset

T$_H$17 cells induce inflammation, which functions to destroy extracellular bacteria and fungi and may contribute to several inflammatory diseases (Fig. 5–17). This subset, which secretes IL-17 and IL-22, was discovered because of its role in animal models of immunologic diseases (multiple sclerosis, inflammatory bowel disease, rheumatoid arthritis) and is increasingly being implicated in these diseases in humans. T$_H$17 cells secrete cytokines that recruit leukocytes, mainly neutrophils but also monocytes, to sites of antigen recognition. Therefore, these cells are important in defense against

FIGURE 5–16 Functions of T$_H$2 cells. T$_H$2 cells produce the cytokines interleukin-4 (IL-4), which stimulates the production of immunoglobulin E (IgE) antibody, and IL-5, which activates eosinophils. IgE participates in the activation of mast cells by protein antigens and coats helminths, and eosinophils destroy the helminths. T$_H$2 cells stimulate the production of other antibody isotypes that may neutralize microbes and toxins, but do not opsonize microbes for phagocytosis or activate complement by the classical pathway. APC, Antigen-presenting cell; IL, interleukin.

extracellular bacterial and fungal infections. Mutations in genes involved in the development and functions of these cells result in increased susceptibility to bacterial and fungal infections, particularly mucocutaneous candidiasis.

Development of T$_H$1, T$_H$2, and T$_H$17 Subsets

The generation of these subsets is regulated by the stimuli that naive CD4$^+$ T cells receive when they encounter microbial antigens (Fig. 5–18). Several important principles

underlie these differentiation pathways. First, each subset is induced best in response to the types of microbes that subset is designed to combat. These are excellent examples of how the adaptive immune response is specialized to protect against an enormous variety of microbes. Second, the most important signals for the differentiation of naive CD4$^+$ T lymphocytes into distinct subsets of effector cells are cytokines produced by APCs and other cells at the time of antigen stimulation. The set of cytokines secreted

FIGURE 5–17 Functions of T$_H$17 cells. T$_H$17 cells produce the cytokine interleukin-17 (IL-17), which induces production of chemokines and other cytokines from various cells, and these recruit neutrophils (and monocytes, not shown) into the site of inflammation. Some of the cytokines made by T$_H$17 cells, notably IL-22, function to maintain epithelial barrier function in the intestinal tract and other tissues. APC, Antigen-presenting cell; CSFs, colony-stimulating factors; TNF, tumor necrosis factor.

by the APCs will vary depending on the types of microbes; therefore the pathways of CD4$^+$ T cell differentiation and the subsets of effector T cells generated are determined by the nature of the infection. Third, each effector T cell subset produces cytokines that amplify itself and inhibit the other subsets. Thus, each type of response becomes increasingly polarized with prolonged stimulation. Fourth, the differentiation of these subsets is associated with the activation of transcription factors that stimulate production of various cytokines. Also, epigenetic changes in cytokine gene loci result in commitment to a

particular cytokine profile and therefore to a distinct subset. Examples of these transcription factors are shown in Figure 5–18. The most important transcription factors for the three subsets are T-bet, GATA-3, and RORγT for T$_H$1, T$_H$2, and T$_H$17, respectively. These work in concert with transcription factors called signal transducers and activators of transcription (STATs) induced by cytokines. Exactly how these transcriptional regulators determine the differentiation pathways and how they can be inhibited therapeutically are topics of intense investigation. Also, although we emphasize unique differentiation pathways, evidence suggests that cells of one subset may convert to another under the influence of cytokines. The extent and significance of such interconversion are not known.

T$_H$1 Differentiation

The differentiation of CD4$^+$ T cells to the T$_H$1 subset is driven by a combination of the cytokines IL-12 and IFN-γ (see Fig. 5–18). In response to many bacteria (especially intracellular bacteria) and viruses, dendritic cells and macrophages produce IL-12, and NK cells produce IFN-γ. When naive T cells recognize the antigens of these microbes, the T cells are exposed to IL-12 and IFN-γ. These two cytokines activate transcription factors that promote the differentiation of the T cells to the T$_H$1 subset. T$_H$1 cells produce IFN-γ, which not only activates macrophages to kill the microbes, but also promotes more T$_H$1 development and inhibits the development of T$_H$2 and T$_H$17 cells. Thus, IFN-γ increasingly polarizes the response to the T$_H$1 subset.

T$_H$2 Differentiation

The development of T$_H$2 cells is stimulated by the cytokine interleukin-4 (see Fig. 5–18). This seems puzzling, because the main source of IL-4 is T$_H$2 cells, so how could the cytokine induce the cells that produce it? It appears that if an infectious microbe does not elicit IL-12 production by APCs, as may occur with helminths, the T cells themselves produce IL-4. Also, helminths may activate cells of the mast cell and eosinophil lineages to secrete IL-4. In antigen-stimulated T cells, IL-4 activates transcription factors that promote differentiation to the T$_H$2 subset, leading to more IL-4 production and thus providing further amplification of the T$_H$2 response.

T$_H$17 Differentiation

The development and maintenance of T$_H$17 cells (see Fig. 5–18) require inflammatory cytokines such as interleukin-6 (IL-6) and IL-1, produced by macrophages and dendritic cells; IL-23, structurally related to IL-12 and made by the same cells; and transforming growth factor β (TGF-β), particularly in mice. IL-6, IL-1, and IL-23 are produced in response to fungi and some bacteria.

Differentiation of CD8⁺ T Cells into CTLs

CD8⁺ T lymphocytes activated by antigen and costimulators differentiate into cytotoxic T lymphocytes that are able to kill infected cells expressing the antigen. CTLs kill infected cells by secreting proteins that insert into the membranes of the infected cells and facilitate the entry of enzymes that induce apoptosis of the infected cells. The differentiation of naive CD8⁺ T cells into fully active CTLs is accompanied by the synthesis of the molecules that make up the killing machinery of these cells (see Chapter 6).

Development of Memory T Lymphocytes

A fraction of antigen-activated T lymphocytes differentiates into long-lived memory cells. Memory cells survive even after the infection is eradicated and antigen is no longer present. These memory T cells can be found in lymphoid organs, in various peripheral tissues, especially mucosa and skin, and in the circulation. Memory T cells require signals delivered by certain cytokines, including IL-7, in order to stay alive. We do not know what factors determine whether the progeny of antigen-stimulated lymphocytes will differentiate into effector cells or memory cells. Memory T cells do not continue to produce cytokines or kill infected cells, but they may be rapidly induced to do so on encountering the antigen that they recognize. Thus, memory cells are a pool of lymphocytes waiting for the infection to return. They can be distinguished from naive and effector cells by several criteria (see Chapter 1). A subset of memory T cells, called central memory cells, populate lymphoid organs and are responsible for rapid clonal expansion after reexposure to antigen. Another subset, called effector memory cells, localize in mucosal and other peripheral tissues and mediate

FIGURE 5–18 Development of T$_H$1, T$_H$2, and T$_H$17 effector cells. After activation by antigen and costimulators, naive helper T cells may differentiate into different subsets under the influence of cytokines produced at the site of activation. Cytokines that induce T$_H$1 development include interleukin-12 (IL-12), which is produced by microbe-activated antigen-presenting cells (APCs), such as dendritic cells and macrophages, and interferon-γ (IFN-γ) made by natural killer (NK) cells. T$_H$2 cells are induced by IL-4, which may be produced by the T cells themselves and by other cells, such as mast cells. T$_H$17 differentiation is triggered by transforming growth factor β (TGF-β), which can be made by many cell types, together with inflammatory cytokines such as IL-6, IL-1, and IL-23, which may be produced by APCs. The major transcription factors involved in helper T cell differentiation include T-bet (for T$_H$1 cells), GATA-3 (for T$_H$2 cells), and RORγt (for T$_H$17 cells), acting in concert with cytokine-activated signal transducer and activator of transcription (STAT) proteins.

rapid effector functions on reintroduction of antigen to these sites.

Decline of the Immune Response

Because of the remarkable expansion of antigen-specific lymphocytes at the peak of an immune response, it is predictable that once the response is over, the system must return to its steady state, called homeostasis, so that it is prepared to respond to the next infectious pathogen (see Fig. 5–12). During the response, the survival and proliferation of T cells are maintained by antigen, costimulatory signals from CD28, and cytokines such as IL-2. Once an infection is cleared and the stimuli for lymphocyte activation disappear, many of the cells that had proliferated in response to antigen are deprived of these survival signals. As a result, these cells die by apoptosis (programmed cell death). The response subsides within 1 or 2 weeks after the infection is eradicated, and the only sign that a T cell–mediated immune response had occurred is the pool of surviving memory lymphocytes.

Numerous mechanisms have evolved to overcome the challenges that T cells face in the generation of a useful cell-mediated immune response. First, naive T cells need to find the antigen. This problem is solved by APCs that capture the antigen and concentrate it in specialized lymphoid organs in the regions through which naive T cells recirculate. Second, the correct type of T lymphocytes (i.e., CD4$^+$ helper T cells or CD8$^+$ CTLs) must respond to antigens from the extracellular and intracellular compartments. This selectivity is determined by the specificity of the CD4 and CD8 co-receptors for class II and class I MHC molecules, and by the segregation of extracellular (vesicular) and intracellular (cytosolic) protein antigens for display by class II and class I MHC molecules, respectively. Third, T cells should respond to microbial antigens but not to harmless proteins. This preference for microbes is maintained because T cell activation requires costimulators that are induced on APCs by microbes. Fourth, antigen recognition by a small number of T cells must lead to a response that is large enough to be effective. This is accomplished by robust clonal expansion after stimulation and by several amplification mechanisms induced by microbes and activated T cells

themselves that enhance the response. Finally, the response must be optimized to combat different types of microbes. This is accomplished largely by the development of specialized subsets of effector T cells.

SUMMARY

* T lymphocytes are the cells of cell-mediated immunity, the arm of the adaptive immune system that combats intracellular microbes, which may be microbes that are ingested by phagocytes and live within these cells or microbes that infect nonphagocytic cells. T lymphocytes also mediate defense against some extracellular microbes and help B lymphocytes to produce antibodies.

* The responses of T lymphocytes consist of sequential phases: recognition of cell-associated microbes by naive T cells, expansion of the antigen-specific clones by proliferation, and differentiation of some of the progeny into effector cells and memory cells.

* T cells use their antigen receptors to recognize peptide antigens displayed by MHC molecules on antigen-presenting cells (APCs), which accounts for the specificity of the ensuing response, and polymorphic residues of the MHC molecules, accounting for the MHC restriction of T cell responses.

* Antigen recognition by the T cell receptor (TCR) triggers signals that are delivered to the interior of the cells by molecules associated with the TCR (CD3 and ζ chains) and by the coreceptors CD4 and CD8, which recognize class II and class I MHC molecules, respectively.

* The binding of T cells to APCs is enhanced by adhesion molecules, notably the integrins, whose affinity for their ligands is increased by antigen recognition by the TCR.

* APCs exposed to microbes or to cytokines produced as part of the innate immune reactions to microbes express costimulators that bind to receptors on T cells and deliver necessary second signals for T cell activation.

- The biochemical signals triggered in T cells by antigen recognition and costimulation result in the activation of various transcription factors that stimulate the expression of genes encoding cytokines, cytokine receptors, and other molecules involved in T cell responses.
- In response to antigen recognition and costimulation, T cells secrete cytokines that induce proliferation of the antigen-stimulated T cells and mediate the effector functions of T cells.
- CD4$^+$ helper T cells may differentiate into subsets of effector cells that produce restricted sets of cytokines and perform different functions. T_H1 cells, which produce IFN-γ, activate phagocytes to eliminate ingested microbes, and stimulate the production of opsonizing and complement-binding antibodies. T_H2 cells, which produce IL-4 and IL-5, stimulate IgE production and activate eosinophils, which function mainly in defense against helminths. T_H17 cells, which produce IL-17, play a role in defense against extracellular bacterial and fungal infections and are implicated in several inflammatory diseases.
- CD8$^+$ T cells recognize peptides of intracellular (cytosolic) protein antigens and may require help from CD4$^+$ T cells to differentiate into effector CTLs. The function of CTLs is to kill cells producing cytoplasmic microbial antigens.

REVIEW QUESTIONS

1. What are the components of the TCR complex? Which of these components are responsible for antigen recognition and which for signal transduction?
2. What are some of the molecules in addition to the TCR that T cells use to initiate their responses to antigens, and what are the functions of these molecules?
3. What is costimulation? What is the physiologic significance of costimulation? What are some of the ligand-receptor pairs involved in costimulation?
4. Summarize the links among antigen recognition, the major biochemical signaling pathways in T cells, and the production of transcription factors.
5. What is the principal growth factor for T cells? Why do antigen-specific T cells expand more than other (bystander) T cells on exposure to an antigen?
6. What are the major subsets of CD4$^+$ helper T cells, and how do they differ?
7. What signals are required to induce the responses of CD8$^+$ T cells?

Answers to and discussion of the Review Questions are available at studentconsult.com.

Effector Mechanisms of T Cell–Mediated Immunity
Functions of T Cells in Host Defense

histocompatibility complex (MHC) molecules in displaying the antigens of intracellular microbes for recognition by T lymphocytes, and in Chapter 5 we discussed how naive T cells recognize these antigens in lymphoid organs and develop into effector cells. In this chapter, we address the following questions:

- How do effector T lymphocytes locate intracellular microbes at any site in the body?
- How do effector T cells eradicate infections by these microbes?
- What are the roles of macrophages and other leukocytes in the destruction of infectious pathogens?

TYPES OF T CELL–MEDIATED IMMUNE REACTIONS

Two types of cell-mediated immune reactions are designed to eliminate different types of microbes. CD4$^+$ helper T cells secrete cytokines that recruit and activate other leukocytes to phagocytose (ingest) and destroy microbes. CD8$^+$ cytotoxic T lymphocytes (CTLs) kill any infected cell containing microbial proteins in the cytosol or nucleus, eliminating cellular reservoirs of infection (Fig. 6–1). Microbial infections may occur anywhere in the body, and some infectious pathogens are able to infect and live within host cells. Pathogenic microbes that infect and survive

Host defense in which T lymphocytes serve as effector cells is called **cell-mediated immunity.** T cells are essential for eliminating microbes that survive and replicate inside cells, and for eradicating infections by some extracellular microbes, often by recruiting other cells to clear the infectious pathogens. Cell-mediated immune responses begin with the activation of naive T cells to proliferate and to differentiate into effector cells. These effector T cells eliminate cell-associated microbes, often working together with macrophages and other leukocytes. In Chapter 3 we described the function of major

FIGURE 6–1 Cell-mediated immunity against intracellular microbes. A, Effector T helper cells of the CD4$^+$ T$_H$1 and T$_H$17 subsets recognize microbial antigens and secrete cytokines that recruit leukocytes (inflammation) and activate phagocytes to kill the microbes. CD8$^+$ T cells also produce cytokines that induce inflammation and activate macrophages (not shown). **B,** CD8$^+$ cytotoxic T lymphocytes (CTLs) kill infected cells with microbes in the cytoplasm.

inside host cells include (1) many bacteria, fungi, and some protozoa that are ingested by phagocytes, but resist the killing mechanisms of these phagocytes and thus survive in vesicles or cytoplasm, and (2) viruses that infect phagocytic and nonphagocytic cells and live and replicate in the cytoplasm of these cells (see Chapter 5, Fig. 5–1). The different classes of T cells differ in the cellular locations of microbes they recognize and in the nature of the reactions they elicit. In general, CD4$^+$ T cells recognize antigens of microbes in phagocytic vesicles and secrete cytokines that recruit and activate leukocytes that kill the microbes, whereas CD8$^+$ cells recognize antigens of microbes that are present in the cytosol and destroy the infected cells.

T cell-mediated immune reactions consist of multiple steps (see Chapter 5, Fig. 5–2). Naive T cells are stimulated by microbial antigens in the lymph nodes and spleen, giving rise to effector T cells whose function is to eradicate intracellular microbes. The differentiated effector T cells then migrate to the site of infection. Phagocytes at these sites that have ingested the microbes into intracellular vesicles display peptide fragments of microbial proteins bound to cell surface class II

MHC molecules for recognition by CD4$^+$ effector T cells. Peptide antigens derived from microbes living in the cytosol of infected cells are displayed by class I MHC molecules for recognition by CD8$^+$ effector T cells. Antigen recognition activates the effector T cells to perform their task of eliminating the infectious pathogens. Thus, in CMI, T cells recognize protein antigens at two stages. First, naive T cells recognize antigens in lymphoid tissues and respond by proliferating and by differentiating into effector cells (see Chapter 5). Second, effector T cells recognize the same antigens anywhere in the body and respond by eliminating these microbes.

This chapter first describes how differentiated effector T cells locate microbes in tissues, then how CD4$^+$ and CD8$^+$ T cells eliminate these microbes.

MIGRATION OF T LYMPHOCYTES IN CELL-MEDIATED IMMUNE REACTIONS

In order for T cell–mediated immune responses to an infection to occur, the T cells must take part in two types of migratory activity. First, naive T cells must migrate between blood and lymphoid tissues throughout the body, until they encounter dendritic cells within a lymph node or the spleen that display the antigens the T cells recognize (see Chapter 3). Second, after the naive T cells are activated and differentiate into expanded clones of effector T cells, these T cells must migrate back to the sites of infection, where they function to kill microbes. The migration of naive and effector T cells are controlled by three families of proteins—selectins, integrins, and chemokines—which regulate the migration of all leukocytes, as described in Chapter 2. The routes of migration of naive and effector T cells differ significantly because of selective expression of different adhesion molecules and chemokine receptors on naive T cells versus effector T cells, together with the selective expression of endothelial adhesion molecules and chemokines in lymphoid tissues and sites of inflammation (Fig. 6–2).

Naive T cells express the adhesion molecule L-selectin (CD62L) and the chemokine receptor CCR7, which mediate their selective migration into lymph nodes through specialized vessels called high endothelial venules (HEVs) (see Fig 6–2). These HEVs are located in the T cell zones of lymphoid tissues and are lined by specialized endothelial cells, which express carbohydrate ligands that bind to L-selectin. HEVs also display chemokines made only in lymphoid tissues that bind CCR7. Naive T cells in the blood engage in L-selectin–mediated rolling interactions with the HEV, allowing chemokines to bind to CCR7 on the T cell. CCR7 transduces intracellular signals that activate the integrin leukocyte function–associated antigen 1 (LFA-1) on the naive T cell to bind tightly to its ligand, intercellular adhesion molecule 1 (ICAM-1) on the HEV, resulting in arrest of the rolling T cells. The T cells then exit the vessel through the endothelial junctions, and remain in the T cell zone of the lymph node because of the chemokines present there. As a result, many naive T cells carried by the blood into an HEV migrate to the T cell zone of the lymph node stroma. This happens constantly in all lymph nodes and mucosal lymphoid tissues in the body. Effector T cells do not express CCR7 or L-selectin, and thus they are not drawn into lymph nodes.

The phospholipid sphingosine 1-phosphate (S1P) plays a key role in the entry and exit of T cells through lymph nodes. The levels of S1P are higher in the blood and lymph than inside lymph nodes. S1P binds to and thereby reduces expression of its receptor, which keeps the expression of the receptor on circulating naive T cells low. When a naive T cell enters the node, it is exposed to lower concentrations of S1P, and expression of the receptor begins to increase. If the T cell does not recognize any antigen, the cell leaves the node through efferent lymphatic vessels, following the gradient of S1P from the node into the lymph. If the T cell does encounter specific antigen and is activated, the surface expression of the S1P receptor is suppressed for several days. As a result, recently activated T cells stay in the lymph node long enough to undergo clonal expansion and differentiation. When this process is completed, S1P receptor is reexpressed on the cell surface; at the same time the cells lose expression of L-selectin and CCR7, which attracted the naive T cells to the lymph nodes. Therefore, activated T cells are drawn out of the nodes into the draining lymph, which then transports the cells to the circulation. The net result of these changes is that differentiated effector T cells leave the lymph nodes and enter the circulation. The importance of the S1P pathway has been highlighted by the development of a drug (fingolimod) that binds to the S1P receptor and blocks the exit of T cells from lymph nodes. This drug is approved for the treatment of the inflammatory disease multiple sclerosis.

Effector T cells migrate to sites of infection because they express adhesion molecules and chemokine receptors that bind to ligands expressed or displayed on vascular endothelium in response to innate immune responses to microbes. The process of differentiation of naive T lymphocytes into effector cells, described in Chapter 5, is accompanied by changes in the collections of adhesion molecules and chemokine receptors expressed on these cells (see Fig. 6–2). The migration of activated T cells into peripheral tissues is controlled by the same interactions involved in the migration of other leukocytes into tissues (see Chapter 2, Fig. 2–16). To summarize, activated T cells express high levels of the glycoprotein ligands for E- and P-selectins and the integrins LFA-1 and VLA-4 (very late antigen 4). The endothelium at the site of infection is exposed to cytokines such as tumor necrosis factor (TNF) and interleukin-1 (IL-1), which act on the endothelial cells to

T cell homing receptor	Ligand on endothelial cell	Function of receptor: ligand pair
Naive T cells		
L-selectin	L-selectin ligand	Adhesion of naive T cells to high endothelial venule (HEV) in lymph node
LFA-1 (β_2-integrin)	ICAM-1	Stable arrest on HEV
CCR7	CCL19 or CCL21	Activation of integrins and chemotaxis
Activated (effector and memory) T cells		
E- and P- selectin ligand	E- or P- selectin	Initial weak adhesion of effector and memory T cells to cytokine-activated endothelium at peripheral site of infection
LFA-1 (β_2-integrin) or VLA-4 (β_1-integrin)	ICAM-1 or VCAM-1	Stable arrest on cytokine-activated endothelium at peripheral site of infection
CXCR3, others	CXCL10, others	Activation of integrins and chemotaxis

FIGURE 6–2 Migration of naive and effector T lymphocytes. A, Naive T lymphocytes home to lymph nodes as a result of L-selectin and integrin binding to their ligands on high endothelial venules (HEVs). Chemokines expressed in lymph nodes bind to receptors on naive T cells, enhancing integrin-dependent adhesion and migration through the HEV. The phospholipid, sphingosine 1-phosphate (S1P), plays a role in the exit of T cells from lymph nodes, by binding to the receptor, called S1PR1 (type 1 sphingosine 1-phosphate receptor). Activated T lymphocytes, including effector cells, home to sites of infection in peripheral tissues, and this migration is mediated by E-selectin and P-selectin, integrins, and chemokines secreted at inflammatory sites. **B,** This table summarizes the functions of the principal T cell homing receptors and their ligands. ICAM-1, Intercellular adhesion molecule 1; LFA-1, leukocyte function–associated antigen 1; VCAM-1, vascular cell adhesion molecule 1; VLA-4, very late antigen 4.

increase expression of E- and P-selectins as well as ligands for integrins, especially ICAM-1 and vascular cell adhesion molecule 1 (VCAM-1), the ligand for the VLA-4 integrin. Effector T cells that are passing through the blood vessels at the infection site bind first to the endothelial selectins, leading to rolling interactions. Effector T cells also express receptors for chemokines that are produced by macrophages and endothelial cells at these inflammatory sites and are displayed on the surface of the endothelium. The rolling T cells recognize these chemokines, leading to increased binding affinity of the integrins for their ligands and firm adhesion of the T cells to the endothelium. After the effector T lymphocytes are arrested on the endothelium, they engage other adhesion molecules at the junctions between endothelial cells, crawling through these junctions into the tissue. Chemokines that were produced by macrophages and other cells in the tissues stimulate the motility of the transmigrating T cells. The net result of these molecular interactions between the T cells and endothelial cells is that the T cells migrate out of the blood vessels to the site of infection. Naive T cells do not express ligands for E- or P-selectin and do not express receptors for chemokines produced at inflammatory sites. Therefore, naive T cells do not migrate into sites of infection or tissue injury.

The homing of effector T cells to a site of infection is independent of antigen recognition, but lymphocytes that recognize microbial antigens are preferentially retained and activated at the site. The homing of effector T cells to sites of infection mainly depends on adhesion molecules and chemokines. Therefore, any effector T cell present in the blood, regardless of antigen specificity, can enter the site of any infection. This nonselective migration presumably maximizes the chances of effector lymphocytes entering tissues where they may encounter the microbes they recognize. The effector T cells that leave the circulation, and that specifically recognize microbial antigen presented by local tissue antigen-presenting cells (APCs), become reactivated and contribute to the killing of the microbe in the APC. One consequence of this reactivation is an increase in the expression of VLA integrins on the T cells. Some of these integrins specifically bind to molecules present in the extracellular matrix, such as hyaluronic acid and fibronectin. Therefore, the antigen-stimulated lymphocytes adhere firmly to the tissue matrix proteins near the antigen, which may serve to keep the cells at the inflammatory sites. This selective retention contributes to accumulation of more and more T cells specific for microbial antigens at the site of infection.

As a result of this sequence of T cell migration events, T cell–mediated immune response to infections are efficiently initiated and carried out, regardless of the location of the infection. In contrast with the activation of naive T cells, which requires antigen presentation and costimulation by dendritic cells, differentiated effector cells are less dependent on costimulation. Therefore, the proliferation and differentiation of naive T cells are confined to lymphoid organs, where dendritic cells (which express abundant costimulators) display antigens, but the functions of effector T cells may be reactivated by any host cell displaying microbial peptides bound to MHC molecules, not just dendritic cells.

Because CD4+ helper T lymphocytes and CD8+ CTLs employ distinct mechanisms to combat infections, we discuss the effector mechanisms of these lymphocyte classes individually. We conclude by describing how the two classes of lymphocytes may cooperate to eliminate intracellular microbes.

EFFECTOR FUNCTIONS OF CD4⁺ HELPER T LYMPHOCYTES

Cell-mediated immunity against pathogens was discovered as a form of immunity to an intracellular bacterial infection that could be transferred from immune animals to naive animals by cells (now known to be T lymphocytes) but not by serum antibodies (Fig. 6–3). It was known from the earliest studies that the specificity of CMI against different microbes was a function of the lymphocytes, but the elimination of the microbes was a function of activated macrophages. The roles of T lymphocytes and phagocytes in CMI are now well understood.

CD4⁺ T lymphocytes of the T_H1 subset enhance the ability of phagocytes to kill microbes, T_H17 cells promote the recruitment of leukocytes to the site of infection, and T_H2 cells activate eosinophils to kill helminthic parasites. Although many of these reactions, such as leukocyte recruitment and phagocyte activation, may occur at the same time and in the same infection, it is convenient to describe the effector functions of these T cells separately.

Role of T_H1 Cells in Host Defense

The major function of T_H1 cells is the activation of macrophages, which is critical for efficient elimination of ingested microbes (see Chapter 5, Fig. 5–15). This reaction was the basis of the original definition of cell-mediated immunity, and remains perhaps the best understood function of CD4⁺ T cells.

Effector T lymphocytes of the T_H1 subset that recognize macrophage-associated antigens activate the macrophages by CD40

FIGURE 6–3 Cell-mediated immunity to an intracellular bacterium, *Listeria monocytogenes.* In these experiments, a sample of lymphocytes or serum (a source of antibodies) was taken from a mouse that had previously been exposed to a sublethal dose of *Listeria* organisms (immune mouse) and transferred to a normal (naive) mouse, and the recipient of the adoptive transfer was challenged with the bacteria. The numbers of bacteria were measured in the spleen of the recipient mouse to determine if the transfer had conferred immunity. Protection against bacterial challenge (seen by reduced recovery of live bacteria) was induced by the transfer of immune lymphoid cells, now known to be T cells **(A)**, but not by the transfer of serum **(B)**. The bacteria were killed in vitro by activated macrophages but not by T cells **(C)**. Therefore, protection depends on antigen-specific T lymphocytes, but bacterial killing is the function of activated macrophages.

ligand–CD40 interactions and by secreting the cytokine interferon-γ (IFN-γ) (Fig. 6–4). As discussed in Chapter 3, macrophages ingest microbes into intracellular vesicles, called phagosomes, which fuse with lysosomes to form phagolysosomes. The microbial proteins in these vesicles are processed, and a few microbial peptides are displayed by class II MHC molecules on the surface of the macrophages. Effector CD4+ T cells specific for these peptides recognize the class II–associated peptides. The T cells respond by expressing on their surface the effector molecule

CD40 ligand (CD40L, or CD154), which binds to the CD40 receptor that is expressed on macrophages. At the same time, the T_H1 cells secrete IFN-γ, which is a potent activator of macrophages. Binding of IFN-γ to its receptor on macrophages functions together with CD40L binding to CD40 to trigger biochemical signaling pathways that lead to the activation of several transcription factors. These transcription factors induce the expression of genes that encode lysosomal proteases and enzymes that stimulate the synthesis of microbicidal reactive oxygen species

FIGURE 6–4 Activation of macrophages by T_H1 lymphocytes. Effector T lymphocytes of the T_H subset recognize the antigens of ingested microbes on macrophages. In response to this recognition, the T lymphocytes express CD40L, which engages CD40 on the macrophages, and the T cells secrete interferon-γ (IFN-γ), which binds to IFN-γ receptors on the macrophages. This combination of signals activates the macrophages to produce microbicidal substances that kill the ingested microbes. Activated macrophages also secrete cytokines that induce inflammation—tumor necrosis factor (TNF), interleukin-1 (IL-1), and chemokines—and activate T cells (IL-12), and they express more major histocompatibility complex (MHC) molecules and costimulators, which enhance T cell responses. **A,** Illustration shows a CD4+ T cell recognizing class II MHC–associated peptides and activating the macrophage. **B,** The table summarizes macrophage responses and their roles in cell-mediated immunity.

and nitric oxide. The net result of CD40L-mediated and IFN-γ–mediated activation is that macrophages become strongly microbicidal and can destroy most ingested microbes. Macrophages that respond in this way to CD40L and IFN-γ are called classically activated macrophages. The critical role of T_H1 cells in defense against intracellular microbes is the reason why individuals with inherited defects in the development or function of this subset are susceptible to infections with such microbes, especially normally harmless atypical mycobacteria. $CD8^+$ T cells also secrete IFN-γ and may contribute to macrophage activation and killing of ingested microbes.

Although macrophage activation is part of the innate immune response to microbes (see Chapter 2, Fig. 2–10), the magnitude of the response is greater in cell-mediated immune reactions, when T cells are involved. This explains why the adaptive immune response can eradicate pathogens that have evolved to resist innate immunity. The requirement for specific antigen recognition by T cells ensures that the cell-mediated immune response is targeted to macrophages carrying microbes, and there is little or no activation of uninfected (bystander) macrophages. The macrophages presenting antigens of phagocytosed microbes to T cells are those with intracellular microbes that need to be killed, and these are the phagocytes that activate effector T cells and are in position to receive help (activating signals) from the responding T_H1 cells.

The interaction between macrophages and T lymphocytes is an excellent example of bidirectional interactions between cells of the innate immune system (macrophages) and adaptive immune systems (T lymphocytes) (Fig. 6–5). Macrophages display microbial antigens to $CD4^+$ T_H1 cells, which stimulates T cell expression of CD40L and IFN-γ. The CD40L and IFN-γ then activate the phagocytes to kill the ingested microbes, thus completing the circle. At the same time, activated macrophages produce IL-12, and this cytokine drives the differentiation of naive $CD4^+$ T cells to T_H1 cells, thus amplifying the response.

Essentially the same reaction, consisting of leukocyte recruitment and activation, may be elicited by injecting a microbial protein into the skin of an individual who has been immunized against the microbe by prior infection or

FIGURE 6–5 Cytokine-mediated interactions between T lymphocytes and macrophages in cell-mediated immunity. Antigen-presenting cells that encounter microbes secrete the cytokine interleukin-12 (IL-12), which stimulates naive $CD4^+$ T cells to differentiate into interferon-γ (IFN-γ)–secreting T_H1 cells and enhances IFN-γ production. IFN-γ activates the macrophages to kill ingested microbes and produce more IL-12, thus amplifying the reaction.

vaccination. This reaction is called **delayed-type hypersensitivity (DTH),** and it is described in Chapter 11 when we discuss injurious immune reactions.

Role of T_H17 Cells in Host Defense

T_H17 cells induce other cells to secrete cytokines that are important for the recruitment of neutrophils and, to a lesser extent, monocytes (see Chapter 5, Fig. 5–17). As a result, leukocytes are brought to the site of infection to assist in eradicating the infection. This T cell–stimulated cellular infiltration, along with an accompanying vascular reaction, is typical of inflammation. Inflammation is a component of T cell–mediated reactions in normal host defense and in many immunologic (hypersensitivity) diseases (see Chapter 11). Recall that inflammation also is one of the major reactions of innate immunity (see Chapter 2). Typically, when T cells stimulate inflammation, the reaction is stronger and more prolonged than when it is elicited by innate immune responses to microbes.

In addition to inflammation, T_H17 cells stimulate the production of anti-microbial substances, called defensins, that function like locally produced endogenous antibiotics. Some cytokines produced by T_H17 cells also help to maintain the functional integrity of epithelial barriers. These reactions of T_H17 cells are critical for defense against fungal and bacterial infections. Rare individuals who have inherited defects in T_H17 responses are prone to developing bacterial abscesses and chronic mucocutaneous candidiasis.

Role of T_H2 Cells in Host Defense

The T_H2 subset of CD4$^+$ T lymphocytes stimulates eosinophil-rich inflammation, which is important in defense against helminthic parasites. When differentiated T_H2 cells recognize antigens, the cells produce the cytokines interleukin-4 and interleukin-5 (as well as IL-10, which is also produced by many other cell populations). IL-4 stimulates the production of IgE antibody, which binds to Fc receptors on mast cells and eosinophils, and IL-5 activates eosinophils (see Fig. 5–16). This reaction is important for defense against helminthic infections, because helminths are killed by the granule proteins of activated eosinophils (see Chapter 8). The cytokines produced by T_H2 cells, as well as by IgE-mediated mast cell activation, stimulate mucus secretion and peristalsis in the intestinal tract, promoting the expulsion of parasites from the gut.

T_H2 cells secrete cytokines that inhibit classical macrophage activation and stimulate the alternative pathway of macrophage activation. IL-4 and IL-10 inhibit the classical pathway of macrophage activation. IL-4 and IL-13 can activate macrophages to express mannose receptors and secrete growth factors that act on fibroblasts to increase collagen synthesis and fibrosis. This type of macrophage response is called alternative macrophage activation, to distinguish it from classical activation, which enhances microbicidal functions (see Chapter 2, Fig. 2–10). Alternative macrophage activation mediated by T_H2 cytokines may play a role in tissue repair following injury and may contribute to fibrosis and tissue damage in patients with chronic parasitic infection or allergic disease.

The relative activation of T_H1 and T_H2 cells in response to an infectious microbe may determine the outcome of the infection (Fig. 6–6). For example, the protozoal parasite *Leishmania major* lives inside macrophages, and its elimination requires the activation of the macrophages by *L. major*–specific T_H1 cells. Most inbred strains of mice make an effective T_H1 response to the parasite and are thus able to eradicate the infection. In some inbred mouse strains, however, the response to *L. major* is dominated by T_H2 cells, and these mice succumb to the infection. *Mycobacterium leprae*, the bacterium that causes leprosy, is a pathogen for humans that also lives inside macrophages and may be eliminated by cell-mediated immune mechanisms. Some people infected with *M. leprae* are unable to eradicate the infection, which, if left untreated, will progress to the classic destructive lesions of lepromatous leprosy. By contrast, in other patients, the bacteria induce strong cell-mediated immune responses with activated T cells and macrophages around the infection and few surviving microbes; this form of less destructive disease is called tuberculoid leprosy. The tuberculoid form is associated with the activation of *M. leprae*–specific T_H1 cells, whereas the destructive lepromatous form is associated with a defect in T_H1 cell activation. The same principle, that the T cell cytokine response to an infectious pathogen is an important determinant of the outcome of the infection, may be true for other infectious diseases.

As mentioned earlier, activated macrophages are best at killing microbes that are confined to vesicles, and microbes that directly enter the cytoplasm (e.g., viruses) or escape from phagosomes into the cytoplasm (e.g., some phagocytosed bacteria) are relatively resistant to the microbicidal mechanisms of phagocytes. Eradication of such pathogens requires another effector mechanism of T cell–mediated immunity, CD8$^+$ CTLs.

EFFECTOR FUNCTIONS OF CD8$^+$ CYTOTOXIC T LYMPHOCYTES

CD8$^+$ cytotoxic T lymphocytes recognize class I MHC–associated peptides on infected cells and kill those cells, thereby eliminating the reservoir of infection (Fig. 6–7). The sources of class I–associated peptides are protein antigens

Infection	Response	Outcome
Leishmania major	Most mouse strains: T$_H$1 ⇒ BALB/c mice: T$_H$2 ⇒	Recovery Disseminated infection
Mycobacterium leprae	Some patients: T$_H$1 ⇒ Some patients: Defective T$_H$1 ⇒	Tuberculoid leprosy Lepromatous leprosy (high bacterial count)

FIGURE 6–6 Balance between T$_H$1 and T$_H$2 cell activation determines outcome of intracellular infections. Naive CD4$^+$ T lymphocytes may differentiate into T$_H$1 cells, which activate phagocytes to kill ingested microbes, and T$_H$2 cells, which inhibit classical macrophage activation. The balance between these two subsets may influence the outcome of infections, as illustrated by *Leishmania* infection in mice and leprosy in humans. IFN, Interferon; IL, interleukin; TNF, tumor necrosis factor.

synthesized in the cytosol and protein antigens of phagocytosed microbes that escape from phagocytic vesicles into the cytosol (see Chapter 3). CD8$^+$ CTLs recognize class I MHC–peptide complexes on the surface of infected cells by their T cell receptor (TCR) and by the CD8 coreceptor. (These infected cells also are called targets of CTLs, because they are destined to be killed by the CTLs.) The TCR and CD8, as well as other signaling proteins, cluster in the CTL membrane at the site of contact with the target cell, and are surrounded by the LFA-1 integrin. These molecules bind their ligands on the target cell, which firmly holds the two cells together, forming an immunologic synapse (see Chapter 5), into which the CTLs secrete cytotoxic proteins.

Antigen recognition by CTLs results in the activation of signal transduction pathways that lead to the exocytosis of the contents of the CTL's granules into the immune synapse between the CTL and target cell. Because CTLs do not require costimulation or T cell help for activation, they can be activated by and are able to kill any infected cell in any tissue. CTLs kill target cells mainly as a result of delivery of granule proteins into the target cells. Two types of granule proteins critical for killing are granzymes (granule enzymes) and perforin. **Granzyme B** cleaves and thereby activates enzymes called caspases (cysteine proteases that cleave proteins after aspartic acid residues) that are present in the cytosol of target cells and whose major function is to induce apoptosis. **Perforin** disrupts the integrity of the target cell plasma membrane and endosomal membranes, thereby facilitating the delivery of granzymes into the cytosol and the initiation of apoptosis.

Activated CTLs also express a membrane protein called Fas ligand, which binds to a death-inducing receptor, called Fas (CD95), on target cells. Engagement of Fas activates caspases and induces target cell apoptosis; this pathway does not require granule exocytosis and probably plays only a minor role in killing by CD8$^+$ CTLs.

FIGURE 6–7 Mechanisms of killing of infected cells by CD8+ cytotoxic T lympho-cytes. CTLs recognize class I MHC–associated peptides of cytoplasmic microbes in infected cells and form tight adhesions (conjugates) with these cells. Adhesion molecules such as integrins stabilize the binding of the CTLs to infected cells (not shown). The CTLs are activated to release (exocytose) their granule contents (perforin and granzymes) toward the infected cell, referred to as target cell. Granzymes are deliv-ered to the cytosol of the target cell by a perforin-dependent mechanism. Granzymes then induce apoptosis. ICAM-1, Intercellular adhesion mole-cule 1; LFA-1, leukocyte function–associated antigen 1.

The net result of these effector mechanisms of CTLs is that the infected cells are killed. Cells that have undergone apoptosis are rapidly phagocytosed and eliminated. The mechanisms that induce fragmentation of target cell DNA, which is the hallmark of apoptosis, also may break down the DNA of microbes living inside the infected cells. Each CTL can kill a target cell, detach, and go on to kill additional targets.

Although we have described the effector func-tions of CD4+ T cells and CD8+ T cells separately, these types of T lymphocytes clearly function cooperatively to eradicate intracellular microbes (Fig. 6–8). If microbes are phagocytosed and remain sequestered in macrophage vesicles, CD4+ T cells may be adequate to eradicate these infections by secreting IFN-γ and activating the microbicidal mechanisms of the macrophages. If the microbes are able to escape from vesicles into the cytoplasm, however, they become insus-ceptible to T cell–mediated macrophage activa-tion, and their elimination requires killing of the infected cells by CD8+ CTLs.

RESISTANCE OF PATHOGENIC MICROBES TO CELL-MEDIATED IMMUNITY

Different microbes have developed diverse mechanisms to resist T lymphocyte–mediated host defense (Fig. 6–9). Many

FIGURE 6–8 Cooperation between CD4+ and CD8+ T cells in eradication of intracellular infections. In a macrophage infected by an intracellular bacterium, some of the bacteria are sequestered in vesicles (phagosomes), and others may escape into the cytoplasm. CD4+ T cells recognize antigens derived from the vesicular microbes and activate the macrophage to kill the microbes in the vesicles. CD8+ T cells recognize anti-gens derived from the cytoplasmic bacteria and are needed to kill the infected cell, thus eliminating the reservoir of infection. CTL, Cytotoxic T lymphocyte; IFN, interferon.

Microbe	Mechanism	
Mycobacteria	Inhibition of phagolysosome fusion	
Herpes simplex virus (HSV)	Inhibition of antigen presentation: an HSV protein interferes with the TAP transporter	
Cytomegalovirus (CMV)	Inhibition of antigen presentation: inhibition of proteasomal activity; removal of class I MHC molecules from endoplasmic reticulum (ER)	
Epstein-Barr virus (EBV)	Inhibition of antigen presentation: inhibition of proteasomal activity	
Epstein-Barr virus (EBV)	Production of IL-10, inhibition of macrophage and dendritic cell activation	
Pox Virus	Inhibition of effector cell activation: production of soluble cytokine receptors	

FIGURE 6–9 Evasion of cell-mediated immunity by microbes. Select examples of different mechanisms by which bacteria and viruses resist the effector mechanisms of CMI. ER, Endoplasmic reticulum; IFN, interferon; IL, interleukin; TAP, transporter associated with antigen processing.

intracellular bacteria, such as *Mycobacterium tuberculosis, Legionella pneumophila,* and *Listeria monocytogenes,* inhibit the fusion of phagosomes with lysosomes or create pores in phagosome membranes, allowing these organisms to escape into the cytosol. Thus, these microbes are able to resist the microbicidal mechanisms of phagocytes and survive and even replicate inside phagocytes. Many viruses inhibit class I MHC–associated antigen presentation, by inhibiting production or expression of class I molecules, by blocking transport of antigenic peptides from the cytosol into the endoplasmic reticulum (ER), and by removing newly synthesized class I molecules from the ERs. All these viral mechanisms reduce the loading of class I MHC molecules by viral peptides. The result of this defective loading is reduced surface expression of class I MHC molecules, because empty class I molecules are unstable and are not expressed on the cell surface. It is interesting that natural killer (NK) cells are activated by class I–deficient cells (see Chapter 2). Thus, host defenses have evolved to combat immune evasion mechanisms of microbes: CTLs recognize class I MHC–associated viral peptides, viruses inhibit class I MHC expression, and NK cells recognize the absence of class I MHC molecules.

Other viruses produce inhibitory cytokines or soluble (decoy) cytokine receptors that bind and neutralize cytokines such as IFN-γ, reducing the amount of cytokines available to trigger cell-mediated immune reactions. Some viruses evade elimination and establish chronic infections by stimulating expression of the inhibitory receptor PD-1 (programmed [cell] death protein 1; see Chapter 9) on CD8+ T cells, thus inhibiting the effector functions of CTLs. Still other viruses directly infect and kill T lymphocytes, the best example being human immunodeficiency virus (HIV), which is able to survive in infected persons by killing CD4+ T cells.

The outcome of infections is influenced by the strength of host defenses and the ability of pathogens to resist these defenses. The same principle is evident when the effector mechanisms of humoral immunity are considered. One approach for tilting the balance between the host and microbes in favor of protective immunity is to vaccinate individuals to enhance cell-mediated immune responses. The principles underlying vaccination strategies are described at the end of Chapter 8, after the discussion of humoral immunity.

SUMMARY

* Cell-mediated immunity is the arm of adaptive immunity that eradicates infections by cell-associated microbes, and utilizes two types of T cells. CD4+ helper T cells recruit and activate phagocytes to kill ingested and some extracellular microbes, and CD8+ cytotoxic T lymphocytes (CTLs) kill cells harboring microbes in their cytosol, eliminating reservoirs of infection.

* Effector T cells are generated in peripheral lymphoid organs, mainly lymph nodes draining sites of microbe entry, by the activation of naive T lymphocytes. The effector T cells are able to migrate to any site of infection.

* The migration of effector T cells is controlled by adhesion molecules and chemokines. Various adhesion molecules are induced on the T cells after activation and bind to their ligands, which themselves are induced on endothelial cells by microbes and by cytokines produced during innate immune responses to microbes. The migration of T cells is independent of antigen, but cells that recognize microbial antigens in tissues are retained at these sites.

* Effector cells of the T_H1 subset of CD4+ helper T cells recognize the antigens of microbes that have been ingested by macrophages. These T cells express CD40 ligand and secrete IFN-γ, which function cooperatively to activate macrophages.

* Activated macrophages produce substances, including reactive oxygen species, nitric oxide, and lysosomal enzymes, that kill ingested microbes. Macrophages also produce cytokines that induce inflammation and some macrophages produce cytokines that promote fibrosis and tissue repair.

* T_H17 cells enhance neutrophil and monocyte recruitment and acute inflammation, which is essential for defense against certain extracellular bacteria and fungi.

* Effector CD4+ T helper cells of the T_H2 subset stimulate eosinophilic inflammation and inhibit the microbicidal functions

of activated macrophages. Eosinophils are important in host defense against helminthic parasites. The balance between activation of T_H1 and T_H2 cells determines the outcomes of many infections, with T_H1 cells promoting and T_H2 cells suppressing defense against intracellular microbes.

* $CD8^+$ T cells differentiate into CTLs that kill infected cells, mainly by inducing DNA fragmentation and apoptosis. $CD4^+$ and $CD8^+$ T cells often function cooperatively to eradicate intracellular infections.

* Many pathogenic microbes have evolved mechanisms to resist cell-mediated immunity. These mechanisms include inhibiting phagolysosome fusion, escaping from the vesicles of phagocytes, inhibiting the assembly of class I MHC–peptide complexes, and producing inhibitory cytokines or decoy cytokine receptors.

REVIEW QUESTIONS

1. What are the types of T lymphocyte–mediated immune reactions that eliminate microbes that are sequestered in the vesicles of phagocytes and microbes that live in the cytoplasm of infected host cells?

2. Why do differentiated effector T cells (which have been activated by antigen) migrate preferentially to tissues that are sites of infection and not to lymph nodes?

3. What are the mechanisms by which T cells activate macrophages, and what are the responses of macrophages that result in the killing of ingested microbes?

4. What are the roles of T_H1, T_H17, and T_H2 cells in defense against intracellular microbes and helminthic parasites?

5. How do $CD8^+$ CTLs kill cells infected with viruses?

6. What are some of the mechanisms by which intracellular microbes resist the effector mechanisms of cell-mediated immunity?

Answers to and discussion of the Review Questions are available at studentconsult.com.

Humoral Immune Responses
Activation of B Lymphocytes and Production of Antibodies

Humoral immunity is mediated by antibodies and is the arm of the adaptive immune response that functions to neutralize and eliminate extracellular microbes and microbial toxins. Humoral immunity is also the principal defense mechanism against microbes with capsules rich in polysaccharides and lipids. This is because B cells respond to, and produce antibodies specific for, many types of extracellular and cell surface molecules, including polysaccharides, lipids, and proteins, but T cells, the mediators of cellular immunity, recognize and respond only to protein antigens that are internalized into or synthesized in cells. Antibodies are produced by B lymphocytes and their progeny. Naive B lymphocytes recognize antigens but do not secrete antibodies, and activation of these cells stimulates their differentiation into antibody-secreting plasma cells.

This chapter describes the process and mechanisms of B cell activation and antibody production, focusing on the following questions:

- How are receptor-expressing naive B lymphocytes activated and converted to antibody-secreting cells?
- How is the process of B cell activation regulated so that the most useful types of antibodies are produced in response to different types of microbes?

Chapter 8 describes how the antibodies that are produced during humoral immune responses function to defend individuals against microbes and toxins.

PHASES AND TYPES OF HUMORAL IMMUNE RESPONSES

Naive B lymphocytes express two classes of membrane-bound antibodies, immunoglobulins M and D (IgM and IgD), that function as receptors for antigens. These naive B cells are activated by antigens binding to membrane Ig and by other signals discussed later in the chapter. The activation of B lymphocytes results in the proliferation of antigen-specific cells, called **clonal expansion,** and in their differentiation into **plasma cells,** which actively secrete antibodies and are thus the effector cells of humoral immunity (Fig. 7–1). The antibodies secreted in response to a microbial antigen have the same specificity as that of the surface receptors on naive B cells that recognize antigen to initiate the response. One activated B cell may generate up

to 4000 plasma cells, which can produce up to 10^{12} antibody molecules per day. In this way, humoral immunity can keep pace with rapidly proliferating microbes. During their differentiation, some B cells may begin to produce antibodies of different heavy-chain isotypes (or classes), which mediate different effector functions and are specialized to combat different types of microbes. This process is called **heavy-chain isotype (or class) switching.** Repeated exposure to a protein antigen results in the production of antibodies with increasing affinity for the antigen. This process is called **affinity maturation,** and it leads to the production of antibodies with improved capacity to bind to and neutralize microbes and their toxins.

Antibody responses to different antigens are classified as T dependent or T independent, based on the requirement for T cell help. B lymphocytes recognize and are activated by a wide variety of chemically distinct antigens, including proteins, polysaccharides, lipids, nucleic acids, and small chemicals. Protein

FIGURE 7–1 Phases of humoral immune responses. Naive B lymphocytes recognize antigens, and under the influence of helper T cells and other stimuli (not shown), the B cells are activated to proliferate, giving rise to clonal expansion, and to differentiate into antibody-secreting plasma cells. Some of the activated B cells undergo heavy-chain isotype switching and affinity maturation, and some become long-lived memory cells.

FIGURE 7–2 Subsets of B cells. Follicular B cells make T-dependent responses to protein antigens, and marginal-zone and B-1 cells account for most of the T-independent antibody responses. In mice, B-1 cells arise earlier in development, from progenitors in the fetal liver, and follicular and marginal-zone B cells arise later, from bone marrow precursors. Note also that the distinctions in the type of response are not absolute; follicular B cells can make T-independent responses, and marginal-zone B cells can make some T-dependent responses. Ig, Immunoglobulin.

antigens are processed in antigen-presenting cells (APCs) and recognized by helper T lymphocytes, which play an important role in B cell activation and induce heavy-chain isotype switching and affinity maturation. (The designation *helper* came from the discovery that some T cells stimulate, or help, B lymphocytes to produce antibodies.) In the absence of T cell help, protein antigens elicit weak or no antibody responses. Therefore, protein antigens, and the antibody responses to these antigens, are called **T dependent.** Polysaccharides, lipids, and other nonprotein antigens stimulate antibody production without the involvement of helper T cells. Therefore, these nonprotein antigens, and the antibody responses to them, are called **T independent.** The antibodies produced in response to T-independent antigens show relatively little heavy-chain isotype switching and affinity maturation. Thus, the most sophisticated and effective antibody responses are generated under the influence of helper T cells, whereas T-independent responses are relatively simple.

Different subsets of B cells respond preferentially to protein and nonprotein

antigens (Fig. 7–2). The majority of B cells are called **follicular B cells** because they reside in and circulate through the follicles of lymphoid organs (see Chapter 1). These follicular B cells make the bulk of T-dependent, class-switched, and high-affinity antibody responses to protein antigens and give rise to long-lived plasma cells. **Marginal-zone B cells,** which are located in the peripheral region of the splenic white pulp, respond to blood-borne polysaccharide antigens, and **B-1 cells** respond to nonprotein antigens in the mucosal tissues and peritoneum. Marginal-zone B cells and B-1 cells express antigen receptors of limited diversity and make predominantly IgM responses, which lack many of the features of T-dependent antibody responses to protein antigens.

Antibody responses to the first and subsequent exposures to an antigen, called primary and secondary responses, differ quantitatively and qualitatively (Fig. 7–3). The amounts of antibody produced after the first encounter with an antigen (in the primary immune response) are smaller than the amounts produced after repeated immunization (in

FIGURE 7–3 Features of primary and secondary antibody responses. Primary and secondary antibody responses differ in several respects, illustrated schematically in **A** and summarized in **B**. In a primary response, naive B cells in peripheral lymphoid tissues are activated to proliferate and differentiate into antibody-secreting plasma cells and memory cells. Some plasma cells may migrate to and survive in the bone marrow for long periods. In a secondary response, memory B cells are activated to produce larger amounts of antibodies, often with more heavy-chain class switching and affinity maturation. These features of secondary responses are seen mainly in responses to protein antigens, because these changes in B cells are stimulated by helper T cells, and only proteins activate T cells. The kinetics of the responses may vary with different antigens and types of immunization. Ig, Immunoglobulin.

secondary immune responses). With protein antigens, secondary responses also show increased heavy-chain isotype switching and affinity maturation, because repeated stimulation by an antigen leads to an increase in the number and activity of helper T lymphocytes.

With this introduction, we now discuss B cell activation and antibody production, beginning with the responses of B cells to the initial encounter with antigen.

STIMULATION OF B LYMPHOCYTES BY ANTIGEN

Humoral immune responses are initiated when antigen-specific B lymphocytes in the spleen, lymph nodes, and mucosal lymphoid tissues recognize antigens. Some of the antigens in tissues or in the blood are transported to and concentrated in the B cell–rich follicles and marginal zones of the peripheral lymphoid organs. In lymph nodes, macrophages lining the subcapsular sinus may capture antigens and take them to the adjacent follicles, where the bound antigens are displayed to B cells. B lymphocytes specific for an antigen use their membrane-bound immunoglobulin (Ig) receptors to recognize the antigen directly, without any need for processing. B cells are capable of recognizing the native (unprocessed) antigen, so that the antibodies that are subsequently secreted (which have the same specificity as the B cell antigen receptors) are able to bind to the native microbe or microbial product.

The recognition of antigen triggers signaling pathways that initiate B cell activation. As with T lymphocytes, B cell activation also requires signals in addition to antigen recognition, and many of these second signals are produced during innate immune reactions to microbes. In the following section, we describe the biochemical mechanisms of B cell activation, followed by a discussion of the functional consequences of antigen recognition.

Antigen-Induced Signaling in B Cells

Antigen-induced clustering of membrane Ig receptors triggers biochemical signals that are transduced by receptor-associated signaling molecules (Fig. 7–4). The process of B lymphocyte activation is, in principle, similar to the activation of T cells (see Chapter 5, Fig. 5–9). In B cells, Ig receptor–mediated signal transduction requires the bringing together (cross-linking) of two or more receptor molecules. Receptor cross-linking occurs when two or more antigen molecules in an aggregate, or repeating epitopes of one antigen molecule, bind to adjacent membrane Ig molecules of a B cell. Polysaccharides, lipids, and other nonprotein antigens often contain multiple identical epitopes in each molecule and are therefore able to bind to numerous Ig receptors on a B cell at the same time. Even protein antigens may be expressed in an array on the surface of microbes and are thus able to cross-link multiple antigen receptors of a B cell.

Signals initiated by antigen receptor cross-linking are transduced by receptor-associated proteins. Membrane IgM and IgD, the antigen receptors of naive B lymphocytes, are membrane bound antibodies and therefore have highly variable extracellular antigen-binding regions (see Chapter 4). However, these membrane receptors have short cytoplasmic tails, so although they recognize antigens, they do not themselves transduce signals. The receptors are noncovalently associated with two proteins, called Igα and Igβ, to form the **B cell receptor (BCR) complex,** analogous to the T cell receptor (TCR) complex of T lymphocytes. The cytoplasmic domains of Igα and Igβ contain conserved immunoreceptor tyrosine-based activation motifs (ITAMs), which are found in signaling subunits of many other activating receptors in the immune system (e.g., CD3 and ζ proteins of the TCR complex; see Chapter 5). When two or more antigen receptors of a B cell are clustered, the tyrosines in the ITAMs of Igα and Igβ are phosphorylated by kinases associated with the BCR complex. These phosphotyrosines recruit the Syk tyrosine kinase (equivalent to ZAP-70 in T cells), which is activated and in turn phosphorylates tyrosine residues on adaptor proteins that then recruit a number of downstream signaling molecules.

The net result of receptor-induced signaling in B cells is the activation of transcription factors that switch on the expression of genes whose protein products are involved in B cell proliferation and differentiation. Some of the important proteins are described below.

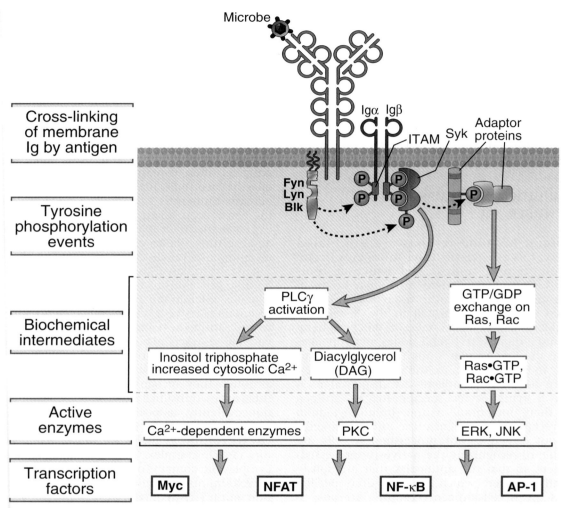

FIGURE 7–4 Antigen receptor–mediated signal transduction in B lymphocytes. Cross-linking of immunoglobulin (Ig) receptors of B cells by antigen triggers biochemical signals that are transduced by the Ig-associated proteins Igα and Igβ. These signals induce early tyrosine phosphorylation events, activation of various biochemical intermediates and enzymes, and activation of transcription factors. Similar signaling events are seen in T cells after antigen recognition. Note that maximal signaling requires cross-linking of at least two Ig receptors by antigens, but only a single receptor is shown for simplicity. AP-1, Activating protein 1; GDP, guanosine diphosphate; GTP, guanosine triphosphate; ITAM, immunoreceptor tyrosine-based activation motif; NFAT, nuclear factor of activated T cells; NF-κB, nuclear factor κB; PKC, protein kinase C; PLC, phospholipase C.

Role of Complement Proteins and Other Innate Immune Signals in B Cell Activation

B lymphocytes express a receptor for a protein of the complement system that provides signals for the activation of these cells (Fig. 7–5). The complement system, introduced in Chapter 2, is a collection of plasma proteins that are activated by microbes and by antibodies attached to microbes and function as effector mechanisms of host defense (see Chapter 8). When the complement system is activated by a microbe, the microbe becomes coated with proteolytic fragments of the most abundant complement protein, C3. One of these fragments is called C3d. B lymphocytes express complement receptor type 2 (CR2, or CD21), which binds C3d. B cells that are specific for a microbe's

FIGURE 7–5 Role of the complement protein C3d in B cell activation. Activation of complement by microbes leads to the binding of a complement breakdown product, C3d, to the microbes. The B cell simultaneously recognizes a microbial antigen (by the immunoglobulin receptor) and bound C3d (by the CR2 receptor). CR2 is attached to a complex of proteins (CD19, CD81) that are involved in delivering activating signals to the B cell.

dendritic cells and other leukocytes, express numerous Toll-like receptors (TLRs; see Chapter 2). TLR engagement on the B cells by microbial products triggers activating signals that work in concert with signals from the antigen receptor. This combination of signals results in optimal B cell proliferation, differentiation, and Ig secretion, thus promoting antibody responses against microbes.

Functional Consequences of B Cell Activation by Antigen

B cell activation by antigen (and other signals) initiates the proliferation and differentiation of the cells and prepares them to interact with helper T lymphocytes, if the antigen is a protein (Fig. 7–6). The activated B lymphocytes enter the cell cycle and begin to proliferate. The cells may also begin to synthesize more IgM and to produce some of this IgM in a secreted form. Thus, antigen stimulation induces the early phase of the humoral immune response. This response is greatest when the antigen is multivalent, cross-links many antigen receptors, and activates complement strongly; all these features are typically seen with polysaccharides and other T-independent antigens, as discussed later. Most soluble protein antigens do not contain multiple identical epitopes, are not capable of cross-linking many receptors on B cells, and by themselves, typically do not stimulate high levels of B cell proliferation and differentiation. However, protein antigens can induce signals in B lymphocytes that lead to important changes in the cells that enhance their ability to interact with helper T lymphocytes.

Activated B cells endocytose protein antigen that binds specifically to the B cell receptor, resulting in degradation of the antigen and display of peptides in a form that can be recognized by helper T cells. Activated B cells reduce their expression of receptors for chemokines that are produced in lymphoid follicles and whose function is to keep the B cells in these follicles. At the same time, there is increased expression of receptors for chemokines that are produced in the T cell zones of lymphoid organs. As a result, the activated B cells migrate out of the follicles and toward the anatomic compartment where helper T cells are concentrated. Because of these changes, the B cells are poised to interact with

antigens recognize the antigen by their Ig receptors and simultaneously recognize the bound C3d via the CR2 receptor. Engagement of CR2 greatly enhances antigen-dependent activation responses of B cells. This role of complement in humoral immune responses again illustrates that microbes or innate immune responses to microbes provide signals in addition to antigen that are necessary for lymphocyte activation. In humoral immunity, complement activation represents one way in which innate immunity facilitates B lymphocyte activation, similar in principle to the role of costimulators of APCs for T lymphocytes.

Microbial products also directly influence B cell activation. B lymphocytes, similar to

	Antigen binding to and cross-linking of membrane Ig	Activation of B lymphocytes	Changes in phenotype, function

Entry into cell cycle: mitosis

Naive B lymphocyte

Increased expression of cytokine receptors

Cytokine receptor

IgM

Low-level IgM secretion

B cell response to antigen	Significance
Entry into cell cycle, mitosis	Clonal expansion
Increased expression of cytokine receptors	Ability to respond to cytokines produced by helper T cells
Migration out of lymphoid follicles	Interaction with helper T cells
Secretion of low levels of IgM	Early phase of humoral immune response

FIGURE 7–6 Functional consequences of immunoglobulin-mediated B cell activation. The activation of B cells by antigen in lymphoid organs initiates the process of B cell proliferation and IgM secretion and prepares the B cell to activate helper T cells and respond to T cell help by stimulating migration of the B cells toward the T cell–rich zones of the lymphoid organs.

and respond to helper T cells that have been activated by the same antigen presented to naive T cells by dendritic cells.

As previously stated, antibody responses to protein antigens require the participation of helper T cells. The next section describes the interactions of helper T cells with B lymphocytes in antibody responses to T-dependent protein antigens. Responses to T-independent antigens are discussed at the end of the chapter.

FUNCTION OF HELPER T LYMPHOCYTES IN HUMORAL IMMUNE RESPONSES TO PROTEIN ANTIGENS

For a protein antigen to stimulate an antibody response, B lymphocytes and helper T lymphocytes specific for that antigen must come together in lymphoid organs and interact in a

way that stimulates B cell proliferation and differentiation. We know this process works efficiently because protein antigens elicit excellent antibody responses within 3 to 7 days after antigen exposure. The efficiency of antigen-induced T-B cell interaction raises many questions. How do B cells and T cells specific for epitopes of the same antigen find one another, considering that both types of lymphocytes specific for any one antigen are rare, probably less than 1 in 100,000 of all the lymphocytes in the body? How do helper T cells specific for an antigen interact with B cells specific for an epitope of the same antigen and not with irrelevant B cells? What signals are delivered by helper T cells that stimulate not only the secretion of antibody but also the special features of the antibody response to proteins, namely, heavy-chain isotype switching and affinity maturation? As discussed next, the answers to these questions are now well understood.

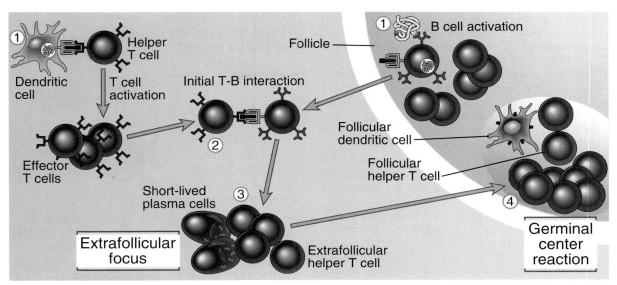

FIGURE 7–7 Sequence of events in helper T cell–dependent antibody responses. T cell–B cell interaction consists of (1) independent activation of two cell types by antigen; (2) migration of cells toward one another and initial interaction between cells; (3) development of extrafollicular focus of activated B cells, in which early antibody responses occur; and (4) formation of germinal centers in which stronger and more effective antibody responses develop.

The process of T-B cell interaction and T cell–dependent antibody responses occurs in a series of sequential steps. It is helpful to summarize these before discussing the individual reactions in more detail. The main events in the process are as follows (Fig. 7–7):

1. CD4$^+$ helper T cells and B cells are independently activated by a protein antigen in different regions of a lymphoid organ and migrate toward each other.
2. These T and B cells initially interact outside the follicles.
3. The initial antigen-specific T-B cell interaction consists of two phases: (a) B cells process and present antigen to the T cells, and (b) the previously activated helper T cells express CD40 ligand and secrete cytokines, which act on the B cells to initiate proliferation and differentiation to plasma cells. The early antibody response, consisting of antibody secretion by plasma cells and some degree of isotype switching, occurs in these extrafollicular foci.
4. Some activated B cells migrate back into the follicle, accompanied by helper T cells that were further activated by the B lymphocytes to develop into follicular helper T cells (T$_{FH}$ cells). In response to signals from the T$_{FH}$

cells, B cells begin to proliferate, forming an organized structure called a germinal center, and the proliferating germinal center B cells undergo extensive somatic mutation of antibody gene variable regions and Ig heavy-chain isotype switching. High-affinity B cells are selected in the germinal center, resulting in the production of high-affinity antibodies. This **germinal center reaction** also results in the generation of long-lived plasma cells (many of which migrate to the bone marrow) and memory B cells. Thus, the events that make the T-dependent antibody response most effective and specialized occur mainly in the germinal center.

Activation and Migration of Helper T Cells

Helper T cells that have been activated by dendritic cells migrate toward the B cell zone and interact with antigen-stimulated B lymphocytes in parafollicular areas of the peripheral lymphoid organs (see Fig. 7–7). The initial activation of T cells requires antigen recognition and costimulation, as described in Chapter 5. The antigens that stimulate CD4$^+$ helper T cells are proteins typically derived from extracellular microbes that are internalized, processed in late endosomes and lysosomes, and displayed bound to class II major histocompatibility complex (MHC) molecules of APCs in the T cell–rich zones of peripheral lymphoid tissues. T cell activation is induced best by microbial antigens, and by protein antigens that are administered with adjuvants, which stimulate the expression of costimulators on APCs. The CD4+ T cells differentiate into effector cells capable of producing various cytokines, and some of these T lymphocytes migrate toward the edges of lymphoid follicles as antigen-stimulated B lymphocytes within the follicles are beginning to migrate outward.

The directed migration of activated B and T cells toward one another depends on changes in the expression of certain chemokine receptors on the activated lymphocytes. On activation, T cells reduce expression of the chemokine receptor CCR7, which recognizes chemokines produced in T cell zones, and increase expression of the chemokine receptor CXCR5, which promotes migration into B cell follicles. B cells, on activation, undergo precisely the opposite changes, decreasing CXCR5 and increasing CCR7 expression. As a result, antigen-activated B and T cells migrate toward one another and meet at the edges of lymphoid follicles or in interfollicular areas. The next step in their interaction occurs here.

Presentation of Antigens by B Lymphocytes to Helper T Cells

The B lymphocytes that bind protein antigens by their membrane Ig antigen receptors endocytose these antigens, process them in endosomal vesicles, and display class II MHC–associated peptides for recognition by CD4+ helper T cells (Fig. 7–8). The membrane Ig of B cells is a high-affinity receptor that enables a B cell to specifically bind a particular antigen, even when the extracellular concentration of the antigen is very low. In addition, antigen bound by membrane Ig is endocytosed efficiently and is delivered to late endosomal vesicles and lysosomes, where proteins are processed into peptides that bind to class II MHC molecules (see Chapter 3). Therefore, B lymphocytes are efficient APCs for the antigens they specifically recognize.

Any one B cell may bind a conformational epitope of a protein antigen, internalize and

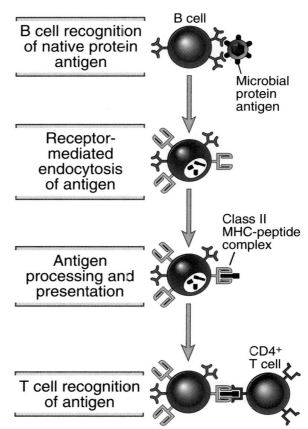

FIGURE 7–8 Antigen presentation by B lymphocytes to helper T cells. B cells specific for a protein antigen bind and internalize that antigen, process it, and present peptides attached to class II major histocompatibility complex (MHC) molecules to helper T cells. The B cells and helper T cells are specific for the same antigen, but the B cells recognize native (conformational) epitopes, and the helper T cells recognize peptide fragments of the antigen. B cells also express costimulators (e.g., B7 molecules) that play a role in T cell activation.

process the protein, and display multiple peptides of that protein for T cell recognition. Therefore, B cells and T cells recognize different epitopes of the same protein antigen. Because B cells present the antigen for which they have specific receptors, and helper T cells specifically recognize peptides derived from the same antigen, the ensuing interaction remains antigen specific. B cells are capable of activating previously differentiated effector T cells but are inefficient at initiating the responses of naive T cells.

The idea that B cells recognize one epitope of the antigen and display different epitopes (peptides) for recognition by helper T cells was first demonstrated by studies using hapten-carrier conjugates. A hapten is a small chemical that is recognized by B cells but stimulates strong antibody responses only if it is attached to a carrier protein. In this situation the B cell binds the hapten portion, ingests the conjugate, and displays peptides derived from the carrier to helper T cells. This concept has been exploited to develop effective vaccines against microbial polysaccharides. Some bacteria have polysaccharide-rich capsules, and the polysaccharides themselves stimulate weak (T-independent) antibody responses, especially in infants and young children. If the polysaccharide is coupled to a carrier protein, however, effective responses are induced against the polysaccharide because helper T cells are engaged in the response. Such **conjugate vaccines** have been very useful for inducing protective immunity against bacteria such as *Haemophilus influenzae*, especially in infants.

Mechanisms of Helper T Cell–Mediated Activation of B Lymphocytes

Helper T lymphocytes that recognize antigen presented by B cells express CD40 ligand (CD40L) and secrete cytokines, which activate the antigen-specific B cells (Fig. 7–9). The process of helper T cell–mediated B lymphocyte activation is analogous to the process of T cell–mediated macrophage activation in cell-mediated immunity (see Chapter 6, Fig. 6–4). CD40L expressed on activated helper T cells binds to CD40 on B lymphocytes. Engagement of CD40 delivers signals to the B cells that stimulate proliferation (clonal expansion) and the synthesis and secretion of antibodies. At the same time, cytokines produced by the helper T cells bind to cytokine receptors on B lymphocytes and stimulate more B cell proliferation and Ig production. The requirement for the CD40L-CD40 interaction ensures that only T and B lymphocytes in physical contact engage in productive interactions. As described previously, the antigen-specific lymphocytes are the cells that physically interact, thus ensuring that the antigen-specific B cells also are the cells that are activated. Helper T cell signals also stimulate heavy-chain isotype switching and affinity maturation, which

FIGURE 7–9 Mechanisms of helper T cell–mediated activation of B lymphocytes. Helper T cells recognize peptide antigens presented by B cells and costimulators (e.g., B7 molecules, not shown) on the B cells. The helper T cells are activated to express CD40 ligand (CD40L) and secrete cytokines, both of which bind to their receptors on the same B cells and activate the B cells. BCR, B cell receptor; TCR, T cell receptor.

typically are seen in antibody responses to T-dependent protein antigens.

Extrafollicular and Germinal Center Reactions

The initial T-B interaction, which occurs at the edge of lymphoid follicles, results in the production of low levels of antibodies, which may be of switched isotypes (described next) but are generally of low affinity (see Fig. 7–7). The plasma cells that are generated in this reaction are typically short-lived and produce antibodies for a few weeks, and few memory B cells are generated.

Some of the helper T cells that are activated by B lymphocytes express high levels of the chemokine receptor CXCR5, which draws these T cells into the adjacent follicles. The CD4+ T cells that migrate into B cell–rich follicles are called **follicular helper T (T$_{FH}$) cells**. The generation and function of T$_{FH}$ cells are dependent on a costimulator of the CD28 family called ICOS (inducible costimulator); inherited mutations in the *ICOS* gene are the cause of some antibody deficiencies (see Chapter 20). T$_{FH}$ cells may develop from uncommitted T cells or from other subsets, including T$_H$1, T$_H$2, and T$_H$17, and may also secrete cytokines, such as IFN-γ, IL-4, or IL-17, which are characteristic of these subsets; the role of these cytokines in B cell responses is described below. In addition, most T$_{FH}$ cells also secrete the cytokine IL-21, whose role in antibody production is a topic of active research.

A few of the activated B cells from the extrafollicular focus migrate back into the lymphoid follicle, and begin to divide rapidly in response to signals from T$_{FH}$ cells. It is estimated that these B cells have a doubling time of approximately 6 hours, so that one cell may produce about 5000 progeny within a week. The region of the follicle containing these proliferating B cells is the **germinal center**, so named because these central lightly staining regions of lymphoid follicles are sites where activated B lymphocytes divide and give rise to progeny with altered B cell receptors. Germinal center B cells undergo extensive isotype switching and somatic mutation of Ig genes, which are described below. The highest affinity B cells are the ones that are selected at the end of the germinal center reaction to differentiate into memory B cells and long-lived plasma cells.

Heavy-Chain Isotype (Class) Switching

Helper T cells stimulate the progeny of IgM and IgD–expressing B lymphocytes to produce antibodies of different heavy-chain isotypes (classes) (Fig. 7–10). Different antibody isotypes perform different functions, and therefore the process of isotype switching broadens the functional capabilities of humoral immune responses. For example, an important defense mechanism against the extracellular stages of most bacteria and viruses is to coat (opsonize) these microbes with antibodies and cause them to be phagocytosed by neutrophils and macrophages. This reaction is best mediated by antibody classes, such as IgG1 and IgG3 (in humans), that bind to high-affinity phagocyte Fc receptors specific for the γ heavy chain (see Chapter 8). Helminths, in contrast, are too large to be phagocytosed, and they are best eliminated by eosinophils. Therefore, defense against these parasites involves coating them with antibodies to which eosinophils bind. The antibody class that is able to do this is IgE, because eosinophils have high-affinity receptors for the Fc portion of the ε heavy chain. Thus, effective host defense requires that the immune system make different antibody isotypes in response to different types of microbes, even though all naive B lymphocytes specific for all these microbes express antigen receptors of the IgM and IgD isotypes.

Another functional consequence of isotype switching is that IgG antibodies produced are able to bind to a specialized Fc receptor called the neonatal Fc receptor (FcRn). FcRn expressed in the placenta mediates the transfer of maternal IgG to the fetus, providing protection to the newborn, and FcRn expressed on endothelial cells and phagocytes plays a special role in protecting IgG antibodies from intracellular catabolism, thereby prolonging its half-life in the blood (see Chapter 8).

Heavy-chain isotype switching is induced by a combination of CD40L-mediated signals and cytokines. These signals act on antigen-stimulated B cells and induce switching in some of the progeny of these cells. In the absence of CD40 or CD40L, B cells secrete only IgM and fail to switch to other isotypes, indicating the essential role of this ligand-receptor pair in class switching. A disease called the **X-linked hyper-IgM syndrome** is caused by mutations in the CD40L gene, which is located on the X chromosome, leading to production of nonfunctional forms of CD40L. In this disease, much of the serum antibody is IgM, because of defective heavy-chain class switching. Patients also have defective cell-mediated immunity against intracellular microbes, because CD40L is important for T cell–mediated activation of macrophages and for the amplification of T cell responses by dendritic cells (see Chapter 6).

The molecular basis of heavy-chain isotype switching is well understood (Fig. 7–11). IgM-producing B cells, which have not undergone switching, contain in their Ig heavy-chain locus a rearranged VDJ gene adjacent to the first

	IgM	IgG subclasses (IgG1, IgG3)	IgE	IgA
Principal effector functions	Complement activation	Fc receptor–dependent phagocyte responses; complement activation; neonatal immunity (placental transfer)	Immunity against helminths Mast cell degranulation (immediate hypersensitivity)	Mucosal immunity (transport of IgA through epithelia)

FIGURE 7–10 Immunoglobulin heavy-chain isotype (class) switching. Antigen-stimulated B lymphocytes may differentiate into IgM antibody-secreting cells, or, under the influence of CD40 ligand (CD40L) and cytokines, some of the B cells may differentiate into cells that produce different Ig heavy-chain isotypes. The principal effector functions of some of these isotypes are listed; all isotypes may function to neutralize microbes and toxins. BAFF is a B cell–activating cytokine that may be involved in switching to IgA, especially in T-independent responses. IFN, Interferon; IL, interleukin; TGF-β, transforming growth factor β.

constant-region cluster, which is C_μ. The heavy-chain mRNA is produced by splicing a VDJ exon to C_μ exons in the initially transcribed RNA, and this mRNA is translated to produce μ heavy chain, which combines with a light chain to give rise to IgM antibody. Thus, the first antibody produced by B cells is IgM. Signals from CD40 and cytokine receptors stimulate transcription through one of the constant regions that is downstream of C_μ. In the intron 5′ of each constant region (except C_δ) is a conserved nucleotide sequence called the switch region. When a downstream constant region becomes transcriptionally active, the switch region 5′ of C_μ recombines with the switch region 5′ of that downstream constant region, and the intervening DNA is deleted. An enzyme called **activation-induced deaminase** (AID), which is induced by CD40 signals, plays a key role in this process. AID converts cytosines (C) in DNA to uracil (U). The sequential action of other enzymes results in the

removal of the U's and the creation of nicks in the DNA. Such a process on both strands leads to double-stranded DNA breaks. When double-stranded DNA breaks in two switch regions are brought together and repaired, the intervening DNA is deleted, and a rearranged VDJ exon that was originally close to C_μ may now be brought immediately upstream of the constant region of a different isotype (e.g., IgG, IgA, IgE). This process is called **switch recombination.** The result is that the B cell begins to produce a new heavy-chain isotype (determined by the C region of the antibody) with the same specificity as that of the original B cell, because specificity is determined by the rearranged VDJ exon.

Cytokines produced by helper T cells determine which heavy-chain isotype is produced by influencing which heavy-chain constant-region gene participates in switch recombination (see Fig. 7–10). For example, the production of opsonizing antibodies, which

FIGURE 7–11 Mechanism of immunoglobulin heavy-chain isotype switching. Left panel, In an IgM-secreting B cell the primary transcript of the rearranged VDJ heavy-chain gene is spliced, combining the VDJ exon with the μ exons to produce an mRNA encoding the μ heavy chain that will form part of an IgM antibody. The VDJ joins with the μ exons because the μ gene is closest to the rearranged VDJ unit. Center and right panels, Signals from helper T cells (CD40 ligand and cytokines) may induce recombination of switch (S) regions such that the rearranged VDJ DNA is moved close to a C gene downstream of $C_μ$. The enzyme activation-induced deaminase (AID) alters nucleotides in the switch regions so that they can be cleaved by other enzymes and joined to downstream switch regions; dashed lines show switch recombination. Subsequently, when the heavy chain gene is transcribed, the VDJ exon is spliced onto the exons of the downstream C gene, producing a heavy chain with a new constant region and thus a new class of Ig. (Exons encoding γ and α heavy chains are not shown for simplicity.) Note that although the C region changes, the VDJ region, and thus the specificity of the antibody, is preserved.

bind to phagocyte Fc receptors, is stimulated by interferon-γ (IFN-γ), the signature cytokine of T_H1 cells (and also produced by some T_{FH} cells derived from these T_H1 cells). These opsonizing antibodies promote phagocytosis, a prelude to microbial killing by phagocytes. IFN-γ also is a phagocyte-activating cytokine, and it stimulates

the microbicidal activities of phagocytes. Thus, the actions of IFN-γ on B cells complement the actions of this cytokine on phagocytes. Many bacteria and viruses stimulate T_H1 and related T_{FH} responses, which activate the effector mechanisms that are best at eliminating these microbes. By contrast, switching to the IgE class is stimulated by interleukin-4 (IL-4), the signature cytokine of T_H2 cells and related T_{FH} cells. IgE functions to eliminate helminths, acting in concert with eosinophils, which are activated by another T_H2 cytokine, IL-5. Predictably, helminths induce strong T_H2 responses, and some of the T_H2 cells may develop into T_{FH} cells that produce IL-4. Thus, the nature of the helper T cell response to a microbe guides the subsequent antibody response, making it optimal for combating that microbe. These are excellent examples of how different components of the immune system are regulated coordinately and function together in defense against different types of microbes, and how helper T cells may function as the master controllers of immune responses.

The nature of antibody isotypes produced is also influenced by the site of immune responses. For example, IgA antibody is the major isotype produced in mucosal lymphoid tissues, probably because cytokines such as TGF-β that promote switching to IgA are made in these tissues. The B cells activated in these lymphoid tissues are also induced to express chemokine receptors and adhesion molecules that favor their migration into the sites just below mucosal epithelial barriers. IgA is the principal antibody isotype that can be actively secreted through mucosal epithelia (see Chapter 8). B-1 cells also appear to be important sources of IgA antibody in mucosal tissues, especially against nonprotein antigens.

Affinity Maturation

Affinity maturation is the process by which the affinity of antibodies produced in response to a protein antigen increases with prolonged or repeated exposure to that antigen. Because of affinity maturation, the ability of antibodies to bind to a microbe or microbial antigen increases if the infection is persistent or recurrent. This increase in affinity is caused by point mutations in the V regions, and particularly in the antigen-binding hypervariable regions, of the genes encoding the antibodies produced (Fig. 7–12). Affinity maturation is seen only in responses to helper T cell–dependent protein antigens, indicating that helper cells are critical in the process. These findings raise two intriguing questions: How do B cells undergo Ig gene mutations, and how are the high-affinity (i.e., most useful) B cells selected to become progressively more numerous?

Affinity maturation occurs in the germinal centers of lymphoid follicles and is the result of somatic hypermutation of Ig genes in dividing B cells, followed by the selection of high-affinity B cells by antigen (Fig. 7–13). In germinal centers the Ig genes of rapidly dividing B cells undergo numerous point mutations. The enzyme AID required for isotype switching also plays a critical role in somatic mutation. The U's that are produced by this enzyme in Ig V-region DNA are frequently converted to T's during DNA replication, or they are removed and repaired by error-prone mechanisms that often lead to mutations. The frequency of Ig gene mutations is estimated to be one in 10^3 base pairs per cell per division, about 100,000-fold to 1 million–fold greater than the mutation rate in most other genes. For this reason, Ig mutation in germinal center B cells is called **somatic hypermutation.** This extensive mutation results in the generation of different B cell clones whose Ig molecules may bind with widely varying affinities to the antigen that initiated the response.

Germinal center B cells undergo apoptosis unless rescued by antigen recognition and T cell help. While somatic hypermutation of Ig genes is taking place in germinal centers, the antibody secreted earlier during the immune response binds residual antigen. The antigen-antibody complexes that are formed may activate complement. These complexes are displayed by **follicular dendritic cells** (FDCs), which reside in the germinal center and express receptors for the Fc portions of antibodies and for complement products, both of which help to display the antigen-antibody complexes. Thus, B cells that have undergone somatic hypermutation are given a chance to bind antigen on FDCs and to be rescued from death. High-affinity B cells most efficiently bind the antigen and are activated to survive. These B cells also internalize the antigen, process it, and present peptides to germinal center T_{FH} cells, which then provide critical survival signals. As the immune response to a protein antigen develops, and especially with repeated antigen exposure, the amount of antibody produced increases. As a result, the amount of available antigen decreases. The B cells that are selected to survive must be able to bind antigen at lower and lower concentrations, and therefore these are cells whose antigen receptors are of higher and higher affinity.

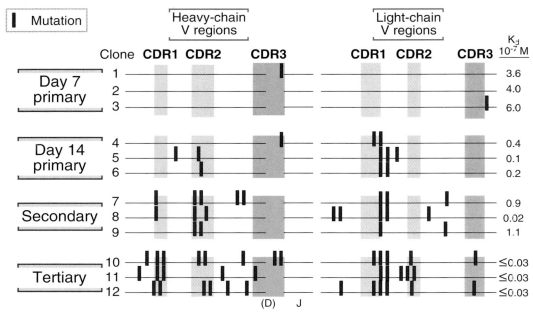

FIGURE 7–12 Affinity maturation in antibody responses. Analysis of several individual antibodies produced by different clones of B cells against one antigen at different stages of primary, secondary, and tertiary immune responses shows that with time and repeated immunization, the antibodies that are produced contain increasing numbers of mutations in their antigen-binding regions, or complementarity-determining region (CDR). The antibodies also show increasing affinities for the antigen, as revealed by the lower dissociation constant (K_d) values at the right. These results imply that the mutations are responsible for the increased affinities of the antibodies for the immunizing antigen. Secondary and tertiary responses refer to responses to the second and third immunizations with the same antigen. *(Modified from Berek C, Milstein C: Mutation drift and repertoire shift in the maturation of the immune response. Immunol Rev 96:23-41, 1987.)*

Antibody-secreting cells that are produced in the germinal centers have also been called plasmablasts because they are not fully differentiated. These cells enter the circulation and tend to migrate to the bone marrow, where they mature into **plasma cells** and may survive for years and continue to produce high-affinity antibodies, even after the antigen is eliminated. It is estimated that more than half of the antibodies in the blood of a normal adult are produced by these long-lived plasma cells; thus, circulating antibodies reflect each individual's history of antigen exposure. These antibodies provide a level of immediate protection if the antigen (microbe or toxin) reenters the body. A fraction of the activated B cells, which often are the progeny of isotype-switched high-affinity B cells, do not differentiate into active antibody secretors but instead become **memory cells.** Memory B cells do not secrete antibodies, but they circulate in the blood and reside in various tissues. They survive for months or years in the absence of additional antigen exposure, ready to respond rapidly if the antigen is reintroduced.

ANTIBODY RESPONSES TO T-INDEPENDENT ANTIGENS

Polysaccharides, lipids, and other nonprotein antigens elicit antibody responses without the participation of helper T cells. Recall that these nonprotein antigens cannot bind to MHC molecules, so they cannot be seen by T cells (see Chapter 3). Many bacteria contain polysaccharide-rich capsules, and defense against such bacteria is mediated primarily by antibodies that bind to capsular polysaccharides and target the bacteria for phagocytosis. Antibody responses to T-independent antigens differ from responses to proteins, and most of these differences are attributable to the roles of helper T cells in antibody responses to proteins (Fig. 7–14). Because polysaccharide and lipid antigens often contain

B cell activation by protein antigen and helper T cells

Naive B cell

Antigen

Migration into germinal center

B cells with somatically mutated Ig V genes and Igs with varying affinities for antigen

B cells with high-affinity membrane Ig bind antigen on follicular dendritic cells (FDCs) and present antigen to helper T cells

FDC

Follicular helper T cell (T_FH)

B cells that recognize antigen on FDCs or interact with helper T cells are selected to survive; other B cells die

High-affinity B cell

FIGURE 7–13 Selection of high-affinity B cells in germinal centers. Some of the B cells that are activated by antigen, with help from T cells, migrate into follicles to form germinal centers, where they undergo rapid proliferation and accumulate mutations in their immunoglobulin (Ig) V genes. The mutations generate B cells with different affinities for the antigen. Follicular dendritic cells (FDCs) display the antigen, and B cells that recognize the antigen are selected to survive. FDCs display antigens by utilizing Fc receptors to bind immune complexes or by using C3 receptors to bind immune complexes with attached C3b and C3d complement proteins (not shown). B cells also bind the antigen, process it, and present it to helper T cells in the germinal centers. As more antibody is produced, the amount of available antigen decreases, so only the B cells that express receptors with higher affinities can bind the antigen and are selected to survive.

	Thymus-dependent antigen	Thymus-independent antigen
Chemical nature	Proteins	Polymeric antigens, especially polysaccharides; also glycolipids, nucleic acids
Features of anitbody response		
Isotype switching	Yes IgM → IgG, IgE, IgA	Low-level switching IgM
Affinity maturation	Yes	Little or no
Secondary response (memory B cells)	Yes	Only seen with some polysaccharide antigens

FIGURE 7–14 Features of antibody responses to T-dependent and T-independent antigens. T-dependent antigens (proteins) and T-independent antigens (nonproteins) induce antibody responses with different characteristics, largely reflecting the influence of helper T cells in the responses to protein antigens. Ig, Immunoglobulin (class).

multivalent arrays of the same epitope, these antigens may be able to cross-link many antigen receptors on a specific B cell. This extensive cross-linking may activate the B cells strongly enough to stimulate their proliferation and differentiation without a requirement for T cell help. Naturally occurring protein antigens usually are not multivalent, possibly explaining why they do not induce full B cell responses themselves but depend on helper T cells to stimulate antibody production. Also, marginal-zone B cells in the spleen are the major contributors to T-independent antibody responses to blood-borne antigens, and B-1 cells make T-independent responses to antigens in mucosal tissues and in the peritoneum.

REGULATION OF HUMORAL IMMUNE RESPONSES: ANTIBODY FEEDBACK

After B lymphocytes differentiate into antibody-secreting cells and memory cells, a fraction of these cells survive for long periods, but most of the activated B cells probably die by a process of programmed cell death. This gradual loss of the activated B cells contributes to the physiologic decline of the humoral immune response. B cells also use a special mechanism for shutting off antibody production. As IgG antibody is produced and circulates throughout the body, the antibody binds to antigen that is still available in the blood and tissues, forming immune complexes. B cells specific for the antigen may bind

Secreted antibody forms complex with antigen

Antigen-antibody complex binds to B cell Ig and Fc receptor

Ig

Igα Igβ

Inhibition of B cell response

ITAM

Fc receptor

ITIM

Block in B cell receptor signaling

FIGURE 7–15 Mechanism of antibody feedback. Secreted IgG antibodies form immune complexes (antigen-antibody complexes) with residual antigen. The complexes interact with B cells specific for the antigen, with the membrane immunoglobulin (Ig) antigen receptors recognizing epitopes of the antigen and a certain type of Fc receptor (FcγRII) recognizing the bound antibody. The Fc receptors block activating signals from the antigen receptor, terminating B cell activation. The cytoplasmic domain of B cell FcγRII contains an ITIM that binds enzymes that inhibit antigen receptor–mediated B cell activation. ITAM, Immunoreceptor tyrosine-based activation motif; ITIM, immunoreceptor tyrosine-based inhibition motif.

the antigen part of the immune complex by their Ig receptors. At the same time, the Fc tail of the attached IgG antibody may be recognized by a special type of Fc receptor expressed on B cells (as well as on many myeloid cells) called FcγRIIB (Fig. 7–15). This Fc receptor delivers inhibitory signals that shut off antigen receptor–induced signals, thereby terminating B cell responses. This process, in which antibody bound to antigen inhibits further antibody production, is called **antibody feedback.** It serves to terminate humoral immune responses once sufficient quantities of IgG antibodies have been produced.

SUMMARY

* Humoral immunity is mediated by antibodies that bind to extracellular microbes

and their toxins, which are neutralized or targeted for destruction by phagocytes and the complement system.

* Humoral immune responses to nonprotein antigens are initiated by recognition of the antigens by specific immunoglobulin receptors of naive B cells. The binding of multivalent antigen cross-links Ig receptors of specific B cells, and biochemical signals are delivered to the inside of the B cells by Ig-associated signaling proteins. These signals induce B cell clonal expansion and IgM secretion.

* Humoral immune responses to a protein antigen, called T-dependent responses, are initiated by binding of the protein to specific Ig receptors of naive B cells in lymphoid follicles. This results in the

generation of signals that prepare the B cell for interaction with helper T cells. In addition, the B cells internalize and process that antigen and present class II MHC–displayed peptides to activated helper T cells also specific for the antigen. The helper T cells express CD40L and secrete cytokines, which function together to stimulate high levels of B cell proliferation and differentiation. Some helper T cells, called follicular helper T cells (T$_{FH}$) migrate into germinal centers and are especially effective at stimulating isotype switching and affinity maturation.

* Heavy-chain isotype switching (or class switching) is the process by which the isotype, but not the specificity, of the antibodies produced in response to an antigen changes as the humoral response proceeds. Isotype switching depends on the combination of CD40L and cytokines, both expressed by helper T cells. Different cytokines induce switching to different antibody isotypes, enabling the immune system to respond in the most effective way to different types of microbes.

* Affinity maturation is the process by which the affinity of antibodies for protein antigens increases with prolonged or repeated exposure to the antigens. The process is initiated by signals from T$_{FH}$ cells, resulting in migration of the B cells into follicles and the formation of germinal centers. Here the B cells proliferate rapidly, and their Ig V genes undergo extensive somatic mutation. The antigen complexed with secreted antibody is displayed by follicular dendritic cells in the germinal centers. B cells that recognize the antigen with high affinity are selected to survive, giving rise to affinity maturation of the antibody response.

* The early T-dependent humoral response occurs in extrafollicular foci and generates low levels of antibodies, with little isotype switching, that are produced by short-lived plasma cells. The later response develops in germinal centers and leads to extensive isotype switching and affinity maturation, generation of long-lived plasma cells that secrete antibodies for many years, and development of long-lived memory B cells, which rapidly respond to reencounter with antigen by proliferation and secretion of high-affinity antibodies.

* Polysaccharides, lipids, and other nonprotein antigens are called T-independent antigens because they induce antibody responses without T cell help. Most T-independent antigens contain multiple identical epitopes that are able to cross-link many Ig receptors on a B cell, providing signals that stimulate B cell responses even in the absence of helper T cell activation. Antibody responses to T-independent antigens show less heavy-chain class switching and affinity maturation than typical for responses to T-dependent protein antigens.

* Secreted antibodies form immune complexes with residual antigen and shut off B cell activation by engaging an inhibitory Fc receptor on B cells.

REVIEW QUESTIONS

1. What are the signals that induce B cell responses to protein antigens and polysaccharide antigens?

2. What are some of the differences between primary and secondary antibody responses to a protein antigen?

3. How do helper T cells specific for an antigen interact with B lymphocytes specific for the same antigen? Where in a lymph node do these interactions mainly occur?

4. What are the mechanisms by which helper T cells stimulate B cell proliferation and differentiation? What are the similarities between these mechanisms and the mechanisms of T cell–mediated macrophage activation?

5. What are the signals that induce heavy-chain isotype switching, and what is the importance of this phenomenon for host defense against different microbes?

6. What is affinity maturation? How is it induced, and how are high-affinity B cells selected to survive?

7. What are the characteristics of antibody responses to polysaccharides and lipids? What types of bacteria stimulate mostly these types of antibody responses?

Answers to and discussion of the Review Questions are available at studentconsult.com

Effector Mechanisms of Humoral Immunity
Elimination of Extracellular Microbes and Toxins

Humoral immunity is the type of host defense mediated by secreted antibodies and necessary for protection against extracellular microbes and their toxins. Antibodies prevent infections by blocking the ability of microbes to bind to and enter host cells. Antibodies also bind to microbial toxins and prevent them from damaging host cells. In addition, antibodies function to eliminate microbes, toxins, and infected cells from the body. Although antibodies are a major mechanism of adaptive immunity against extracellular microbes, they cannot reach microbes that live inside cells. However, humoral immunity is vital even for defense against microbes that live and divide inside cells, such as viruses, because antibodies can bind to these microbes before they enter host cells or during passage from infected to uninfected cells, thus preventing spread of infection. Defects in antibody production are associated with increased susceptibility to infections by many bacteria, viruses, and parasites. Most effective vaccines work by stimulating the production of antibodies.

This chapter describes how antibodies provide defense against infections, addressing the following questions:

- What are the mechanisms used by secreted antibodies to combat different types of infectious agents and their toxins?
- What is the role of the complement system in defense against microbes?
- How do antibodies combat microbes that enter through the gastrointestinal and respiratory tracts?
- How do antibodies protect the fetus and newborn from infections?

Before describing the mechanisms by which antibodies function in host defense, we summarize the features of antibody molecules that are important for these functions.

PROPERTIES OF ANTIBODIES THAT DETERMINE EFFECTOR FUNCTION

Several features of the production and structure of antibodies contribute in important ways to the functions of these molecules in host defense.

Antibodies function throughout the body and in the lumens of mucosal organs. Antibodies are produced after stimulation of B lymphocytes by antigens in peripheral lymphoid organs (lymph nodes, spleen, mucosal lymphoid tissues) and at tissue sites of inflammation. Many of the antigen-stimulated B lymphocytes differentiate into antibody-secreting plasma cells, some of which remain in lymphoid organs or inflamed tissues while others migrate to and reside in the bone marrow. Plasma cells synthesize and secrete antibodies of different heavy-chain isotypes (classes). These secreted antibodies enter the blood, from where they may reach any peripheral site of infection, and enter mucosal secretions, where they prevent infections by microbes that try to enter through the epithelia. Thus, antibodies are able to perform their functions throughout the body.

Protective antibodies are produced during the first (primary) response to a microbe and in larger amounts during subsequent (secondary) responses (see Chapter 7, Fig. 7–3). Antibody production begins within the first week after infection or vaccination. The plasma cells that migrate to the bone marrow continue to produce antibodies for months or years. If the microbe again tries to infect the host, the continuously secreted antibodies provide immediate protection. Some of the antigen-stimulated B lymphocytes differentiate into memory cells, which do not secrete antibodies but are ready to respond if the antigen appears again. On encounter with the microbe, these memory cells rapidly differentiate into antibody-producing cells, providing a large burst of antibody for more effective defense against the infection. A goal of vaccination is to stimulate the development of long-lived plasma cells and memory cells.

Antibodies use their antigen-binding (Fab) regions to bind to and block the harmful effects of microbes and toxins, and they use their Fc regions to activate diverse effector mechanisms that eliminate these microbes and toxins (Fig. 8–1). This spatial segregation of the antigen recognition and effector functions of antibody molecules was introduced in Chapter 4. Antibodies sterically block the infectivity of microbes and the injurious effects of microbial toxins simply by binding to the microbes and toxins, using only their Fab regions to do so. Other functions of antibodies require the participation of various components of host defense, such as phagocytes and the complement system. The Fc portions of immunoglobulin (Ig) molecules, made up of the heavy-chain constant regions, contain the binding sites for Fc receptors on phagocytes and for complement proteins. The binding of antibodies to Fc and complement receptors occurs only after several Ig molecules recognize and become attached to a microbe or microbial antigen. Therefore, even the Fc-dependent functions of antibodies require antigen recognition by the Fab regions. This feature of antibodies ensures that they activate effector mechanisms only when needed, that is, when they recognize their target antigens.

Heavy-chain isotype (class) switching and affinity maturation enhance the protective functions of antibodies. Isotype switching and affinity maturation are two changes that occur in the antibodies produced by antigen-stimulated B lymphocytes, especially during responses to protein antigens (see Chapter 7). Heavy-chain isotype switching results in the production of antibodies with distinct Fc regions, capable of different effector functions (see Fig. 8–1). By switching to different antibody isotypes in response to various microbes, the humoral immune system is able to engage host mechanisms that are optimal for combating these microbes. Affinity maturation is induced by prolonged or repeated stimulation with protein antigens, and it leads to the production of antibodies with higher and higher affinities for the antigen. This change increases the ability of antibodies to bind to and neutralize or eliminate microbes, especially if the microbes are persistent or capable of recurrent infections. This is one of the reasons for the recommended practice of giving multiple rounds of immunizations with

Antibody isotype	Effector functions
IgG	Neutralization of microbes and toxins
	Opsonization of antigens for phagocytosis by macrophages and neutrophils
	Activation of the classical pathway of complement
	Antibody-dependent cellular cytotoxicity mediated by NK cells
	Neonatal immunity: transfer of maternal antibody across placenta and gut
	Feedback inhibition of B cell activation
IgM	Activation of the classical pathway of complement
IgA	Mucosal immunity: secretion of IgA into lumens of gastrointestinal and respiratory tracts, neutralization of microbes and toxins
IgE	Defense against helminths
	Mast cell degranulation (immediate hypersensitivity reactions)

FIGURE 8–1 Effector functions of antibodies. Antibodies are produced by the activation of B lymphocytes by antigens and other signals (not shown). Antibodies of different heavy-chain classes (isotypes) perform different effector functions, as illustrated schematically in **A** and summarized in **B.** (Some properties of antibodies are listed in Figure 4–3.) Ig, Immunoglobulin; NK, natural killer.

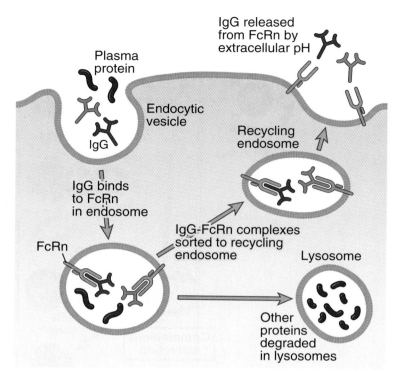

FIGURE 8–2 Neonatal Fc receptor (FcRn) contributes to the long half-life of IgG molecules. Circulating IgG molecules are ingested by endothelial cells and bind the FcRn, an IgG-binding receptor present in the acidic environment of endosomes. In endothelial cells, FcRn sequesters IgG molecules in endosomal vesicles (pH ~4). The FcRn-IgG complexes recycle back to the cell surface, where they are exposed to the neutral pH (~7) of the blood, which releases the bound antibody back into the circulation.

the same antigen for generating protective immunity.

Switching to the IgG isotype prolongs the duration an antibody lasts in the blood and therefore increases the functional activity of the antibody. The **neonatal Fc receptor** (FcRn) is expressed in placenta, endothelium, phagocytes, and a few other cell types. In the endothelium, FcRn plays a special role in protecting IgG antibodies from intracellular catabolism (Fig. 8–2). FcRn is found in the endosomes of endothelial cells, where it binds to IgG that has been taken up by the cells. Once bound to the FcRn, the IgG is recycled back into the circulation, thus avoiding lysosomal degradation. This unique mechanism for protecting a blood protein is the reason why IgG antibodies have a half-life of about 3 weeks, much longer than that of other Ig isotypes and most other plasma proteins. This property of Fc regions of IgG has been exploited to increase the half-life of other proteins by coupling the proteins to an IgG Fc region. One of several therapeutic agents based on this principle is the tumor necrosis factor (TNF) receptor–Fc fusion protein, which functions as an antagonist of TNF and is used to treat various

inflammatory diseases. By coupling the soluble receptor to the Fc portion of a human IgG molecule, the half-life of the protein becomes much greater than that of the receptor by itself.

With this introduction, we proceed to a discussion of the mechanisms used by antibodies to combat infections. Much of the chapter is devoted to effector mechanisms that are not influenced by anatomic considerations; that is, they may be active anywhere in the body. At the end of the chapter, we describe the special features of antibody functions at particular anatomic locations.

NEUTRALIZATION OF MICROBES AND MICROBIAL TOXINS

Antibodies bind to and block, or neutralize, the infectivity of microbes and the interactions of microbial toxins with host cells (Fig. 8–3). Most microbes use molecules in their envelopes or cell walls to bind to and gain entry into host cells. Antibodies may attach to these microbial surface molecules, thereby preventing the

FIGURE 8–3 Neutralization of microbes and toxins by antibodies. A, Antibodies at epithelial surfaces, such as in the gastrointestinal and respiratory tracts, block the entry of ingested and inhaled microbes, respectively. **B,** Antibodies prevent the binding of microbes to cells, thereby blocking the ability of the microbes to infect host cells. **C,** Antibodies inhibit the spread of microbes from an infected cell to an adjacent uninfected cell. **D,** Antibodies block the binding of toxins to cells, thereby inhibiting the pathologic effects of the toxins.

microbes from infecting the host. The most effective vaccines available today work by stimulating the production of neutralizing antibodies, which bind microbes and prevent them from infecting cells. Microbes that are able to enter host cells may be released from these infected cells and go on to infect other neighboring cells. Antibodies can neutralize the microbes during their transit from cell to cell and thus limit the spread of infection. If an infectious microbe does colonize the host, its harmful effects may be caused by endotoxins or exotoxins, which often bind

to specific receptors on host cells in order to mediate their effects. Antibodies against toxins prevent binding of the toxins to host cells and thus block the harmful effects of the toxins. Emil von Behring's demonstration of this type of protection mediated by the administration of antibodies against diphtheria toxin was the first formal demonstration of therapeutic immunity against a microbe or its toxin, then called serum therapy, and the basis for awarding von Behring the first Nobel Prize in Physiology or Medicine in 1901.

FIGURE 8–4 Antibody-mediated opsonization and phagocytosis of microbes. A, Antibodies of certain IgG subclasses bind to microbes and are then recognized by Fc receptors on phagocytes. Signals from the Fc receptors promote the phagocytosis of the opsonized microbes and activate the phagocytes to destroy these microbes. **B,** Table lists the different types of human Fc receptors and their cellular distribution and principal functions. DCs, Dendritic cells; Ig, immunoglobulin; NK, natural killer.

OPSONIZATION AND PHAGOCYTOSIS

Antibodies coat microbes and promote their ingestion by phagocytes (Fig. 8–4). The process of coating particles for subsequent phagocytosis is called **opsonization,** and the molecules that coat microbes and enhance their phagocytosis are called **opsonins.** When several antibody molecules bind to a microbe, an array of Fc regions is formed projecting away from the microbial surface. If the antibodies belong to certain isotypes (IgG1 and IgG3 in humans), their Fc regions bind to a high-affinity receptor for the Fc regions of γ heavy chains, called FcγRI (CD64), which is expressed on neutrophils and macrophages. The phagocyte extends its plasma membrane around the attached microbe and ingests the microbe into a vesicle called a phagosome, which fuses with lysosomes. The binding of antibody Fc tails to FcγRI also activates the phagocytes, because the FcγRI contains a signaling chain that triggers numerous biochemical pathways in the phagocytes. The activated neutrophil or macrophage produces, in its lysosomes, large amounts of reactive oxygen species, nitric oxide, and proteolytic enzymes, all of which combine to destroy the ingested microbe. Antibody-mediated phagocytosis is the major mechanism of defense against encapsulated bacteria, such as pneumococci. The polysaccharide-rich capsules of these bacteria protect the organisms from phagocytosis in the absence of antibody, but opsonization by antibody promotes phagocytosis and destruction of the bacteria. The spleen contains large numbers of phagocytes and is an important site of phagocytic clearance of opsonized bacteria. This is why patients who have undergone splenectomy for traumatic rupture of the organ are susceptible to disseminated infections by encapsulated bacteria.

One of the Fcγ receptors, FcγRIIB, is important not for the effector function of antibodies but for shutting down antibody production and reducing inflammation. The role of FcγRIIB in feedback inhibition of B cell activation was discussed in Chapter 7 (see Fig. 7–15). FcγRIIB also inhibits activation of macrophages and dendritic cells and may thus serve an antiinflammatory function as well. Pooled IgG from healthy donors is given intravenously to patients with various inflammatory diseases. This preparation is called **intravenous immune**

FIGURE 8–5 Antibody-dependent cellular cytotoxicity (ADCC). Antibodies of certain immunoglobulin G (IgG) subclasses bind to cells (e.g., infected cells), and the Fc regions of the bound antibodies are recognized by an Fcγ receptor on natural killer (NK) cells. The NK cells are activated and kill the antibody-coated cells.

globulin (IVIG), and its beneficial effect in these diseases may be partly mediated by its binding to FcγRIIB on various cells.

ANTIBODY-DEPENDENT CELLULAR CYTOTOXICITY

Natural killer (NK) cells and other leukocytes may bind to antibody-coated cells and destroy these cells (Fig. 8–5). NK cells express an Fcγ receptor called FcγRIII (CD16), which is one of several kinds of NK cell–activating receptors (see Chapter 2). FcγRIII binds to arrays of IgG antibodies attached to the surface of a cell, generating signals that cause the NK cell to discharge its granule proteins, which kill the opsonized cell. This process is called **antibody-dependent cellular cytotoxicity** (ADCC). Cells infected with enveloped viruses typically express viral glycoproteins on their surface that can be recognized by specific antibodies and this may facilitate ADCC-mediated destruction of the infected cells. ADCC is also one of the mechanisms by which therapeutic antibodies used to treat cancers eliminate tumor cells.

IMMUNOGLOBULIN E– AND EOSINOPHIL/ MAST CELL–MEDIATED REACTIONS

Immunoglobulin E antibodies activate mast cell and eosinophil–mediated reactions that provide defense against helminthic parasites and are involved in allergic diseases. Most helminths are too large to be phagocytosed,

FIGURE 8–6 IgE- and eosinophil-mediated killing of helminths. IgE antibody binds to helminths and recruits and activates eosinophils via FcεRI, leading to degranulation of the cells and release of toxic mediators. IL-5 secreted by T$_H$2 cells enhances the ability of eosinophils to kill the parasites.

and their thick integument makes them resistant to many of the microbicidal substances produced by neutrophils and macrophages. The humoral immune response to helminths is dominated by IgE antibodies. The IgE antibody binds to the worms and promotes the attachment of eosinophils through the high-affinity Fc receptor for IgE, FcεRI, expressed on eosinophils and mast cells. Engagement of FcεRI, together with the cytokine interleukin-5 (IL-5) produced by T$_H$2 helper T cells reacting against the helminths, leads to activation of the eosinophils, which release their granule contents, including proteins that can kill the worms (Fig. 8–6). IgE antibodies may also bind to and activate mast cells, which secrete cytokines, including chemokines, that attract more leukocytes that function to destroy the helminths.

This IgE-mediated reaction illustrates how Ig isotype switching optimizes host defense. B cells respond to helminths by switching to IgE, which is useful against helminths, but B cells respond to most bacteria and viruses by switching to IgG antibodies, which promote phagocytosis by FcγRI. As discussed in Chapters 5 and 7, these patterns of isotype switching are determined by the cytokines produced by helper T cells responding to the different types of microbes.

IgE antibodies also are involved in allergic diseases (see Chapter 11).

THE COMPLEMENT SYSTEM

The complement system is a collection of circulating and cell membrane proteins that play important roles in host defense against microbes

and in antibody-mediated tissue injury. The term **complement** refers to the ability of these proteins to assist, or complement, the antimicrobial activity of antibodies. The complement system may be activated by microbes in the absence of antibody, as part of the innate immune response to infection, and by antibodies attached to microbes, as part of adaptive immunity (see Fig. 2–13).

The activation of complement proteins involves sequential proteolytic cleavage of these proteins, leading to the generation of effector molecules that participate in eliminating microbes in different ways. This cascade of complement protein activation, as with all enzymatic cascades, is capable of achieving tremendous amplification; therefore an initially small number of activated complement molecules produced early in the cascade may generate a large number of effector molecules. Activated complement proteins become covalently attached to the cell surfaces where the activation occurs, ensuring that complement effector functions are limited to the correct sites. The complement system is tightly regulated by molecules present on normal host cells, and this regulation prevents uncontrolled and potentially harmful complement activation.

Pathways of Complement Activation

Of the three major pathways of complement activation, two, called the alternative and lectin pathways, are initiated by microbes in the absence of antibody, and the third, called the classical pathway, is initiated by certain isotypes of antibodies attached to antigens (Fig. 8–7). Several proteins in each pathway interact in a precise sequence. The most abundant complement protein in the plasma, C3, plays a central role in all three pathways. C3 is spontaneously hydrolyzed in plasma at a low level, but its products are unstable, rapidly broken down, and lost.

The **alternative pathway** of complement activation is triggered when a breakdown product of C3 hydrolysis, called C3b, is deposited on the surface of a microbe. Here, the C3b forms stable covalent bonds with microbial proteins or polysaccharides and is thus protected from further degradation. (As described later, C3b is prevented from binding stably to normal host cells by several regulatory proteins present on host cells but absent from microbes.) The

FIGURE 8–7 Early steps of complement activation. A, Table illustrates the steps in the activation of the alternative, classical, and lectin pathways. Although the sequence of events is similar, the three pathways differ in their requirement for antibody and the proteins used.

Continued

B

Protein	Serum conc. (µg/mL)	Function
C3	1000-1200	C3b binds to the surface of a microbe, where it functions as an opsonin and as a component of C3 and C5 convertases C3a stimulates inflammation
Factor B	200	Bb is a serine protease and the active enzyme of C3 and C5 convertases
Factor D	1-2	Plasma serine protease that cleaves factor B when it is bound to C3b
Properdin	25	Stabilizes the C3 convertase (C3bBb) on microbial surfaces

C

Protein	Serum conc. (µg/mL)	Function
C1 (C1qr$_2$s$_2$)		Initiates the classical pathway; C1q binds to Fc portion of antibody; C1r and C1s are proteases that lead to C4 and C2 activation
C4	300-600	C4b covalently binds to surface of microbe or cell where antibody is bound and complement is activated C4b binds to C2 for cleavage by C1s C4a stimulates inflammation
C2	20	C2a is a serine protease functioning as an active enzyme of C3 and C5 convertases
Mannose-binding lectin (MBL)	0.8-1	Initiates the lectin pathway; MBL binds to terminal mannose residues of microbial carbohydrates. An MBL-associated protease activates C4 and C2, as in the classical pathway.

FIGURE 8–7, cont'd. B, Table summarizes the important properties of the proteins involved in the early steps of the alternative pathway of complement activation. **C,** Table summarizes the important properties of the proteins involved in the early steps of the classical and lectin pathways. Note that C3, which is listed among the alternative pathway proteins **(B),** also is the central component of the classical and lectin pathways.

microbe-bound C3b binds another protein called factor B, which is then broken down by a plasma protease to generate the Bb fragment. This fragment remains attached to C3b, and the C3bBb complex enzymatically breaks down more C3, functioning as the alternative pathway C3 convertase. As a result of this convertase activity, many more C3b and C3bBb molecules are produced and become attached to the microbe. Some of the C3bBb molecules bind an additional C3b molecule, and the C3bBb3b complex functions as a C5 convertase, to break down the complement protein C5 and initiate the late steps of complement activation.

The **classical pathway** of complement activation is triggered when IgM or certain subclasses of IgG (IgG1, IgG2, and IgG3 in humans) bind to antigens (e.g., on a microbial cell surface). As a result of this binding, adjacent Fc regions of the antibodies become accessible to and bind the C1 complement protein (which is made up of a binding component called C1q and two proteases called C1r and C1s). The attached C1 becomes enzymatically active, resulting in the binding and sequential cleavage of two proteins, C4 and C2. C4b (one of the C4 fragments) becomes covalently attached to the antibody and to the microbial surface where the antibody is bound, then binds C2, which is cleaved by active C1 to yield the C4b2a complex. This complex is the classical pathway C3 convertase, which functions to break down C3, and the C3b that is generated again becomes attached to the microbe. Some of the C3b binds to the C4b2a complex, and the resultant C4b2a3b complex functions as a C5 convertase, which cleaves the C5 complement protein.

The **lectin pathway** of complement activation is initiated not by antibodies but by the attachment of plasma mannose-binding lectin (MBL) to microbes. MBL is structurally similar to a component of C1 of the classical pathway and serves to activate C4. The subsequent steps are essentially the same as in the classical pathway.

The net result of these early steps of complement activation is that microbes acquire a coat of covalently attached C3b. Note that the alternative and lectin pathways are effector mechanisms of innate immunity, whereas the classical pathway is a mechanism of adaptive humoral immunity. These pathways differ in their initiation, but once triggered, their late steps are the same.

The late steps of complement activation are initiated by the binding of C5 to the C5 convertase and subsequent proteolysis of C5, generating C5b (Fig. 8–8). The remaining components, C6, C7, C8, and C9, bind sequentially to a complex nucleated by C5b. The final protein in the pathway, C9, polymerizes to form a pore in the cell membrane through which water and ions can enter, causing death of the microbe. This poly-C9 is the key component of the **membrane attack complex** (MAC), and its formation is the end result of complement activation.

Functions of the Complement System

The complement system plays an important role in the elimination of microbes during innate and adaptive immune responses. The main effector functions of the complement system are illustrated in Figure 8–9.

Microbes coated with C3b are phagocytosed by virtue of C3b being recognized by complement receptor type 1 (CR1, or CD35), which is expressed on phagocytes. Thus, C3b functions as an opsonin. Opsonization is probably the most important function of complement in defense against microbes. The MAC can induce osmotic lysis of cells, including microbes. MAC-induced lysis is effective only against microbes that have thin cell walls and little or no glycocalyx, such as the *Neisseria* species of bacteria. Small peptide fragments of C3, C4, and especially C5 which are produced by proteolysis, are chemotactic for neutrophils, stimulate the release of inflammatory mediators from various leukocytes, and act on endothelial cells to enhance movement of leukocytes and plasma proteins into tissues. In this way, complement fragments induce inflammatory reactions that also serve to eliminate microbes.

In addition to its antimicrobial effector functions, the complement system provides stimuli for the development of humoral immune responses. When C3 is activated by a microbe by the alternative pathway, one of its breakdown products, C3d, is recognized by complement receptor type 2 (CR2) on B lymphocytes. Signals delivered by this receptor stimulate B cell responses against the microbe. This process is described in Chapter 7 (see Fig. 7–5) and is an example of an innate immune response to a microbe (complement activation) enhancing an adaptive immune response to the same microbe (B cell activation and antibody production). Complement proteins bound to antigen-antibody complexes are recognized by follicular dendritic cells in germinal centers, allowing the antigens to be displayed for further B cell activation and selection of high-affinity B cells. This complement-dependent antigen display is another way in which the complement system promotes antibody production.

Inherited deficiencies of complement proteins are the cause of human diseases. Deficiency of C3 results in profound

FIGURE 8–8 Late steps of complement activation. A, The late steps of complement activation start after the formation of the C5 convertase and are identical in the alternative and classical pathways. Products generated in the late steps induce inflammation (C5a) and cell lysis (membrane attack complex). **B,** Table summarizes properties of the proteins in the late steps of complement activation.

susceptibility to infections and usually is fatal early in life. Deficiencies of the early proteins of the classical pathway, C2 and C4, may have no clinical consequence, or may result in increased susceptibility to infections, or are associated with an increased incidence of systemic lupus erythematosus, an immune complex disease. The increased incidence of lupus may be because the classical pathway functions to eliminate immune complexes from the circulation and this process is impaired in individuals lacking C2 and C4. Deficiencies of C9 and MAC formation result in increased susceptibility to *Neisseria* infections. Some individuals inherit polymorphisms in the gene encoding MBL, leading to production of a protein that is functionally defective; such defects are associated with increased susceptibility to infections. Inherited deficiency of the alternative pathway protein properdin also causes increased susceptibility to bacterial infection.

FIGURE 8–9 The functions of complement. A, C3b opsonizes microbes and is recognized by the type 1 complement receptor (CR1) of phagocytes, resulting in ingestion and intracellular killing of the opsonized microbes. Thus, C3b is an opsonin. CR1 also recognizes C4b, which may serve the same function. Other complement products, such as the inactivated form of C3b (iC3b), also bind to microbes and are recognized by other receptors on phagocytes (e.g., type 3 complement receptor, a member of integrin family of proteins). **B,** Membrane attack complex creates pores in cell membranes and induces osmotic lysis of the cells. **C,** Small peptides released during complement activation bind to receptors on neutrophils and stimulate inflammatory reactions. The peptides that serve this function are C5a, C3a, and C4a (in decreasing order of potency).

Regulation of Complement Activation

Mammalian cells express regulatory proteins that inhibit complement activation, thus preventing complement-mediated damage to host cells (Fig. 8–10). Many such regulatory proteins have been described. Decay-accelerating factor (DAF) is a lipid-linked cell surface protein that disrupts the binding of Bb to C3b and the binding of C4b to C2a, thus blocking C3 convertase formation and terminating complement activation by both the alternative and the classical pathways. Membrane cofactor protein (MCP) serves as a cofactor for the proteolysis of C3b into inactive fragments, a process mediated by a plasma enzyme called factor I. CR1 may displace C3b and promote its degradation. A regulatory protein called C1 inhibitor (C1 INH) stops complement activation early, at the stage of C1 activation. Additional regulatory proteins limit complement activation at the late steps, such as MAC formation.

FIGURE 8–10 Regulation of complement activation. A, The lipid-linked cell surface protein decay-accelerating factor (DAF) and the type 1 complement receptor (CR1) interfere with the formation of the C3 convertase by removing Bb (in alternative pathway) or C4b (in classical pathway; not shown). Membrane cofactor protein (MCP, or CD46) and CR1 serve as cofactors for cleavage of C3b by a plasma enzyme called factor I, thus destroying any C3b that may be formed. **B,** C1 inhibitor (C1 INH) prevents the assembly of the C1 complex, which consists of C1q, C1r, and C1s proteins, thereby blocking complement activation by the classical pathway.

The presence of these regulatory proteins is an adaptation of mammals. Microbes lack the regulatory proteins and are therefore susceptible to complement. Even in mammalian cells, the regulation can be overwhelmed by too much complement activation. Therefore, mammalian cells can become targets of complement if they are coated with large amounts of antibodies, as in some hypersensitivity diseases (see Chapter 11).

Inherited deficiencies of regulatory proteins cause uncontrolled and pathologic complement activation. Deficiency of C1 INH is the cause of a disease called **hereditary angioneurotic edema,** in which excessive C1 activation and the production of vasoactive protein fragments lead to leakage of fluid (edema) in the larynx and many other tissues. A disease called **paroxysmal nocturnal hemoglobinuria** results from the acquired deficiency in hematopoietic stem cells of an enzyme that synthesizes the glycolipid anchor for several cell surface proteins, including the complement regulatory protein DAF and CD59. In these patients, unregulated complement activation occurs on erythrocytes, leading to their lysis. Deficiency of the regulatory protein factors H and I results in increased complement activation and reduced levels of C3, causing increased susceptibility to infection.

FUNCTIONS OF ANTIBODIES AT SPECIAL ANATOMIC SITES

The effector mechanisms of humoral immunity described so far may be active at any site in the body to which antibodies gain access. As mentioned previously, antibodies are produced in peripheral lymphoid organs and bone marrow

C

Plasma proteins

Protein	Plasma concentration	Function
C1 inhibitor (C1 INH)	200 µg/mL	Inhibits C1r and C1s serine protease activity
Factor I	35 µg/mL	Proteolytically cleaves C3b and C4b
Factor H	480 mg/mL	Causes dissociation of alternative pathway C3 convertase subunits Cofactor for factor I–mediated cleavage of C3b
C4 binding protein (C4BP)	300 µg/mL	Causes dissociation of classical pathway C3 convertase subunits Cofactor for factor I–mediated cleavage of C4b

Membrane proteins

Protein	Distribution	Function
Membrane cofactor protein (MCP, CD46)	Leukocytes, epithelial cells, endothelial cells	Cofactor for factor I–mediated cleavage of C3b and C4b
Decay-accelerating factor (DAF)	Blood cells, endothelial cells, epithelial cells	Blocks formation of C3 convertase
CD59	Blood cells, endothelial cells, epithelial cells	Blocks C9 binding and prevents formation of the MAC
Type 1 complement receptor (CR1, CD35)	Mononuclear phagocytes, neutrophils, B and T cells, erythrocytes, eosinophils, FDCs	Causes dissociation of C3 convertase subunits Cofactor for factor I–mediated cleavage of C3b and C4b

FIGURE 8–10, cont'd. C, Table lists the major regulatory proteins of the complement system and their functions. FDCs, Fo icular dendritic cells; MAC, membrane attack complex.

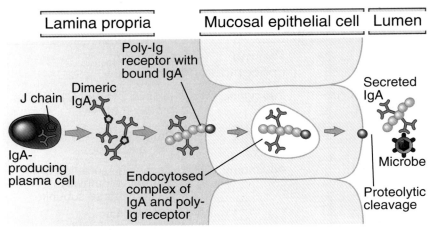

FIGURE 8–11 Transport of IgA through epithelium. In the mucosa of the gastrointestinal and respiratory tracts, IgA is produced by plasma cells in the lamina propria and is actively transported through epithelial cells by an IgA-specific Fc receptor, called the poly-Ig receptor because it recognizes IgM as well. On the luminal surface, the IgA with a portion of the bound receptor is released. Here the antibody recognizes ingested or inhaled microbes and blocks their entry through the epithelium.

and readily enter the blood, from where they may go anywhere. Antibodies also serve protective functions at two special anatomic sites, the mucosal organs and the fetus. There are special mechanisms for transporting antibodies across epithelia and across the placenta, and antibodies play vital roles in defense in these locations.

Mucosal Immunity

Immunoglobulin A is produced in mucosal lymphoid tissues, transported across epithelia, and binds to and neutralizes microbes in the lumens of the mucosal organs (Fig. 8–11). Microbes often are inhaled or ingested, and antibodies that are secreted into the lumens of the respiratory or gastrointestinal tract bind to these microbes and prevent them from colonizing the host. This type of immunity is called mucosal immunity (or secretory immunity). The principal class of antibody produced in mucosal tissues is IgA. In fact, because of the vast surface area of the intestines, IgA accounts for 60% to 70% of the approximately 3 grams of antibody produced daily by a healthy adult. The propensity of B cells in mucosal epithelial tissues to produce IgA is because the cytokines that induce switching to this isotype, including transforming growth factor β (TGF-β), are produced at high levels in mucosa-associated lymphoid tissues, and the IgA-producing B cells are predisposed to home back to mucosal tissues. Also, some of the IgA is produced by a subset

of B cells, called B-1 cells, which also have a propensity to migrate to mucosal tissues; these cells secrete IgA in response to nonprotein antigens without T cell help.

Intestinal mucosal B cells are located in the lamina propria, beneath the epithelial barrier, and IgA is produced in this region. To bind and neutralize microbial pathogens in the lumen before they invade, the IgA must be transported across the epithelial barrier into the lumen. Transport through the epithelium is carried out by a special Fc receptor, the poly-Ig receptor, which is expressed on the basal surface of the epithelial cells. This receptor binds IgA, endocytoses it into vesicles, and transports it to the luminal surface. Here the receptor is cleaved by a protease, and the IgA is released into the lumen still carrying a portion of the bound poly-Ig receptor (the secretory component). The attached secretory component protects the antibody from degradation by proteases in the gut. The antibody can then recognize microbes in the lumen and block their binding to and entry through the epithelium. Mucosal immunity is the mechanism of protective immunity against poliovirus infection that is induced by oral immunization with the attenuated virus.

Neonatal Immunity

Maternal antibodies are actively transported across the placenta to the fetus and across the gut epithelium of neonates,

Mechanism of immune evasion	Example(s)	
Antigenic variation	Many viruses, e.g., influenza, HIV Bacteria, e.g. *Neisseria gonorrhoeae, E. coli*	
Inhibition of complement activation	Many bacteria	
Resistance to phagocytosis	Pneumococcus	

FIGURE 8–12 Evasion of humoral immunity by microbes. This table lists the principal mechanisms by which microbes evade humoral immunity, with illustrative examples. HIV, Human immunodeficiency virus.

protecting the newborn from infections. Newborn mammals have incompletely developed immune systems and are unable to mount effective immune responses against many microbes. During their early life, they are protected from infections by antibodies acquired from their mothers. This is the only example of naturally occurring passive immunity. Neonates acquire maternal IgG antibodies by two routes, both of which rely on the **neonatal Fc receptor** (FcRn). During pregnancy, some classes of maternal IgG bind to FcRn expressed in the placenta, and the IgG is actively transported into the fetal circulation. After birth, neonates ingest maternal antibodies in their mothers' colostrum and milk. Ingested IgA antibodies provide mucosal immune protection to the neonate. The neonate's intestinal epithelial cells also express FcRn, which binds ingested IgG antibody and carries it across the epithelium. Thus, neonates acquire the IgG antibody profiles of their mothers and are protected from infectious microbes to which the mothers were exposed or vaccinated.

EVASION OF HUMORAL IMMUNITY BY MICROBES

Microbes have evolved numerous mechanisms to evade humoral immunity (Fig. 8–12). Many bacteria and viruses mutate their antigenic surface molecules so that they can no longer be recognized by antibodies produced in response to previous infections. Antigenic variation typically is seen in viruses, such as influenza virus, human immunodeficiency virus (HIV), and rhinovirus. There are so many variants of the major antigenic surface glycoprotein of HIV, called gp120, that antibodies against one HIV isolate may not protect against other HIV isolates. This is one reason why gp120 vaccines are not effective in protecting people from HIV infection. Bacteria such as *Escherichia coli* vary the antigens contained in their pili and thus evade antibody-mediated defense. The trypanosome parasite, which causes sleeping sickness, expresses new surface glycoproteins whenever it encounters antibodies against the original glycoprotein. As a result, infection with this protozoan parasite

Type of vaccine	Examples	Form of protection
Live attenuated, or killed, bacteria	BCG, cholera	Antibody response
Live attenuated viruses	Polio, rabies	Antibody response; cell-mediated immune response
Subunit (antigen) vaccines	Tetanus toxoid, diphtheria toxoid	Antibody response
Conjugate vaccines	*Haemophilus influenzae* infection	Helper T cell–dependent antibody response to polysaccharide antigens
Synthetic vaccines	Hepatitis (recombinant proteins)	Antibody response
Viral vectors	Clinical trials of HIV antigens in canary pox vector	Cell-mediated and humoral immune responses
DNA vaccines	Clinical trials ongoing for several infections	Cell-mediated and humoral immune responses

FIGURE 8–13 Vaccination strategies. This table lists different types of vaccines in use or tried, as well as the nature of the protective immune responses induced by these vaccines. BCG, Bacille Calmette-Guérin; HIV, human immunodeficiency virus.

is characterized by waves of parasitemia, each wave consisting of an antigenically new parasite that is not recognized by antibodies produced against the parasites in the preceding wave. Other microbes inhibit complement activation or resist phagocytosis.

VACCINATION

Vaccination is the process of stimulating protective adaptive immune responses against microbes by exposure to nonpathogenic forms or components of the microbes. The development of vaccines against infections has been one of the great successes of immunology. The only human disease to be intentionally eradicated from the earth is smallpox, and this was achieved by a worldwide program of vaccination. Polio is likely to be the second such disease, and as mentioned in Chapter 1, many other diseases have been largely controlled by vaccination (see Fig. 1–2).

Several types of vaccines are in use and being developed (Fig. 8–13). Some of the most effective vaccines are composed of attenuated microbes, which are treated to abolish their infectivity and pathogenicity while retaining their antigenicity. Immunization with these attenuated microbes stimulates the production of neutralizing antibodies against microbial antigens that protect vaccinated individuals from subsequent infections. For some infections, such as polio, the vaccines are given orally, to stimulate mucosal IgA responses that protect individuals from natural infection, which occurs by the oral route. Vaccines composed of microbial proteins and polysaccharides, called subunit vaccines, work in the same way. Some microbial polysaccharide antigens (which cannot stimulate T cell help) are chemically coupled to proteins so that helper T cells are activated and high-affinity antibodies are produced against the polysaccharides. These are called conjugate vaccines, and they are excellent examples of the practical application of our knowledge of helper T cell–B cell interactions. Immunization with inactivated microbial toxins and with microbial proteins synthesized in the laboratory stimulates antibodies that bind to and neutralize the native toxins and the microbes, respectively.

One of the continuing challenges in vaccination is to develop vaccines that stimulate cell-mediated immunity (CMI) against intracellular microbes. Injected or orally administered antigens are extracellular antigens, and they induce mainly antibody responses. To elicit T cell–mediated (e.g., cytotxic T lymphocyte) responses, it may be necessary to deliver the antigens to the interior of antigen-presenting cells (APCs), particularly dendritic cells. Attenuated viruses can achieve this goal, but only a few viruses have been successfully treated such that they remain able to infect cells, retain immunogenicity, yet are safe. Many newer approaches are being tried to stimulate CMI by vaccination. One of these approaches is to incorporate microbial antigens into viral vectors, which will infect host cells and produce the antigens inside the cells. Another technique is to immunize individuals with DNA encoding a microbial antigen in a bacterial plasmid. The plasmid is ingested by host APCs, and the antigen is produced inside the cells. Yet another approach is to link protein antigens to monoclonal antibodies that direct the antigens into dendritic cells that are particularly efficient at cross-presentation and may thus induce CTL activation. Many of these strategies are now undergoing clinical trials for different infections.

SUMMARY

* Humoral immunity is the type of adaptive immunity that is mediated by antibodies. Antibodies prevent infections by blocking the ability of microbes to invade host cells, and they eliminate microbes by activating several effector mechanisms.
* In antibody molecules, the antigen-binding (Fab) regions are spatially separate from the effector (Fc) regions. The ability of antibodies to neutralize microbes and toxins is entirely a function of the antigen-binding regions. Even Fc-dependent effector functions are activated after antibodies bind antigens.

* Antibodies are produced in lymphoid tissues and bone marrow, but they enter the circulation and are able to reach any site of infection. Heavy-chain isotype switching and affinity maturation enhance the protective functions of antibodies.
* Antibodies neutralize the infectivity of microbes and the pathogenicity of microbial toxins by binding to and interfering with the ability of these microbes and toxins to attach to host cells.
* Antibodies coat (opsonize) microbes and promote their phagocytosis by binding to Fc receptors on phagocytes. The binding of antibody Fc regions to Fc receptors also stimulates the microbicidal activities of phagocytes.
* The complement system is a collection of circulating and cell surface proteins that play important roles in host defense. The complement system may be activated on microbial surfaces without antibodies (alternative and lectin pathways, components of innate immunity) and after the binding of antibodies to antigens (classical pathway, a component of adaptive humoral immunity). Complement proteins are sequentially cleaved, and active components, in particular C4b and C3b, become covalently attached to the surfaces on which complement is activated. The late steps of complement activation lead to the formation of the cytolytic membrane attack complex. Different products of complement activation promote phagocytosis of microbes, induce cell lysis, and stimulate inflammation. Mammals express cell surface and circulating regulatory proteins that prevent inappropriate complement activation on host cells.
* IgA antibody is produced in the lamina propria of mucosal organs and is actively transported by a special Fc receptor across the epithelium into the lumen, where it blocks the ability of microbes to invade the epithelium.
* Neonates acquire IgG antibodies from their mothers through the placenta and from the milk through gut epithelium, using the neonatal Fc receptor to capture and transport the maternal antibodies.

- Microbes have developed strategies to resist or evade humoral immunity, such as varying their antigens and becoming resistant to complement and phagocytosis.
- Most vaccines in current use work by stimulating the production of neutralizing antibodies. Many approaches are being tested to develop vaccines that can stimulate protective cell-mediated immune responses.

REVIEW QUESTIONS

1. What regions of antibody molecules are involved in the functions of antibodies?
2. How do heavy-chain isotype (class) switching and affinity maturation improve the abilities of antibodies to combat infectious pathogens?
3. In what situations does the ability of antibodies to neutralize microbes protect the host from infections?
4. How do antibodies assist in the elimination of microbes by phagocytes?
5. How is the complement system activated?
6. Why is the complement system effective against microbes, but does not react against host cells and tissues?
7. What are the functions of the complement system, and what components of complement mediate these functions?
8. How do antibodies prevent infections by ingested and inhaled microbes?
9. How are neonates protected from infection before their immune system has reached maturity?

Answers to and discussion of the Review Questions are available at studentconsult.com

Immunological Tolerance and Autoimmunity
Self-Nonself Discrimination in the Immune System and Its Failure

One of the remarkable properties of the normal immune system is that it can react to an enormous variety of microbes but does not react against the individual's own (self) antigens. This unresponsiveness to self antigens, also called **immunological tolerance,** is maintained despite the fact that the molecular mechanisms by which lymphocyte receptor specificities are generated are not biased to exclude receptors for self antigens. In other words, lymphocytes with the ability to recognize self antigens are constantly being generated during the normal process of lymphocyte maturation. Furthermore, many self antigens have ready access to the immune system, so that unresponsiveness to these antigens cannot be maintained simply by concealing them from lymphocytes. It follows that there must exist mechanisms that prevent immune responses to self antigens. These mechanisms are responsible for one of the cardinal features of the immune system, namely, its ability to discriminate between self and nonself (usually microbial) antigens. If these mechanisms fail, the immune system may attack the individual's own cells and tissues. Such reactions are called **autoimmunity,** and the diseases they cause are called autoimmune diseases.

In this chapter we address the following questions:

- How does the immune system maintain unresponsiveness to self antigens?
- What are the factors that may contribute to the loss of self-tolerance and the development of autoimmunity?

This chapter begins with a discussion of the important principles and features of self-tolerance. Then we discuss the different mechanisms that maintain tolerance to self antigens, and how each mechanism may fail, resulting in autoimmunity.

IMMUNOLOGICAL TOLERANCE: SIGNIFICANCE AND MECHANISMS

Immunological tolerance is a lack of response to antigens that is induced by exposure of lymphocytes to these antigens. When lymphocytes with receptors for a particular antigen encounter this antigen, any of several outcomes is possible. The lymphocytes may be activated to proliferate and to differentiate into effector and memory cells, leading to a productive immune response; antigens that elicit such a response are said to be **immunogenic.** The lymphocytes may be functionally inactivated or killed, resulting in tolerance; antigens that induce tolerance are said to be **tolerogenic.** In some situations, the antigen-specific lymphocytes may not react in any way; this phenomenon has been called immunological ignorance, implying that the lymphocytes simply ignore the presence of the antigen. Normally, microbes are immunogenic and self antigens are tolerogenic. The choice between lymphocyte activation and tolerance is determined largely by the nature of the antigen and the additional signals present when the antigen is displayed to the immune system. In fact, the same antigen may be administered in different ways to induce an immune response or tolerance. This experimental observation has been exploited to analyze what factors determine whether activation or tolerance develops as a consequence of encounter with an antigen.

The phenomenon of immunological tolerance is important for several reasons. First, as we stated at the outset, self antigens normally induce tolerance, and failure of self-tolerance is the underlying cause of autoimmune diseases. Second, if we learn how to induce tolerance in lymphocytes specific for a particular antigen, we may be able to use this knowledge to prevent or control unwanted immune reactions. Strategies for inducing tolerance are being tested to treat allergic and autoimmune diseases and to prevent the rejection of organ transplants. The same strategies may be valuable in gene therapy, to prevent immune responses against the products of newly expressed genes or vectors, and even for stem cell transplantation if the stem cell donor is genetically different from the recipient. **Immunological tolerance to different self antigens may be induced when developing lymphocytes encounter these antigens in** the generative (central) lymphoid organs, a process called central tolerance, or when mature lymphocytes encounter self antigens in secondary lymphoid organs or peripheral tissues, called peripheral tolerance (Fig. 9–1). Central tolerance is a mechanism of tolerance only to self antigens that are present in the generative lymphoid organs, namely, the bone marrow and thymus. Tolerance to self antigens that are not present in these organs must be induced and maintained by peripheral mechanisms. We have only limited knowledge of how many and which self antigens induce central or peripheral tolerance or are ignored by the immune system.

With this brief background, we proceed to a discussion of the mechanisms of immunological tolerance and how the failure of each mechanism may result in autoimmunity. Tolerance in T cells, especially CD4$^+$ helper T lymphocytes, is discussed first because many of the mechanisms of self-tolerance were defined by studies of these cells. In addition, CD4$^+$ helper T cells orchestrate virtually all immune responses to protein antigens, so tolerance in these cells may be enough to prevent both cell-mediated and humoral immune responses against self protein antigens. Conversely, failure of tolerance in helper T cells may result in autoimmunity manifested by T cell–mediated attack against self antigens or by the production of autoantibodies against self proteins.

CENTRAL T LYMPHOCYTE TOLERANCE

The principal mechanisms of central tolerance in T cells are cell death and the generation of CD4$^+$ regulatory T cells (Fig. 9–2). The lymphocytes that develop in the thymus consist of cells with receptors capable of recognizing many antigens, both self and foreign. If an immature lymphocyte interacts strongly with a self antigen, displayed as a peptide bound to a self major histocompatibility complex (MHC) molecule, that lymphocyte receives signals that trigger apoptosis, and the cell dies before it can complete its maturation. This process, called **negative selection** (see Chapter 4), is a major mechanism of central tolerance. The process of negative selection affects self-reactive CD4$^+$ T cells and CD8$^+$ T cells, which recognize self peptides displayed by class II MHC

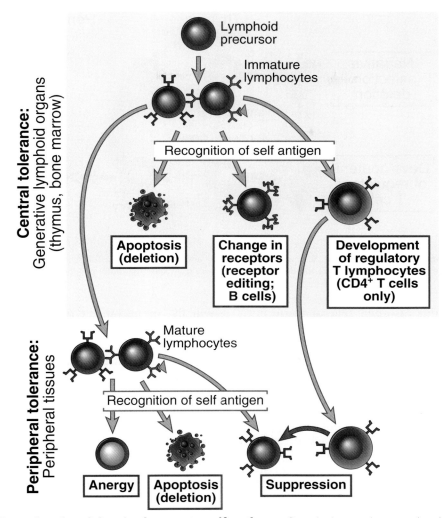

FIGURE 9–1 Central and peripheral tolerance to self antigens. Central tolerance: Immature lymphocytes specific for self antigens may encounter these antigens in the generative (central) lymphoid organs and are deleted; B lymphocytes change their specificity (receptor editing); and some T lymphocytes develop into regulatory T cells. Some self-reactive lymphocytes may complete their maturation and enter peripheral tissues. Peripheral tolerance: Mature self-reactive lymphocytes may be inactivated or deleted by encounter with self antigens in peripheral tissues, or suppressed by regulatory T cells.

and class I MHC molecules, respectively. It is not known why strong T cell receptor (TCR) signaling in response to antigen recognition by immature lymphocytes in the thymus leads to apoptosis rather than cellular activation and proliferation.

Immature lymphocytes may interact strongly with an antigen if the antigen is present at high concentrations in the thymus, and if the lymphocytes express receptors that recognize the antigen with high affinity. Antigens that induce

negative selection may include proteins that are abundant throughout the body, such as plasma proteins and common cellular proteins. Surprisingly, many self proteins that are normally present in peripheral tissues are also expressed in some of the epithelial cells of the thymus. A protein called AIRE (autoimmune regulator) is responsible for the thymic expression of some peripheral tissue antigens. Mutations in the *AIRE* gene are the cause of a rare disorder called autoimmune polyendocrine (polyglandular)

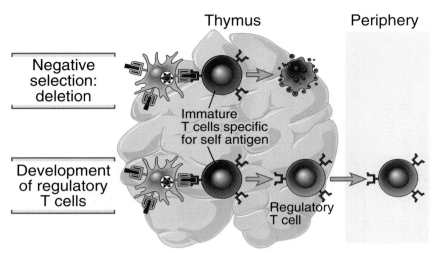

FIGURE 9–2 Central T cell tolerance. Strong recognition of self antigens by immature T cells in the thymus may lead to death of the cells (negative selection, or deletion), or the development of regulatory T cells that enter peripheral tissues.

syndrome. In this disorder, several tissue antigens are not expressed in the thymus because of a lack of functional AIRE, so immature T cells specific for these antigens are not eliminated. These antigens are expressed normally in the appropriate peripheral tissues (since only thymic expression is under the control of AIRE). Therefore, T cells specific for these antigens emerge from the thymus, encounter the antigens in the peripheral tissues, and attack the tissues and cause disease. It is not known why endocrine organs are the major targets of this autoimmune attack; this may be because AIRE specifically facilitates the expression in thymic epithelial cells of genes mainly expressed in these organs. Although this rare syndrome illustrates the importance of negative selection in the thymus for maintaining self-tolerance, it is not known if defects in negative selection contribute to common autoimmune diseases. Negative selection is imperfect, and numerous self-reactive lymphocytes are present in healthy individuals. As discussed next, peripheral mechanisms may prevent the activation of these lymphocytes.

Some immature CD4$^+$ T cells that recognize self antigens in the thymus with high affinity do not die but develop into regulatory T cells and enter peripheral tissues (see Fig. 9–2). The functions of regulatory T cells are described later in the chapter. What determines whether a thymic CD4$^+$ T cell that recognizes a self antigen

will die or become a regulatory T cell is also not known.

PERIPHERAL T LYMPHOCYTE TOLERANCE

Peripheral tolerance is induced when mature T cells recognize self antigens in peripheral tissues, leading to functional inactivation (anergy) or death, or when the self-reactive lymphocytes are suppressed by regulatory T cells (Fig. 9–3). Each of these mechanisms of peripheral T cell tolerance is described in this section. Peripheral tolerance is clearly important for preventing T cell responses to self antigens that are not present in the thymus, and also may provide backup mechanisms for preventing autoimmunity in situations where central tolerance is incomplete.

Antigen recognition without adequate costimulation results in T cell anergy or death, or makes T cells sensitive to suppression by regulatory T cells. As noted in previous chapters, naive T lymphocytes need at least two signals to induce their proliferation and differentiation into effector and memory cells: Signal 1 is always antigen, and signal 2 is provided by costimulators that are expressed on antigen-presenting cells (APCs) typically as part of the innate immune response to microbes (or to damaged host cells). It is believed that dendritic cells in normal uninfected tissues and

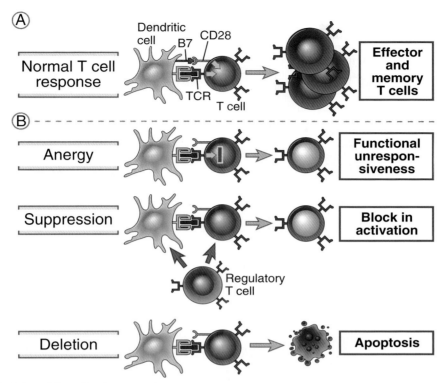

FIGURE 9–3 Peripheral T cell tolerance. A, Normal T cell responses require antigen recognition and costimulation. **B,** Three major mechanisms of peripheral T cell tolerance: cell-intrinsic anergy, suppression by regulatory T cells, and deletion (apoptotic cell death).

peripheral lymphoid organs are in a resting (or immature) state, in which they express little or no costimulators, such as B7 proteins (see Chapter 5). These dendritic cells may constantly process and display the self antigens that are present in the tissues. T lymphocytes with receptors for the self antigens are able to recognize the antigens and thus receive signals from their antigen receptors (signal 1), but the T cells do not receive strong costimulation because there is no accompanying innate immune response. The presence or absence of costimulation is a major factor determining whether T cells are activated or tolerized. Some examples illustrating this concept are discussed below.

Anergy

Anergy in T cells refers to long-lived functional inactivation that occurs when these cells recognize antigens without adequate levels of the costimulators that are needed for full T cell activation (Fig. 9–4). Anergic cells survive but are incapable of responding to the antigen. The two best-defined mechanisms of cell-intrinsic unresponsiveness are a block in signaling by the TCR complex and the delivery of inhibitory signals from receptors other than the TCR complex.

When T cells recognize antigens without costimulation, the TCR complex may lose its ability to transmit activating signals. In some cases, this is related to the activation of enzymes (ubiquitin ligases) that modify signaling proteins and target them for intracellular destruction by proteases.

On recognition of self antigens, T cells also may preferentially engage one of the inhibitory receptors of the CD28 family, cytotoxic T lymphocyte–associated antigen 4 (CTLA-4, or CD152) or programmed death protein 1 (PD-1), both of which function to terminate T cell activation (see Chapter 5). The net result is long-lasting T cell anergy (see Fig. 9–4). It is intriguing

FIGURE 9–4 T cell anergy. An antigen presented by costimulator-expressing antigen-presenting cells (APCs) induces a normal T cell response. If the T cell recognizes antigen without strong costimulation, the T cell receptors may lose their ability to deliver activating signals, or the T cell may engage inhibitory receptors, such as cytotoxic T lymphocyte–associated protein 4 (CTLA-4), that block activation.

that CTLA-4, which is involved in shutting off T cell responses, recognizes the same B7 costimulators that bind to CD28 and initiate T cell activation. One theory to explain how T cells choose to use CD28 or CTLA-4, with these very different outcomes, is based on the fact that CTLA-4 has a higher affinity for B7 molecules than does CD28. Thus, when B7 levels are low (as would be expected normally when APCs are displaying self antigens), the receptor that is preferentially engaged is the high-affinity CTLA-4, but when B7 levels are high (as in infections), the low-affinity activating receptor CD28 is engaged to a greater extent. CTLA-4 works by blocking and removing B7 molecules from the surface of APCs, thus further reducing costimulation and preventing the activation of T cells; CTLA-4 might also deliver inhibitory signals to T cells. This is an interesting example of how the level of available costimulation (in this case, B7 molecules) influences the balance of T cell activation or tolerance. As discussed below, CTLA-4 also is used by regulatory T cells to suppress immune responses.

Several experimental animal models and clinical observations support the importance of T cell anergy and inhibitory receptors in the maintenance of self-tolerance. Forced expression of

FIGURE 9–5 Development and function of regulatory T cells. CD4⁺ T cells that recognize self antigens may differentiate into regulatory cells in the thymus or peripheral tissues, in a process that is dependent on the transcription factor FoxP3. (The larger arrow from the thymus, compared to the one from peripheral tissues, indicates that most of these cells probably arise in the thymus.) These regulatory cells inhibit the activation of naive T cells and their differentiation into effector T cells, by contact-dependent mechanisms or by secreting cytokines that inhibit T cell responses. The generation and maintenance of regulatory T cells also require interleukin-2 (not shown). APC, Antigen-presenting cell.

high levels of B7 costimulators in a tissue in a mouse, using transgenic technology, results in autoimmune reactions against antigens in that tissue. Thus, artificially providing second signals breaks anergy and activates autoreactive T cells. If CTLA-4 or PD-1 molecules are blocked (by treatment with antibodies) or eliminated (by gene knockout) in a mouse, that mouse develops autoimmune reactions against its own tissues. Cancer patients treated with antibodies that block CTLA-4 or PD-1, in order to remove inhibition and boost their antitumor immune responses, also develop autoimmune reactions against multiple tissues. These results suggest that the inhibitory receptors are constantly functioning to keep autoreactive T cells in check. Polymorphisms in the *CTLA4* gene have been associated with some autoimmune diseases in humans.

Immune Suppression by Regulatory T Cells

Regulatory T cells develop in the thymus or peripheral tissues on recognition of self antigens and block the activation of potentially harmful lymphocytes specific for these self antigens (Fig. 9–5). A majority of self-reactive regulatory T cells probably develop in the thymus (see Fig. 9–2), but they may also arise in peripheral lymphoid organs. Most regulatory T cells are CD4⁺ and express high levels of CD25, the α chain of the interleukin-2 (IL-2) receptor. The development and function of these cells require a transcription factor called FoxP3. Mutations of the gene encoding FoxP3 in humans or in mice cause a systemic, multiorgan autoimmune disease, demonstrating the importance of regulatory T cells for the maintenance of self-tolerance. The human disease is known by the acronym IPEX, for *i*mmune dysregulation, *p*olyendocrinopathy, *e*nteropathy, *X*-linked syndrome. This genetic proof of the ability of FoxP3⁺ cells to prevent autoimmunity is perhaps the best evidence for the critical importance of this cell population in maintaining self-tolerance. The survival and function of regulatory T cells are dependent on the cytokine IL-2, and this role of IL-2 accounts for the severe autoimmune disease that develops in mice in which the gene encoding IL-2 or the α or β chain of the IL-2 receptor is deleted. The cytokine transforming growth factor β (TGF-β) also plays a role in the generation of regulatory T cells, perhaps by stimulating expression of the FoxP3 transcription factor. Many cell types can produce TGF-β, but the source of TGF-β for inducing regulatory T cells in the thymus or peripheral tissues is not defined.

Regulatory T cells may suppress immune responses by several mechanisms. Some regulatory cells produce cytokines (e.g., IL-10, TGF-β) that inhibit the activation of lymphocytes, dendritic cells, and macrophages. Regulatory cells express CTLA-4, which, as discussed earlier, may block or deplete B7 molecules from APCs and make these APCs incapable of providing costimulation via CD28 and activating T cells. Regulatory T cells, by virtue of the high level of expression of the IL-2 receptor, may capture this essential T cell growth factor and reduce its availability for responding T cells.

The great interest in regulatory T cells has in part been driven by the hypothesis that the underlying abnormality in some autoimmune diseases in humans is defective regulatory T cell function or the resistance of pathogenic T cells to regulation. However, convincing evidence for the importance of defective regulation in common human autoimmune diseases is lacking, perhaps because it has proved difficult to define the maintenance, heterogeneity, and functions of regulatory T cells in humans. There is also growing interest in cellular therapy with regulatory T cells to treat graft-versus-host disease, graft rejection, and autoimmune disorders.

Deletion: Apoptosis of Mature Lymphocytes

Recognition of self antigens may trigger pathways of apoptosis that result in elimination (deletion) of the self-reactive lymphocytes (Fig. 9–6). There are two likely mechanisms of death of mature T lymphocytes induced by self antigens. First, antigen recognition induces the production of pro-apoptotic proteins in T cells that induce cell death by the mitochondrial pathway, in which various mitochondrial proteins leak out and activate caspases, cytosolic enzymes that induce apoptosis. In normal immune responses, the activity of these pro-apoptotic proteins is counteracted by anti-apoptotic proteins that are induced by costimulation and by growth factors produced during the responses. However, self antigens, which are recognized without strong costimulation, do not stimulate production of anti-apoptotic proteins, and the relative deficiency of survival signals induces death of the cells that recognize these antigens. Second, recognition of self antigens may lead to the coexpression of death receptors and their ligands. This ligand-receptor interaction generates signals through the death receptor that culminate in the activation of caspases and apoptosis by what is called the death receptor pathway. The best-defined death receptor–ligand pair involved in self-tolerance is a protein called Fas (CD95), which is expressed on many cell types, and Fas ligand (FasL), which is expressed mainly on activated T cells. FasL binding to Fas may induce death of both T and B cells exposed to self antigens.

Evidence from genetic studies supports the role of apoptosis in self-tolerance. Eliminating the mitochondrial pathway of apoptosis in mice results in a failure of deletion of self-reactive T cells in the thymus and also in peripheral tissues. Mice with mutations in the *fas* and *fasl* genes and children with mutations in *FAS* all develop autoimmune diseases with lymphocyte accumulation. Children with mutations in the genes encoding caspase 8 or 10, which are downstream of FAS signaling, also have similar autoimmune diseases. The human diseases, collectively called the autoimmune lymphoproliferative syndrome, are rare and are the only known examples of defects in apoptosis causing a complex autoimmune phenotype.

From this discussion of the mechanisms of T cell tolerance, it should be clear that self antigens differ from foreign microbial antigens in several ways, which contribute to the choice between tolerance induced by the former and activation by the latter (Fig. 9–7). Self antigens are present

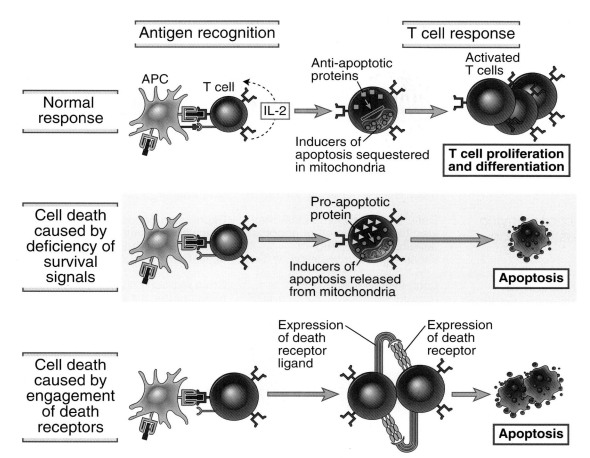

FIGURE 9–6 Mechanisms of apoptosis of T lymphocytes. T cells respond to antigen presented by normal antigen-presenting cells (APCs) by secreting interleukin-2 (IL-2), expressing anti-apoptotic (pro-survival) proteins, and undergoing proliferation and differentiation. The anti-apoptotic proteins prevent the release of mediators of apoptosis from mitochondria. Self antigen recognition by T cells without costimulation (which may provide survival signals) may lead to relative deficiency of intracellular anti-apoptotic proteins, and the excess of pro-apoptotic proteins causes cell death by inducing release of mediators of apoptosis from mitochondria (death by the mitochondrial [intrinsic] pathway of apoptosis). Alternatively, self antigen recognition may lead to expression of death receptors and their ligands, such as Fas and Fas ligand (FasL), on lymphocytes, and engagement of the death receptor leads to apoptosis of the cells by the death receptor (extrinsic) pathway.

in the thymus, where they induce deletion and generate regulatory T cells; by contrast, most microbial antigens tend to be excluded from the thymus, because the lymphatics in which these antigens are transported do not drain into the thymus. Self antigens are displayed by resting APCs in the absence of innate immunity and second signals, thus favoring the induction of T cell anergy or death, or suppression by regulatory T cells. By contrast, microbes elicit innate immune reactions, leading to the expression of costimulators and cytokines that promote T cell proliferation and differentiation into effector cells. Self antigens are present throughout life

and may therefore cause prolonged or repeated TCR engagement, again promoting anergy and apoptosis.

Our understanding of the mechanisms of T cell tolerance and their role in preventing autoimmunity is largely based on experimental animal models. Extending these studies to humans remains an important challenge.

B LYMPHOCYTE TOLERANCE

Self polysaccharides, lipids, and nucleic acids are T-independent antigens that are not recognized

Feature of antigen	Tolerogenic self antigens	Immunogenic foreign antigens
	Tissue	Microbe
Location of antigen	Presence in generative organs (some self antigens) induces negative selection and other mechanisms of central tolerance	Presence in blood and peripheral tissues (most microbial antigens) permits concentration in secondary lymphoid organs
Accompanying costimulation	Deficiency of costimulators may lead to T cell anergy or apoptosis, development of Treg, or sensitivity to suppression by Treg	Expression of costimulators, typically seen with microbes, promotes lymphocyte survival and activation
Duration of antigen exposure	Long-lived persistence (throughout life); prolonged TCR engagement may induce anergy and apoptosis	Short exposure to microbial antigen reflects effective immune response.

FIGURE 9–7 Features of protein antigens that influence the choice between T cell tolerance and activation. This table summarizes some of the characteristics of self and foreign (e.g., microbial) protein antigens that determine why the self antigens induce tolerance and microbial antigens stimulate T cell–mediated immune responses. TCR, T cell receptor; Treg, T regulatory cells.

by T cells. These antigens must induce tolerance in B lymphocytes to prevent autoantibody production. Self proteins may fail to elicit autoantibody responses because of tolerance in helper T cells and in B cells. It is suspected that diseases associated with autoantibody production, such as systemic lupus erythematosus, are caused by defective tolerance in both B lymphocytes and helper T cells.

Central B Cell Tolerance

When immature B lymphocytes interact strongly with self antigens in the bone marrow, the B cells either change their receptor specificity (receptor editing) or are killed (negative selection) (Fig. 9–8). Some immature B cells that recognize self antigens in the bone marrow may reexpress RAG genes, resume immunoglobulin (Ig) light-chain gene recombination, and express a new Ig light chain (see Chapter 4). This new light chain associates with the previously expressed Ig heavy chain to produce a new antigen receptor that is no longer specific for the self antigen. This process of changing receptor specificity, called **receptor editing,** reduces the chance that potentially harmful self-reactive B cells will leave the marrow. It is estimated that 25% to 50% of mature B cells in a normal individual may have undergone receptor editing during their maturation. (There is no evidence that developing T cells can undergo receptor editing.)

If editing fails, immature B cells that recognize self antigens with high avidity receive death signals and die by apoptosis. This process of deletion is similar to negative selection of immature T lymphocytes. As in the T cell compartment, negative selection of B cells eliminates lymphocytes with high-affinity receptors for abundant, and usually widely expressed, cell membrane or soluble self antigens.

If antigens, such as soluble proteins, are recognized in the bone marrow with low avidity, the B cells survive but antigen receptor expression is reduced, and the cells become functionally unresponsive (anergic).

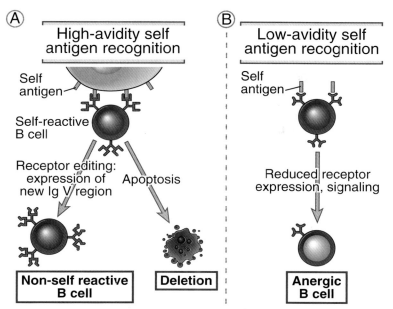

FIGURE 9–8 Central tolerance in immature B lymphocytes. A, An immature B cell that recognizes multivalent self antigens with high avidity in the bone marrow either changes its antigen receptor (receptor editing) or dies by apoptosis (negative selection, or deletion). **B,** If the self antigen is recognized weakly (with low avidity), the B cell reduces antigen receptor expression and becomes functionally unresponsive.

Peripheral B Cell Tolerance

Mature B lymphocytes that encounter self antigens in peripheral lymphoid tissues become incapable of responding to that antigen (Fig. 9–9). According to one hypothesis, if B cells recognize an antigen and do not receive T cell help (because helper T cells have been eliminated or are tolerant), the B cells become anergic because of a block in signaling from the antigen receptor. Anergic B cells may leave lymphoid follicles and are subsequently excluded from the follicles. These excluded B cells may die because they do not receive necessary survival stimuli. B cells that recognize self antigens in the periphery may also undergo apoptosis, or inhibitory receptors on the B cells may be engaged, thus preventing activation.

Now that we have described the principal mechanisms of self-tolerance, we consider the consequences of the failure of self-tolerance, namely, the development of autoimmunity. The mechanisms of tissue injury in autoimmune diseases and therapeutic strategies for these disorders are described in Chapter 11.

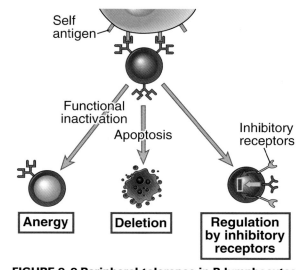

FIGURE 9–9 Peripheral tolerance in B lymphocytes.
A mature B cell that recognizes a self antigen without T cell help is functionally inactivated and becomes incapable of responding to that antigen (anergy), or dies by apoptosis (deletion), or its activation is suppressed by engagement of inhibitory receptors.

AUTOIMMUNITY

Autoimmunity is defined as an immune response against self (autologous) antigens. It is an important cause of disease, estimated to affect 2% to 5% of the population in developed countries, and the prevalence of several autoimmune diseases is increasing. A cautionary note is that in many cases, diseases associated with uncontrolled immune responses are called autoimmune without formal evidence that the responses are directed against self antigens.

Pathogenesis

The principal factors in the development of autoimmunity are the inheritance of susceptibility genes and environmental triggers, such as infections (Fig. 9–10). Tissue injury in autoimmune diseases may be caused by antibodies against self antigens or by T cells reactive with self antigens (see Chapter 11). Much has been learned from experimental animal models about how tolerance in self-reactive T and B cells may fail and how these lymphocytes may become pathogenic. It is

FIGURE 9–10 Postulated mechanisms of autoimmunity. In this proposed model of organ-specific T cell–mediated autoimmunity, various genetic loci may confer susceptibility to autoimmunity, probably by influencing the maintenance of self-tolerance. Environmental triggers, such as infections and other inflammatory stimuli, promote the influx of lymphocytes into tissues and the activation of antigen-presenting cells (APCs) and subsequently of self-reactive T cells, resulting in tissue injury.

postulated that susceptibility genes interfere with pathways of self-tolerance and lead to the persistence of self-reactive T and B lymphocytes. Environmental stimuli may cause cell and tissue injury and inflammation, resulting in the entry and activation of these self-reactive lymphocytes. The activated lymphocytes injure the tissues and cause the disease.

However, despite our growing knowledge of the immunological abnormalities that may result in autoimmunity, we still do not know the etiology of common human autoimmune diseases. This lack of understanding results from several factors: autoimmune diseases in humans usually are heterogeneous and multifactorial; the self antigens that are the inducers and targets of the autoimmune reactions often are unknown; and the diseases may manifest clinically long after the autoimmune reactions have been initiated. Recent advances, including the identification of disease-associated genes, better techniques for studying antigen-specific immune responses in humans, and the analysis of animal models that can be extrapolated to clinical situations, hold promise for providing answers to the enigma of autoimmunity.

Genetic Factors

Inherited risk for most autoimmune diseases is attributable to multiple gene loci, of which the largest contribution is made by MHC genes. If an autoimmune disease develops in one of two twins, the same disease is more likely to develop in the other twin than in an unrelated member of the general population. Furthermore, this increased incidence is greater among monozygotic (identical) twins than among dizygotic twins. These findings prove the importance of genetics in the susceptibly to autoimmunity. Genome-wide association studies, linkage analyses in families, and interbreeding studies in animals have revealed some of the common variations (polymorphisms) of genes that may contribute to different autoimmune diseases. Emerging results suggest that these common variants are more frequent (predisposing) or less frequent (protective) in patients than in healthy controls. Their importance is reinforced by the finding that many of these polymorphisms may affect immune responses, and the same genetic polymorphisms are associated with different autoimmune

diseases. However, these polymorphisms are present in healthy individuals, and the individual contribution of each of these genes to the development of autoimmunity is very small. In some cases, autoimmunity-associated genes are variants (mutations) that are rare or nonexistent in healthy individuals, rather than commonly detected polymorphisms. Such rare variants could have a large impact on the development of autoimmunity.

Many autoimmune diseases in humans and inbred animals are linked to particular MHC alleles (Fig. 9–11). The association between HLA alleles and autoimmune diseases in humans was recognized many years ago and was one of the first indications that T cells played an important role in these disorders (because the only known function of MHC molecules is to present peptide antigens to T cells). The incidence of a particular autoimmune disease often is greater among individuals who inherit a particular HLA allele(s) than in the general population. This increased incidence is called the odds ratio or relative risk of an HLA-disease association; the same nomenclature is applicable to the association of any gene with any disease. It is important to point out that although an HLA allele may increase the risk of developing a particular autoimmune disease, the HLA allele is not, by itself, the cause of the disease. In fact, the disease never develops in the vast majority of people who inherit an HLA allele that does confer increased risk of the disease. Despite the clear association of MHC alleles with several autoimmune diseases, the role of these alleles in the development of the diseases remains unknown. Some hypotheses are that particular MHC alleles may contribute to the development of autoimmunity because they are required to present pathogenic self peptides to autoreactive T cells, or they are inefficient at displaying certain self antigens in the thymus, leading to defective negative selection of T cells, or because peptide antigens presented by these MHC alleles may fail to stimulate regulatory T cells.

Polymorphisms in non-HLA genes are associated with various autoimmune diseases and may contribute to failure of self-tolerance or abnormal activation of lymphocytes (Fig. 9–12, A). Many such disease-associated variants have been described. Polymorphisms in the gene encoding the

Disease	MHC allele	Relative risk
Ankylosing spondylitis	HLA-B27	90
Rheumatoid arthritis	HLA-DRB1*01/*04/*10	4-12
Type 1 diabetes mellitus	HLA-DRB1*0301/0401	35
Pemphigus vulgaris	HLA-DR4	14

FIGURE 9–11 Association of autoimmune diseases with alleles of the major histocompatibility complex (MHC) locus. Family and linkage studies show a greater likelihood of developing certain autoimmune diseases in persons who inherit particular human leukocyte antigen (HLA) alleles than in persons who lack these alleles (odds ratio or relative risk). Selected examples of HLA-disease associations are listed. For instance, in people who have the HLA-B27 allele, the risk of development of ankylosing spondylitis, an autoimmune diseases of the spine, is 90 to 100 times higher than in B27-negative people; other diseases show various degrees of association with other HLA alleles. Breeding studies in animals have also shown that the incidence of some autoimmune diseases correlates strongly with the inheritance of particular MHC alleles (e.g., type 1 diabetes mellitus with a mouse class II allele called I-A^{g7}).

tyrosine phosphatase PTPN22 (protein tyrosine phosphatase N22) may regulate both B and T cell activation and are associated with numerous autoimmune diseases, including rheumatoid arthritis, systemic lupus erythematosus, and type 1 diabetes mellitus. Genetic variants of the cytoplasmic microbial sensor NOD-2 that may provide reduced resistance to intestinal microbes are associated with about 25% of cases of Crohn's disease, an inflammatory bowel disease, in some ethnic populations. Other polymorphisms associated with multiple autoimmune diseases include genes encoding the IL-2 receptor α chain CD25, believed to influence the balance of effector and regulatory T cells; the receptor for the cytokine IL-23, which promotes the development of proinflammatory T_H17 cells; and CTLA-4, a key inhibitory receptor in T cells discussed earlier. It is hoped that elucidation of these genetic associations will reveal pathogenic mechanisms or provide new ideas for better prediction and treatment.

Some rare autoimmune disorders are mendelian in origin, caused by mutations in single genes that have high penetrance and lead to autoimmunity in most or all individuals who inherit these mutations. These genes, alluded to earlier, include *AIRE*, *FOXP3*, and *FAS* (Fig. 9–12, B). Mutations in these genes have been valuable for identifying key molecules and pathways involved in self-tolerance. These mendelian forms of autoimmunity are exceedingly rare,

however, and common autoimmune diseases are not caused by mutations in any of these known genes.

Role of Infections and Other Environmental Influences

Infections may activate self-reactive lymphocytes, thereby triggering the development of autoimmune diseases. Clinicians have recognized for many years that the clinical manifestations of autoimmunity sometimes are preceded by infectious prodromes. This association between infections and autoimmune tissue injury has been formally established in animal models.

Infections may contribute to autoimmunity in several ways (Fig. 9–13). An infection of a tissue may induce a local innate immune response, which may lead to increased production of costimulators and cytokines by tissue APCs. These activated tissue APCs may be able to stimulate self-reactive T cells that encounter self antigens in the tissue. In other words, infection may break T cell tolerance and promote the activation of self-reactive lymphocytes. Some infectious microbes may produce peptide antigens that are similar to, and cross-react with, self antigens. Immune responses to these microbial peptides may result in an immune attack against self antigens. Such cross-reactions between microbial and self antigens are termed

Immune Responses against Tumors and Transplants
Immunity to Noninfectious Transformed and Foreign Cells

Cancer and organ transplantation are two clinical situations in which the role of the immune system has received a great deal of attention. In cancer, it is widely believed that enhancing immunity against tumors holds much promise for treatment. In organ transplantation, of course, the situation is precisely the reverse: Immune responses against the transplants are a barrier to successful transplantation, and learning how to suppress these responses is a major goal of transplant immunologists. Because of the importance of the immune system in host responses to tumors and transplants, tumor immunology and transplantation immunology have become subspecialties in which researchers and clinicians come together to address both fundamental and clinical questions.

Immune responses against tumors and transplants share several characteristics. These are situations in which the immune system is not responding to microbes, as it usually does, but to noninfectious cells that are perceived as foreign. The antigens that mark tumors and transplants as foreign may be expressed in virtually any cell type that is the target of malignant transformation or is grafted from one individual to another. Therefore, the mechanisms for inducing immune responses against tumors must be effective for diverse cell types. Also, a major mechanism by which the immune system kills both tumor cells and the cells of tissue transplants is by cytotoxic T lymphocytes (CTLs). For all these reasons, immunity to tumors and to transplants is discussed together in this chapter. We focus on the following questions:

- What are the antigens in tumors and tissue transplants that are recognized as foreign by the immune system?
- How does the immune system recognize and react to tumors and transplants?
- How can immune responses to tumors and grafts be manipulated to enhance tumor rejection and inhibit graft rejection?

We discuss tumor immunity first, then transplantation, with an emphasis on the principles common to both.

IMMUNE RESPONSES AGAINST TUMORS

For over a century it has been proposed that a physiologic function of the adaptive immune system is to prevent the outgrowth of transformed cells or to destroy these cells before they become harmful tumors. Control and elimination of malignant cells by the immune system is called **immune surveillance.** Several lines of evidence support the idea that immune surveillance against tumors is important for preventing tumor growth (Fig. 10–1). However, the fact that common malignant tumors develop in immunocompetent individuals indicates that tumor immunity is often incapable of preventing tumor growth or is easily overwhelmed by rapidly growing tumors. Immunologists have been interested in defining the types of tumor antigens against which the immune system reacts and developing strategies for maximally enhancing antitumor immunity.

Tumor Antigens

Malignant tumors express various types of molecules that may be recognized by the immune system as foreign antigens (Fig. 10–2). If the immune system is able to react against a tumor in the individual, the tumor must express antigens that are seen as nonself by the individual's immune system.

In experimental tumors induced by chemical carcinogens or radiation, the tumor antigens may be mutants of normal cellular proteins. Virtually any gene may be mutagenized randomly in different tumors, and most of the mutated genes play no role in tumorigenesis. Recent sequencing of tumor genomes has revealed that common human tumors harbor a large number of mutations in diverse genes, and the products of many of these altered genes may function as tumor antigens. Some tumor antigens are products of mutated or translocated oncogenes or tumor suppressor genes that presumably are involved in the process of malignant transformation, called driver mutations. Other mutations may result from defects in DNA repair that are common in cancers, and

Evidence	Conclusion
Lymphocytic infiltrates around some tumors and enlargement of draining lymph nodes correlate with better prognosis	Immune responses against tumors inhibit tumor growth
Transplants of a tumor are rejected by animals, and more rapidly if the animals have been previously exposed to that tumor; immunity to tumor transplants can be transferred by lymphocytes from a tumor-bearing animal	Tumor rejection shows features of adaptive immunity (specificity, memory) and is mediated by lymphocytes
Immunodeficient individuals have an increased incidence of some types of tumors	The immune system protects against the growth of tumors
Therapeutic blockade of inhibitory receptors such as PD-1 and CTLA-4 leads to tumor remission	Tumors evade immune surveillance in part by activating inhibitory receptors on T cells

FIGURE 10–1 Evidence supporting the concept that the immune system reacts against tumors. Several lines of clinical and experimental evidence indicate that defense against tumors is mediated by reactions of the adaptive immune system.

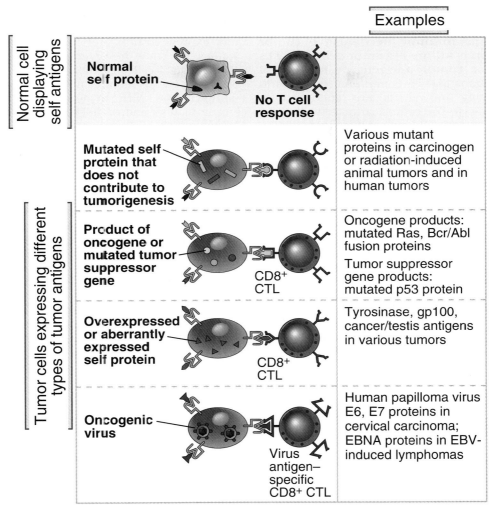

FIGURE 10–2 Types of tumor antigens recognized by T cells. Tumor antigens that are recognized by tumor-specific CD8+ T cells may be mutated forms of random self proteins that do not contribute to malignant behavior of the tumor products of oncogenes or tumor suppressor genes, overexpressed or aberrantly expressed self proteins, or products of oncogenic viruses. Tumor antigens also may be recognized by CD4+ T cells, but less is known about the role that CD4+ T cells play in tumor immunity. CTL, Cytotoxic T lymphocyte; EBNA, Epstein-Barr virus nuclear antigen; EBV, Epstein-Barr virus; gp100, glycoprotein of 100 kD.

may represent passenger mutations that are not directly involved in malignant transformation. However, both types of mutations may encode proteins that are seen as foreign, and therefore both may be relevant from an immunologic standpoint.

Surprisingly, in several human tumors, the antigens that elicit immune responses appear to be normal (unmutated) proteins that are overexpressed, or whose expression normally is limited to particular tissues or stages of development but is dysregulated in the tumors. These structurally normal self antigens would not be expected to elicit immune responses, but their aberrant expression may be enough to make them immunogenic. For example, self proteins that are expressed only in embryonic tissues may not induce tolerance in adults; thus the same proteins expressed in tumors may be recognized as foreign by the immune system. In tumors caused by oncogenic viruses, the tumor antigens may be products of the viruses.

Immune Mechanisms of Tumor Rejection

The principal immune mechanism of tumor eradication is killing of tumor cells by CTLs specific for tumor antigens. A majority of tumor antigens that elicit immune responses in tumor-bearing individuals are endogenously synthesized cytosolic or nuclear proteins that are displayed as class I major histocompatibility complex (MHC)–associated peptides. Therefore, these antigens are recognized by class I MHC–restricted CD8+ CTLs, whose function is to kill cells producing the antigens. The role of CTLs in tumor rejection has been established in animal models: Transplants of tumors can be destroyed by transferring tumor-reactive CD8+ T cells into the tumor-bearing animals. Studies of some human tumors indicate that abundant CTL infiltration predicts a more favorable clinical course compared with tumors with sparse CTLs.

CTL responses against tumors often are induced by recognition of tumor antigens on host antigen-presenting cells (APCs), which ingest tumor cells or their antigens and present the antigens to T cells (Fig. 10–3). Tumors may arise from virtually any nucleated cell type, which are able to display class I MHC–associated peptides (because all nucleated cells express class I MHC molecules), but often the tumor cells do not express costimulators or class II MHC molecules. We know, however, that the activation of naive CD8+ T cells to proliferate and differentiate into active CTLs requires not only recognition of antigen (class I MHC–associated peptide) but also costimulation and/or help from class II MHC–restricted CD4+ T cells (see Chapter 5). How, then, can tumors of different cell types stimulate CTL responses? The likely answer is that tumor cells or their proteins are ingested by the host's dendritic cells, and the antigens of the tumor cells are processed and displayed by class I MHC molecules on the host dendritic cells. This process is called **cross-presentation** or cross-priming, because one cell type (the dendritic cell) presents antigens of another cell (the tumor cell) and activates (or primes) CD8+ T lymphocytes specific for the second cell type. The phenomenon of cross-presentation, and how it differs from typical pathways of antigen presentation, were introduced in Chapter 3 (see Fig. 3–16). Thus, tumor antigens may be recognized by CD8+ T cells and by CD4+ T cells in much the same manner as any other protein antigens displayed by dendritic cells. At the same time, these APCs express

FIGURE 10–3 Induction of CD8+ T cell responses against tumors. CD8+ T cell responses to tumors may be induced by cross-priming (also called cross-presentation), in which the tumor cells or tumor antigens (or both) are taken up by dendritic cells, processed, and presented to T cells. In some cases, B7 costimulators expressed by these antigen-presenting cells (APCs) provide the second signals for the differentiation of the CD8+ T cells. The APCs may also stimulate CD4+ helper T cells, which may provide signals for CTL development (see Chapter 5, Fig. 5–7). Differentiated CTLs kill tumor cells without a requirement for costimulation or T cell help. CTL, Cytotoxic T lymphocyte.

costimulators that provide signals for the activation of the T cells.

It is not known how tumors induce the expression of costimulators on APCs because, as discussed in Chapter 5, the physiologic stimuli for the induction of costimulators are usually microbes, and tumors are generally sterile. One possibility is that tumor cells die if their growth outstrips their blood and nutrient supply, and dying cells release products that stimulate innate responses (damage-associated molecular patterns; see Chapter 2). The activation of APCs to express costimulators is part of these responses.

Once naive CD8+ T cells have differentiated into effector CTLs, they are able to kill tumor cells expressing the relevant antigens without a requirement for costimulation or T cell help. Thus, CTL differentiation may be induced by cross-presentation of tumor antigens by host APCs, but the CTLs are effective against the tumor itself.

Immune mechanisms in addition to CTLs may play a role in tumor rejection. Antitumor CD4+ T cell responses and antibodies have been detected in patients, but whether these responses actually protect individuals against tumor growth has not been established. Experimental studies have shown that activated macrophages and natural killer (NK) cells are capable of killing tumor cells in vitro, but the protective role of these effector mechanisms in tumor-bearing individuals is also largely unknown.

Evasion of Immune Responses by Tumors

Immune responses often fail to check tumor growth because tumors evolve in the host to evade immune recognition or resist immune effector mechanisms. The immune system faces daunting challenges in combating malignant tumors, because immune responses must kill all the tumor cells in order to be effective, and tumors can grow rapidly. Often, the growth of the tumor simply outstrips immune defenses. Immune responses against tumors may be weak because many tumor antigens are weakly immunogenic.

Tumor cells develop several mechanisms of resistance to immune recognition and destruction (Fig. 10–4). Not surprisingly, tumor cells that have mutated to evade the host immune response are selected to survive and grow. Therefore, the ability to avoid destruction by the

FIGURE 10–4 How tumors evade immune responses. Antitumor immunity develops when T cells recognize tumor antigens and are activated. Tumor cells may evade immune responses by losing expression of antigens or major histocompatibility complex (MHC) molecules or by producing immunosuppressive cytokines or ligands such as PD-L1 for inhibitory receptors on T cells.

immune system is now considered one of the hallmarks of cancer. Some tumors stop expressing the antigens that are the targets of immune attack. These tumors are called antigen loss variants. If the lost antigen is not involved in maintaining the malignant properties of the tumor, the variant tumor cells continue to grow and spread. Other tumors stop expressing class I MHC molecules, so they cannot display antigens to CD8+ T cells. NK cells recognize molecules expressed on tumor cells, but not on normal cells, and are activated when their target cells lack class I MHC molecules. Therefore, NK cells may provide a mechanism for killing class I MHC–negative tumors. Still other tumors may secrete cytokines, such as transforming growth factor β, that suppress immune responses. Some tumors express ligands for T cell inhibitory receptors such as PD-1. Tumors may also induce low levels of B7 costimulators on APCs, resulting in preferential engagement of the inhibitory receptor CTLA-4 on T cells rather than the stimulatory receptor CD28 (see Chapter 9). The net result may be reduced T cell activation upon recognition of tumor antigens. Some tumors may induce regulatory T cells, which also suppress antitumor immune responses.

Immunologic Approaches for Cancer Therapy

The main strategies for cancer immunotherapy aim to provide antitumor effectors (antibodies and T cells) to patients, actively immunize patients against their tumors, and stimulate the patients' own antitumor immune responses (Fig. 10–5). At present, most treatment protocols for disseminated cancers, which cannot be cured surgically, rely on chemotherapy and irradiation, both of which damage normal nontumor tissues and are associated with serious toxicities. Because the immune response is highly specific, it has long been hoped that tumor-specific immunity may be used to selectively eradicate tumors without injuring the patient. Immunotherapy remains a major goal of tumor immunologists, and many approaches have been tried in experimental animals and in humans.

One of the earliest strategies for tumor immunotherapy relied on various forms of passive immunization, in which immune effectors are injected into cancer patients. Monoclonal antibodies against various tumor antigens, sometimes coupled to potent toxins, have been tried in many cancers. The antibodies bind to tumor antigens and either activate host effector mechanisms, such as phagocytes or the complement system, or deliver the toxins to the tumor cells. For example, an antibody specific for CD20, which is expressed on B cells, is used to treat B cell tumors, usually in combination with chemotherapy. Because CD20 is not expressed by hematopoietic stem cells, normal B cells are replenished after the antibody treatment is stopped. Other monoclonal antibodies that are used in cancer therapy may work by blocking growth factor signaling (e.g., anti-Her2/Neu for breast cancer and anti-EGF-receptor antibody for various tumors) or by inhibiting angiogenesis (e.g., antibody against the vascular endothelial growth factor for colon cancer and other tumors). T lymphocytes may be isolated from the blood or tumor infiltrates of a patient, expanded by culture with growth factors, and injected back into the same patient. The T cells presumably contain tumor-specific CTLs, which find the tumor and destroy it. This approach, called adoptive cellular immunotherapy, has been tried as a therapy for several types of metastatic cancers, but results have been variable among different patients and tumors.

Many new strategies for cancer immunotherapy rely on boosting the host's own immune responses against tumors. One way of stimulating active immunity against tumors is to vaccinate patients with their own tumor cells or with antigens from these cells. An important reason for defining tumor antigens is to produce and use these antigens to vaccinate individuals against their own tumors. Vaccines may be administered as recombinant proteins with adjuvants. More recently, there has been great interest in growing dendritic cells from individuals (by isolating precursors from the blood and expanding them by culture with growth factors), exposing the dendritic cells to tumor cells or tumor antigens, and using these tumor-pulsed dendritic cells as vaccines (see Fig. 10–5). It is hoped that the dendritic cells bearing tumor antigens will mimic the normal pathway of cross-presentation and will generate CTLs against the tumor cells. Tumors caused by oncogenic viruses can be prevented by vaccinating against these viruses. Two such vaccines that are proving to be remarkably effective are against hepatitis B virus (the cause of a common form of liver cancer) and human papillomavirus (the cause of cervical cancer).

The realization that tumors activate regulatory mechanisms that suppress immune responses has led to promising recent approaches, and a new paradigm in tumor immunotherapy. The principle of this strategy is to boost host immune responses against tumors by blocking normal inhibitory signals for lymphocytes, thus removing the brakes on the immune response. An antibody against CTLA-4 is now approved for the treatment of melanoma, and clinical trials

A **Passive immunity by transfer of tumor-specific T cells or antibodies**

Tumor-antigen specific T cells removed from patient and expanded *in vitro*

Monoclonal antibodies specific for tumor antigen

Transfer of tumor-specific T cells or antibodies into cancer patients

Tumor cell

Antibody or T cell recognition and killing of tumor cells

B **Active T cell immunity enhanced by dendritic cell vaccines**

Dendritic cells pulsed with tumor antigens

Vaccinate with tumor-antigen pulsed dendritic cell

CD8+ T cell

Tumor antigen presentation to patient's tumor-specific T cells

Activation of tumor-specific T cells and killing of tumor cells

C **Active immunity enhanced by blockade of T cell inhibitory molecules**

Monoclonal antibodies specific for inhibitory receptors (e.g., PD-1, CTLA-4) on T cells

Transfer of antibodies into cancer patient

Antibody blockade of inhibitory receptor

Tumor-specific T cells

Inhibitory ligand   Inhibitory receptor

Activation of tumor-specific T cells and killing of tumor cells

FIGURE 10–5 Strategies for enhancing antitumor immune responses. The major approaches currently used for the immunotherapy of cancers are transfer of antitumor antibodies or T cells, a form of passive immunity **(A)**, immunization with various cancer vaccines, such as autologous dendritic cells incubated with tumor cells or antigens **(B)**, and blockade of inhibitory pathways (whose normal role is illustrated in the lower part of the figure) to boost endogenous antitumor responses **(C)**.

of antibodies that block PD-1 have shown impressive efficacy in a variety of cancers. Predictably, patients treated with these antibodies, especially anti–CTLA-4, develop manifestations of autoimmunity, because the physiologic function of the inhibitory receptors is to maintain tolerance to self antigens (see Chapter 9).

Other ways of boosting antitumor immune responses include treating patients with cytokines that promote lymphocyte activation. The first cytokine to be used in this way was interleukin-2 (IL-2), but its clinical use is limited by serious toxic effects at the high doses that are needed to stimulate antitumor T cell responses. IL-2 also enhances the numbers and functions of regulatory T cells, which may interfere with antitumor immunity. Many other cytokines have been tried for systemic therapy or local administration at sites of tumors, with mostly unimpressive results thus far.

IMMUNE RESPONSES AGAINST TRANSPLANTS

From the initial attempts to replace damaged tissues by tissue transplantation, it was realized that individuals reject grafts from other individuals. Rejection results from inflammatory reactions that damage the transplanted tissues. Studies since the 1940s and 1950s established that graft rejection is mediated by the adaptive immune system, because it shows specificity and memory and it is dependent on lymphocytes (Fig. 10–6). Much of the knowledge about the immunology of transplantation came from studies with inbred strains of rodents, particularly mice. All members of an inbred strain are genetically identical to each other and different from the members of other strains. The earliest experiments showed that grafts among members of one inbred strain are accepted and grafts from one strain to another are rejected, firmly establishing rejection as a process controlled by the animal's genes. Later experiments defined the nature of the genes that are responsible for graft rejection, and showed that the products of these genes are expressed in all tissues.

As we mentioned in Chapter 3, the genes that contribute the most to the rejection of grafts exchanged between mice of different inbred strains were called **major histocompatibility complex (MHC)** genes. The language of transplantation immunology evolved from the experimental studies. The individual that provides the graft is called the **donor,** and the individual in whom the graft is placed is the **recipient** or **host.** Animals that are identical to one another (and grafts exchanged among these animals) are said to be **syngeneic;** animals (and grafts) of one species that differ from other animals of the same species are said to be **allogeneic;** and animals (and grafts) of different species are **xenogeneic.** Allogeneic and xenogeneic grafts, also called **allografts** and **xenografts,** are always rejected by a recipient with a normal immune system. The antigens that serve as the targets of rejection are called alloantigens and xenoantigens, and the antibodies and T cells that react against these antigens are alloreactive and xenoreactive, respectively. In the clinical situation, transplants are exchanged between allogeneic individuals, who are members of an outbred species who differ from one another (except for identical twins). Most of the following discussion focuses on immune responses to allografts.

Transplantation Antigens

The antigens of allografts that serve as the principal targets of rejection are proteins encoded in the MHC. Homologous MHC genes and molecules are present in all mammals; the human MHC is called the **human leukocyte antigen** (HLA) complex. It took more than 20 years after the discovery of the MHC to show that the physiologic function of MHC molecules is to display peptide antigens for recognition by

Evidence	Conclusion
Prior exposure to donor MHC molecules leads to accelerated graft rejection	Graft rejection shows memory and specificity, two cardinal features of adaptive immunity
The ability to reject a graft rapidly can be transferred to a naive individual by lymphocytes from a sensitized individual	Graft rejection is mediated by lymphocytes
Depletion or inactivation of T lymphocytes by drugs or antibodies results in reduced graft rejection	Graft rejection requires T lymphocytes

FIGURE 10–6 Evidence indicating that the rejection of tissue transplants is an immune reaction. Clinical and experimental evidence indicates that rejection of grafts is a reaction of the adaptive immune system. MHC, Major histocompatibility complex.

T lymphocytes (see Chapter 3). Recall that every person expresses six class I MHC alleles (one allele of HLA-A, -B, and -C from each parent) and at least six class II MHC alleles (one allele of HLA-DQ and -DP and one or two of -DR from each parent, and some combinations of these). MHC genes are highly polymorphic, with over 5000 HLA alleles among all humans, including about 1800 HLA-A alleles, 2500 HLA-B alleles, and 1000 DR alleles. Because these alleles can be inherited and expressed in virtually any combination, every individual is likely to express some MHC proteins that differ from those of another individual and that therefore appear foreign to another individual's immune system, except in the case of identical twins.

The response to MHC antigens on another individual's cells is one of the strongest immune responses known. T cell receptors (TCRs) for antigens have evolved to recognize MHC molecules, which is essential for surveillance of cells harboring infectious microbes. Recall that as a result of positive selection of developing T cells in the thymus, mature T cells that have some affinity for self MHC molecules survive, and many of these will have high affinity for self MHC displaying foreign peptides. Allogeneic MHC molecules containing peptides derived from the allogeneic cells may look like self MHC molecules plus bound foreign peptides (Fig. 10–7). Therefore, recognition of allogeneic MHC molecules in allografts is an example of an immunologic cross-reaction. Many clones of T cells specific for different foreign peptides bound to the same self MHC molecule may cross-react with any one allogeneic MHC molecule, as long as the allogeneic MHC molecule resembles complexes of self MHC plus foreign peptides. As a result, many self MHC–restricted T cells specific

(A) Normal

Self MHC molecule presents foreign peptide to T cell selected to recognize self MHC weakly, but may recognize self MHC–foreign peptide complexes as well

(B) Allorecognition

The self MHC–restricted T cell recognizes the allogeneic MHC molecule whose structure resembles a self MHC–foreign peptide complex

(C) Allorecognition

The self MHC–restricted T cell recognizes a structure formed by both the allogeneic MHC molecule and the bound peptide

FIGURE 10–7 Recognition of allogeneic major histocompatibility complex (MHC) molecules by T lymphocytes. Recognition of allogeneic MHC molecules may be thought of as a cross-reaction in which a T cell specific for a self MHC molecule–foreign peptide complex (**A**) also recognizes an allogeneic MHC molecule whose structure resembles that of a self MHC molecule–foreign peptide complex (**B** and **C**). Peptides derived from the graft (labeled self peptide) may not contribute to allorecognition (**B**), or they may form part of the complex that the T cell recognizes (**C**). The type of T cell recognition depicted in **B** and **C** is direct allorecognition.

for different peptide antigens may recognize any one allogeneic MHC molecule. Also, the process of negative selection in the thymus eliminates cells that strongly recognize self MHC, but there is no mechanism for selectively eliminating T cells whose TCRs have a high affinity for allogeneic MHC molecules, because these are never present in the thymus. Furthermore, a single allogeneic graft cell will express thousands of MHC molecules, every one of which may be recognized as foreign by a graft recipient's T cells. By contrast, in the case of an infected cell, only a small fraction of the self MHC molecules on the cell surface will carry a foreign microbial peptide recognized by the host's T cells. The net result of these features of allorecognition is that as many as 0.1% to 1% of all T cells in a normal individual may react against an allogeneic MHC molecule, much more than the 1 in 10^5 or 10^6 T cells that recognize any microbial antigen.

Although MHC proteins are the major antigens that stimulate graft rejection, other polymorphic proteins also may play a role in rejection. Non-MHC antigens that induce graft rejection are called minor histocompatibility antigens, and most are allelic forms of normal cellular proteins that happen to differ between donor and recipient. The rejection reactions that minor histocompatibility antigens elicit usually are not as strong as reactions against foreign MHC proteins. Two clinical situations in which minor antigens are important targets of rejection are blood transfusion and hematopoietic stem cell transplantation, discussed later.

Induction of Immune Responses Against Transplants

The induction of T cell–mediated immune responses against tissue transplants has to overcome the same problem as in responses against tumors: Because a graft may contain many cell types, often including epithelial and connective tissue cells, how can the immune system recognize and react against all these cells? The answer is that T cells in the recipient may recognize donor alloantigens in the graft in different ways, depending on what cells in the graft are displaying these alloantigens.

T cells may recognize allogeneic MHC molecules in the graft displayed by donor dendritic cells in the graft, or graft alloantigens may be processed and presented by the host's dendritic cells (Fig. 10–8). Many tissues contain dendritic cells, and when the tissues are transplanted, the dendritic cells are carried into the graft recipients. When T cells in the recipient recognize donor allogeneic MHC molecules on graft dendritic cells, the T cells are activated; this process is called **direct recognition** (or direct presentation) of alloantigens. Direct recognition stimulates the development of alloreactive T cells (e.g., CTLs) that recognize and attack the cells of the graft.

Alloantigens may be recognized by the recipient by a second pathway, which is much like that for recognition of any foreign antigen. If graft cells (or alloantigens) are ingested by recipient dendritic cells, donor alloantigens are processed and presented by the self MHC molecules on recipient APCs. This process is called **indirect recognition** (or indirect presentation) and is similar to the cross-presentation of tumor antigens discussed earlier. The dendritic cells that present alloantigens by the direct or indirect pathway also provide costimulators and can stimulate helper T cells as well as alloreactive CTLs. However, if alloreactive CTLs are induced by the indirect pathway, these CTLs are specific for donor alloantigens displayed by the recipient's self MHC molecules on the recipient's APCs, and they cannot recognize and kill cells in the graft (which, of course, express donor MHC molecules). When graft alloantigens are recognized by the indirect pathway, the subsequent rejection of the graft likely is mediated mainly by alloreactive $CD4^+$ T cells. These T cells may enter the graft together with host APCs, recognize graft antigens displayed by the APCs, and secrete cytokines that injure the graft by an inflammatory reaction.

We do not know the relative importance of the direct and indirect pathways of allorecognition in the rejection of allografts. The direct pathway may be most important for CTL-mediated acute rejection, and the indirect pathway may play a greater role in chronic rejection, described later.

T cell responses to allografts require costimulation, but how grafts stimulate the expression of costimulators on APCs is unclear. As with tumors, graft cells may undergo necrosis, perhaps in the period of ischemia before the transplant is done, and substances released from the injured and dead cells activate APCs by innate immune mechanisms. As we discuss later, blocking costimulation is one therapeutic strategy for promoting graft survival.

The **mixed lymphocyte reaction** (MLR) is an in vitro model of T cell recognition

(A) Direct allorecognition

Allogeneic antigen-presenting cell (dendritic cell)

Allogeneic MHC

Alloreactive T cell

T cell recognizes unprocessed allogeneic MHC molecule on graft APCs

(B) Indirect allorecognition

Allogeneic MHC

Dendritic cell in recipient

Self MHC

Allogeneic tissue cell

Uptake and processing of allogeneic MHC molecules by recipient APC

Alloreactive T cell

Peptide derived from allogeneic MHC molecule

T cell recognizes processed peptide of allogeneic MHC molecule bound to self MHC molecule on host APC

FIGURE 10–8 Direct and indirect recognition of alloantigens. A, Direct alloantigen recognition occurs when T cells bind directly to intact allogeneic major histocompatibility complex (MHC) molecules on antigen-presenting cells (APCs) in a graft, as illustrated in Figure 10–7. **B,** Indirect alloantigen recognition occurs when allogeneic MHC molecules from graft cells are taken up and processed by recipient APCs, and peptide fragments of the allogeneic MHC molecules are presented by recipient (self) MHC molecules. Recipient APCs also may process and present graft proteins other than allogeneic MHC molecules.

of alloantigens. In this model, T cells from one individual are cultured with leukocytes of another individual, and the responses of the T cells are assayed. The magnitude of this response is proportional to the extent of the MHC differences between these individuals and is a rough predictor of the outcomes of grafts exchanged between these individuals.

Although much of the emphasis on allograft rejection has been on the role of T cells, it is clear that alloantibodies also contribute to rejection. Most of these antibodies are helper T cell–dependent high-affinity antibodies. In order to produce alloantibodies, recipient B cells recognize donor alloantigens and then process and present peptides derived from these antigens to helper T cells (that may have been previously activated by recipient DCs presenting the same donor alloantigen), thus initiating the process of antibody production. This is a good example of indirect presentation of alloantigens, in this case by B lymphocytes.

Immune Mechanisms of Graft Rejection

Graft rejection is classified into hyperacute, acute, and chronic, on the basis of clinical and pathologic features (Fig. 10–9). This historical classification was devised by clinicians and has stood the test of time remarkably well. It also has become apparent that each type of rejection is mediated by a particular type of immune response.

Hyperacute rejection occurs within minutes of transplantation and is characterized by thrombosis of graft vessels and ischemic necrosis of the graft. Hyperacute rejection is mediated by circulating antibodies that are specific for antigens on graft endothelial cells and that are present before transplantation. These preformed antibodies may be natural IgM antibodies specific for blood group antigens or may be antibodies, specific for allogeneic MHC molecules, that are induced by exposure to allogeneic cells due to previous blood transfusions, pregnancy, or organ transplantation. Almost immediately after transplantation, the antibodies bind to antigens on the graft vascular endothelium and activate the complement and clotting systems, leading to injury to the endothelium and thrombus formation. Hyperacute rejection is not a common problem in clinical transplantation, because every donor and recipient are matched for blood type and potential recipients are tested for antibodies against the cells of the prospective donor. (The test for antibodies is called a cross-match.)

(A) **Hyperacute rejection**

Endothelial cell
Blood vessel
Circulating alloantigen-specific antibody
Alloantigen (e.g., blood group antigen)

Complement activation, endothelial damage, inflammation, and thrombosis

(B) **Acute rejection**

Parenchymal cells

Parenchymal cell damage, interstitial inflammation

i

Alloreactive antibody
Endothelial cell

Endothelialitis

ii

(C) **Chronic rejection**

Cytokines
APC
Macrophage
Cytokines
Alloantigen-specific CD4+ T cell
Vascular smooth muscle cell

Chronic inflammatory reaction in vessel wall, intimal smooth muscle cell proliferation, vessel occlusion

FIGURE 10–9 Mechanisms and histopathology of graft rejection. A representative histologic appearance of each type of rejection is shown on the right. **A,** In hyperacute rejection, preformed antibodies react with alloantigens on the vascular endothelium of the graft, activate complement, and trigger rapid intravascular thrombosis and necrosis of the vessel wall. **B,** In acute rejection, CD8+ T lymphocytes reactive with alloantigens on graft endothelial cells and parenchymal cells or antibodies reactive with endothelial cells cause damage to these cell types. Inflammation of the endothelium is called endothelialitis. The histology shows acute cellular rejection in **i** and humoral (antibody-mediated) rejection in **ii. C,** In chronic rejection with graft arteriosclerosis, T cells reactive with graft alloantigens may produce cytokines that induce inflammation and proliferation of intimal smooth muscle cells, leading to luminal occlusion.

However, hyperacute rejection is the major barrier to xenotransplantation, as discussed later.

Acute rejection occurs within days or weeks after transplantation, is due to an active immune response of the host stimulated by alloantigens in the graft, and is the principal cause of early graft failure. Acute rejection is mediated by T cells and antibodies specific for alloantigens in the graft. The T cells may be CD8+ CTLs that directly destroy graft cells, or CD4+ cells that secrete cytokines and induce inflammation, which destroys the graft. T cells may also react against cells in graft vessels, leading to vascular damage. Antibodies contribute especially to the vascular component of acute rejection. Antibody-mediated injury to graft vessels is caused mainly by complement activation by the classical pathway. Current immunosuppressive therapy is designed mainly to prevent and reduce acute rejection by blocking the activation of alloreactive T cells.

Chronic rejection is an indolent form of graft damage that occurs over months or years, leading to progressive loss of graft function. Chronic rejection may be manifested as fibrosis of the graft and by gradual narrowing of graft blood vessels, called graft arteriosclerosis. In both lesions, the culprits are believed to be T cells that react against graft alloantigens and secrete cytokines, which stimulate the proliferation and activities of fibroblasts and vascular smooth muscle cells in the graft. Alloantibodies also contribute to chronic rejection. Although treatments to prevent or curtail acute rejection have steadily improved, chronic rejection is refractory to most of these therapies and is becoming the principal cause of graft failure.

Prevention and Treatment of Graft Rejection

The mainstay of preventing and treating the rejection of organ transplants is immunosuppression, designed mainly to inhibit T cell activation and effector functions (Fig. 10–10). One of the most useful class of immunosuppressive drugs in clinical transplantation has been the calcineurin inhibitors cyclosporine and tacrolimus (FK506), which function by blocking the T cell phosphatase calcineurin. This enzyme is required to activate the transcription factor NFAT (nuclear factor of activated T cells), and blocking its activity inhibits the transcription of cytokine genes in the T cells. The advent of cyclosporine as a clinically useful drug opened up a new era in transplantation medicine and has allowed the transplantation of heart, liver, and lung. Another widely used drug is rapamycin, which inhibits a kinase called mTOR, which is required for T cell responses to cytokine growth factors. Many other immunosuppressive agents are now used as adjuncts to or instead of calcineurin and mTOR inhibitors (see Fig. 10–10). All these immunosuppressive drugs carry the problem of nonspecific immunosuppression (i.e., the drugs inhibit responses to more than the graft). Therefore, patients receiving these drugs as part of their posttransplantation regimen become susceptible to infections, particularly infections by intracellular microbes, and demonstrate an increased incidence of cancer, especially tumors caused by oncogenic viruses.

The matching of donor and recipient HLA alleles by tissue typing had an important role in minimizing graft rejection before cyclosporine became available for clinical use. Although MHC matching is critical for the success of transplantation of some types of tissues (e.g., allogeneic bone marrow grafts) and improves survival of other types of organ grafts (e.g., renal allografts), modern immunosuppression is so effective that HLA matching is not considered necessary for many types of organ transplants (e.g., heart), especially because the number of donors is limited and the recipients often are

Drug	Mechanism of action
Cyclosporine and tacrolimus	Block T cell cytokine production by inhibiting the phosphatase calcineurin and thus blocking activation of the NFAT transcription factor
Mycophenolate mofetil	Blocks lymphocyte proliferation by inhibiting guanine nucleotide synthesis in lymphocytes
Rapamycin	Blocks lymphocyte proliferation by inhibiting mTOR and IL-2 signaling
Corticosteroids	Reduce inflammation by effects on multiple cell types
Antithymocyte globulin	Binds to and depletes T cells by promoting phagocytosis or complement-mediated lysis (used to treat acute rejection)
Anti–IL-2 receptor(CD25) antibody	Inhibits T cell proliferation by blocking IL-2 binding; may also opsonize and help eliminate activated IL-2R–expressing T cells
CTLA4-Ig (belatacept)	Inhibits T cell activation by blocking B7 costimulator binding to T cell CD28
Anti-CD52 (alemtuzumab)	Depletes lymphocytes by complement-mediated lysis

FIGURE 10–10 Treatments for graft rejection. Table lists agents used to treat rejection of organ grafts and their mechanisms of action. Like cyclosporine, tacrolimus (FK506) is a calcineurin inhibitor, but it is not as widely used. CTLA4-Ig, Cytotoxic T lymphocyte–associated protein 4–immunoglobulin (fusion protein); IL, interleukin; NFAT, nuclear factor of activated T cells.

too sick to wait for well-matched organs to become available.

The long-term goal of transplant immunologists is to induce immunological tolerance specifically for the graft alloantigens. If this is achieved, it will allow graft acceptance without shutting off other immune responses in the host. Experimental and clinical attempts to induce graft-specific tolerance are ongoing.

A major problem in transplantation is the shortage of suitable donor organs. **Xenotransplantation** is a possible solution for this problem. Experimental studies show that hyperacute rejection is a frequent cause of xenotransplant loss. The reasons for the high incidence of hyperacute rejection of xenografts are that individuals often contain antibodies that react with cells from other species and the xenograft cells lack regulatory proteins that can inhibit human complement activation. These antibodies, similar to antibodies against blood group antigens, are called natural antibodies because their production does not require prior exposure to the xeno-antigens. It is thought that these antibodies are produced against bacteria that normally inhabit the gut, and that the antibodies cross-react with cells of other species. Xenografts also are subject to acute rejection, much like allografts. Attempts are ongoing to modify xenogeneic tissues genetically in ways that reduce their rejection by recipients of other species.

Transplantation of Blood Cells and Hematopoietic Stem Cells

Transplantation of blood cells, called **transfusion,** is the oldest form of transplantation in clinical medicine. The major barrier to transfusion is the presence of foreign **blood group antigens,** the prototypes of which are the ABO antigens (Fig. 10–11). These antigens are expressed on red blood cells, endothelial cells, and many other cell types. ABO antigens are carbohydrates on membrane glycoproteins or glycosphingolipids; they contain a core glycan that may have an additional terminal sugar. Blood group antigens A and B have different terminal sugars (*N*-acetylgalactosamine and galactose, respectively); AB individuals express both terminal sugars on different glycolipid molecules; and individuals with blood group O express the core glycan but neither of the terminal sugars. Individuals expressing one blood group antigen are tolerant of that antigen but have antibodies against the other; O group individuals make both anti-A and anti-B antibodies. These antibodies are produced against antigens that are expressed by intestinal microbes and that cross-react with the ABO blood group

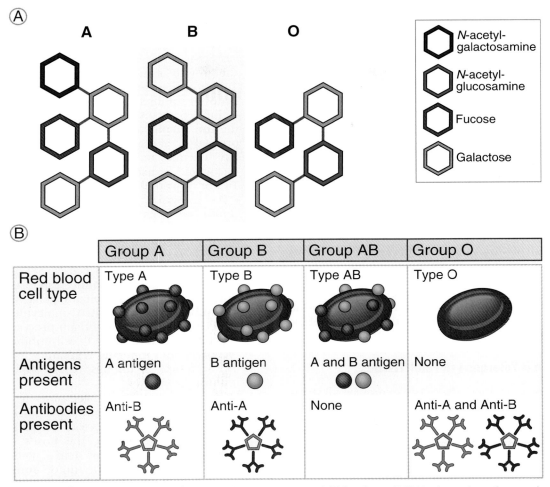

FIGURE 10–11 ABO blood group antigens. A, Chemical structure of ABO antigens. **B,** Table shows the antigens and antibodies present in people with the major ABO blood groups.

antigens. The preformed antibodies react against transfused blood cells expressing the target antigens, and the result may be a severe **transfusion reaction.** This problem is avoided by matching blood donors and recipients, a standard practice in medicine. Because the blood group antigens are sugars, they do not elicit T cell responses. Blood group antigens other than the ABO antigens also are involved in transfusion reactions, and these usually are less severe. One important example is the Rh antigen, which is a red cell membrane protein that can be the target of maternal antibodies that may attack a developing fetus when the fetus expresses paternal Rh and the mother lacks the protein.

Hematopoietic stem cell transplantation is being used increasingly to correct hematopoietic defects, to restore bone marrow cells damaged by irradiation and chemotherapy for cancer, and to treat leukemias. Either bone marrow cells or, more often, hematopoietic stem cells mobilized in a donor's blood are injected into the circulation of a recipient, and the cells home to the marrow. The transplantation of hematopoietic stem cells poses many special problems. Before transplantation, some of the bone marrow of the recipient has to be destroyed to create space to receive the transplanted stem cells, and this depletion of the recipient's marrow inevitably causes deficiency of blood cells, including immune cells. The immune system reacts strongly against allogeneic hematopoietic stem cells, so successful transplantation requires careful HLA matching of donor and recipient. If mature allogeneic T cells are transplanted with the stem cells, these mature T cells can attack the recipient's tissues, resulting in a serious clinical reaction called **graft-versus-host disease.** Since HLA matching is always done for these transplants, this reaction is likely directed against minor histocompatibility antigens. The same reaction is exploited to kill leukemia cells, and hematopoietic stem cell transplantation is now commonly used to treat leukemias resistant to chemotherapy. NK cells in the marrow inoculum may also contribute to the destruction of leukemia cells.

Even if the graft is successful, recipients often are severely immunodeficient while their immune systems are being reconstituted. Despite these problems, hematopoietic stem cell transplantation is a successful therapy for a wide variety of diseases affecting the hematopoietic and lymphoid systems.

Maternal Tolerance to Fetal Tissues

During pregnancy, the fetus expresses alloantigens encoded by paternally inherited genes, but the fetus is not immunologically rejected by the mother. There has been great interest in trying to understand the mechanisms responsible for immunologic acceptance of the fetus, and why these mechanisms might fail, resulting in pregnancy failures. It is clear that the anatomy of the trophoblast and placenta plays a key role in tolerance to the fetus, because pregnant animals that do not react against paternal MHC antigens in the fetus readily reject paternal tissues placed at other sites. The placenta may be a tissue that does not allow T cells to enter the fetus or that actively suppresses immune responses by the action of abundant regulatory T cells or immunosuppressive molecules. The maternal trophoblast expresses low levels of conventional class I MHC molecules, which may prevent CD8+ T cell–mediated immune responses, and also expresses unique atypical class I MHC molecules, which likely prevent maternal NK cell recognition and attack. All these mechanisms have been demonstrated in experimental animals, but which of these is involved in maternal tolerance of the fetus in humans remains unknown.

SUMMARY

- A physiologic function of the immune system is to eradicate tumors and prevent the growth of tumors.
- Tumor antigens may be products of oncogenes or tumor suppressor genes, mutated cellular proteins that do not contribute to the malignant phenotype, overexpressed or aberrantly expressed structurally normal molecules, or products of oncogenic viruses.
- Tumor rejection is mediated mainly by CTLs recognizing peptides derived from tumor antigens. The induction of CTL responses against tumor antigens often involves ingestion of tumor cells or their antigens by dendritic cells and presentation of the antigens to T cells.
- Tumors may evade immune responses by losing expression of their antigens, shutting off expression of MHC molecules or molecules involved in antigen processing, expressing ligands for T cell inhibitory receptors, and inducing regulatory T cells or secreting cytokines that suppress immune responses.
- Immunotherapy for cancer aims to enhance antitumor immunity by passively providing immune effectors to patients or by actively boosting the host's own effectors. Approaches for active boosting include vaccination with tumor antigens or with tumor antigen-pulsed dendritic cells, and treatment of cancer patients with antibodies that block T cell inhibitory receptors.
- Tissue transplants are rejected by the immune system, and the major antigen targets of rejection are MHC molecules.
- The antigens of allografts that are recognized by T cells are allogeneic MHC molecules that resemble peptide-loaded self MHC molecules that the T cells are selected to recognize. Graft antigens either are directly presented to recipient T cells or are picked up and presented by host APCs.
- Grafts may be rejected by different mechanisms. Hyperacute rejection is mediated by preformed antibodies to blood group antigens or HLA molecules, which cause endothelial injury and thrombosis of blood

vessels in the graft. Acute rejection is mediated by T cells, which injure graft cells and endothelium, and by antibodies that bind to the endothelium. Chronic rejection is caused by T cells that produce cytokines that stimulate growth of vascular smooth muscle cells and tissue fibroblasts.

* Treatment for graft rejection is designed to suppress T cell responses and inflammation. The mainstay of treatment has been immunosuppressive drugs, including corticosteroids and cyclosporine; many other agents are in clinical use now.
* Hematopoietic stem cell transplants elicit strong rejection reactions, carry the risk of graft-versus-host disease, and often lead to temporary immunodeficiency in recipients.
* The mammalian fetus expresses paternally derived antigens that are allogeneic to the pregnant mother, but the fetus is not rejected because of various local immunosuppressive mechanisms intrinsic to the placenta.

REVIEW QUESTIONS

1. What are the main types of tumor antigens that the immune system reacts against?
2. What is the evidence that tumor rejection is an immunologic phenomenon?
3. How do naive CD8+ T cells recognize tumor antigens, and how are these cells activated to differentiate into effector CTLs?
4. What are some of the mechanisms by which tumors may evade the immune response?
5. What are some strategies for enhancing host immune responses to tumor antigens?
6. Why do normal T cells, which recognize foreign peptide antigens bound to self MHC molecules, react strongly against the allogeneic MHC molecules of a graft?
7. What are the principal mechanisms of rejection of allografts?
8. How is the likelihood of graft rejection reduced in clinical transplantation?
9. What are some of the problems associated with the transplantation of bone marrow cells?

Answers to and discussion of the Review Questions are available at studentconsult.com.

Hypersensitivity
Disorders Caused by Immune Responses

The concept that the immune system is required for defending the host against infections has been emphasized throughout this book. However, immune responses are themselves capable of causing tissue injury and disease. Injurious, or pathologic, immune reactions are called **hypersensitivity reactions.** An immune response to an antigen may result in sensitivity to challenge with that antigen, and therefore hypersensitivity is a reflection of excessive or aberrant immune responses. Hypersensitivity reactions may occur in two situations. First, responses to foreign antigens (microbes and noninfectious environmental antigens) may be dysregulated or uncontrolled, resulting in tissue injury. Second, the immune responses may be directed against self (autologous) antigens, as a result of the failure of self-tolerance (see Chapter 9). Responses against self antigens are termed **autoimmunity,** and disorders caused by such responses are called **autoimmune diseases.**

This chapter describes the important features of hypersensitivity reactions and the resulting diseases, focusing on their pathogenesis. Their clinicopathologic features are described only briefly and can be found in other medical textbooks. The following questions are addressed:

- What are the mechanisms of different types of hypersensitivity reactions?
- What are the major clinical and pathologic features of diseases caused by these reactions, and what principles underlie treatment of such diseases?

TYPES OF HYPERSENSITIVITY REACTIONS

Hypersensitivity reactions are classified on the basis of the principal immunologic mechanism that is responsible for tissue injury and disease (Fig. 11–1). We prefer the more informative descriptive designations rather than numeric terms, so these descriptors

Type of hypersensitivity	Pathologic immune mechanisms	Mechanisms of tissue injury and disease
Immediate hypersensitivity (Type I)	T_H2 cells, IgE antibody, mast cells, eosinophils	Mast cell–derived mediators (vasoactive amines, lipid mediators, cytokines) Cytokine-mediated inflammation (eosinophils, neutrophils)
Antibody-mediated diseases (Type II)	IgM, IgG antibodies against cell surface or extracellular matrix antigens	Complement- and Fc receptor–mediated recruitment and activation of leukocytes (neutrophils, macrophages) Opsonization and phagocytosis of cells Abnormalities in cellular function, e.g. hormone receptor signaling
Immune complex–mediated diseases (Type III)	Immune complexes of circulating antigens and IgM or IgG antibodies deposited in vascular basement membrane	Complement- and Fc receptor–mediated recruitment and activation of leukocytes
T cell–mediated diseases (Type IV)	1. CD4+ T cells (cytokine-mediated inflammation) 2. CD8+ CTLs (T cell–mediated cytolysis)	1. Macrophage activation, cytokine-mediated inflammation 2. Direct target cell lysis, cytokine-mediated inflammation

FIGURE 11–1 Types of hypersensitivity reactions. In the four major types of hypersensitivity reactions, different immune effector mechanisms cause tissue injury and disease. CTLs, Cytotoxic T lymphocytes; Ig, immunoglobulin.

are used throughout this chapter. Immediate hypersensitivity, or type I hypersensitivity, is a type of pathologic reaction that is caused by the release of mediators from mast cells. This reaction is most often triggered by the production of immunoglobulin E (IgE) antibody against environmental antigens and the binding of IgE to mast cells in various tissues. Antibodies other than IgE may cause diseases in two ways. Antibodies directed against cell or tissue antigens can damage these cells or tissues or can impair their function. These diseases are said to be antibody mediated and represent type II hypersensitivity. Sometimes, antibodies against soluble antigens may form complexes with the antigens, and the immune complexes may deposit in blood vessels in various tissues, causing inflammation and tissue injury. Such diseases are called immune complex diseases and represent type III hypersensitivity. Lastly, some diseases result from the reactions of T lymphocytes, often against self antigens in tissues. These T cell–mediated diseases represent type IV hypersensitivity.

This classification scheme is useful because it distinguishes the mechanisms of immune-mediated tissue injury. In many human immunologic diseases, however, the damage may result from a combination of antibody-mediated and T cell–mediated reactions, so it is often difficult to classify these diseases neatly into one type of hypersensitivity.

IMMEDIATE HYPERSENSITIVITY

Immediate hypersensitivity is an IgE antibody– and mast cell–mediated reaction to certain antigens that causes rapid vascular leakage and mucosal secretions, often followed by inflammation. IgE-mediated immediate hypersensitivity reactions are also called **allergy,** or **atopy,** and individuals with a strong propensity to develop these reactions are said to be atopic. Such reactions may affect various tissues and may be of varying severity in different individuals. Common types of these reactions include hay fever, food allergies, bronchial asthma, and anaphylaxis. Allergies are the most frequent disorders of the immune system, estimated to affect about 20% of people and the incidence of allergic diseases has been increasing in industrialized societies.

The sequence of events in the development of immediate hypersensitivity reactions begins with the activation of T$_H$2 cells and the production of IgE antibodies in response to an antigen, binding of the IgE to Fc receptors of mast cells, then on subsequent exposure to the antigen, cross-linking of the bound IgE by the antigen and release of mast cell mediators (Fig. 11–2). Some mast cell mediators cause a rapid increase in vascular permeability and smooth muscle contraction, resulting in many of the symptoms of these reactions (Fig. 11–3). This vascular and smooth muscle reaction may occur within minutes of reintroduction of antigen into a previously sensitized individual—thus the name **immediate hypersensitivity.** Other mast cell mediators are cytokines that recruit neutrophils and eosinophils to the site of the reaction over several hours. This inflammatory component is called the **late-phase reaction,** and it is mainly responsible for the tissue injury that results from repeated bouts of immediate hypersensitivity.

With this background, we proceed to a discussion of the steps in immediate hypersensitivity reactions.

Activation of T$_H$2 Cells and Production of IgE Antibody

In individuals who are prone to allergies, exposure to some antigens results in the activation of T$_H$2 cells and the production of IgE antibody (see Fig. 11–2). Most individuals do not mount strong T$_H$2 responses to foreign antigens. For unknown reasons, when some individuals encounter certain antigens, such as proteins in pollen, certain foods, insect venoms, or animal dander, or if they are treated with certain drugs such as penicillin, there is a strong T$_H$2 response. Immediate hypersensitivity develops as a consequence of the activation of T$_H$2 cells in response to protein antigens or chemicals that bind to proteins. Antigens that elicit immediate hypersensitivity (allergic) reactions often are called allergens. Any atopic individual may be allergic to one or more of these antigens. It is not understood why only a small subset of common environmental antigens causes them to elicit T$_H$2-mediated reactions and IgE production, or what characteristics of these antigens are responsible for their behavior as allergens.

FIGURE 11–2 The sequence of events in immediate hypersensitivity. Immediate hypersensitivity reactions are initiated by the introduction of an allergen, which stimulates T_H2 reactions and immunoglobulin E (IgE) production. IgE binds to Fc receptors (FcεRI) on mast cells, and subsequent exposure to the allergen activates the mast cells to secrete the mediators that are responsible for the pathologic reactions of immediate hypersensitivity.

FIGURE 11–3 Immediate hypersensitivity. A, Kinetics of the immediate and late-phase reactions. The immediate vascular and smooth muscle reaction to allergen develops within minutes after challenge (allergen exposure in a previously sensitized individual), and the late-phase reaction develops 2 to 24 hours later. **B,** Morphology of the immediate reaction is characterized by vasodilation, congestion, and edema. **C,** Late-phase reaction is characterized by an inflammatory infiltrate rich in eosinophils, neutrophils, and T cells. *(Micrographs courtesy Dr. Daniel Friend, Department of Pathology, Brigham and Women's Hospital, Boston.)*

Two of the cytokines secreted by T_H2 cells, interleukin-4 (IL-4) and IL-13, stimulate B lymphocytes specific for the foreign antigens to switch to IgE-producing plasma cells. Therefore, atopic individuals produce large amounts of IgE antibody in response to antigens that do not elicit IgE responses in other people. The propensity toward T_H2 development, IgE production, and immediate hypersensitivity has a strong genetic basis; the major known risk for developing allergies is a family history of atopic disease. Many different genes appear to play contributory roles, but the mechanisms by which these genes influence the development of allergies are poorly understood.

Activation of Mast Cells and Secretion of Mediators

IgE antibody produced in response to an allergen binds to high-affinity Fc receptors, specific for the ε heavy chain, that are expressed on mast cells (see Fig. 11–2). Thus, in an atopic individual, mast cells are coated with IgE antibody specific for the antigen(s) to which the individual is allergic. This process of coating mast cells with IgE is called **sensitization,** because coating with IgE specific for an antigen makes the mast cells sensitive to activation by subsequent encounter with that antigen. In normal individuals, by contrast, mast cells may carry IgE molecules of many different specificities, because many antigens may elicit small IgE

responses, and the amount of IgE specific for any one antigen is not enough to cause immediate hypersensitivity reactions upon exposure to that antigen. Mast cells are present in all connective tissues, especially under epithelia, and they are usually located adjacent to blood vessels. Which of the body's mast cells are activated by cross-linking of allergen-specific IgE often depends on the route of entry of the allergen. For example, inhaled allergens activate mast cells in the submucosal tissues of the bronchus, whereas ingested allergens activate mast cells in the wall of the intestine.

The high-affinity receptor for IgE, called FcεRI, consists of three polypeptide chains, one of which binds the Fc portion of the ε heavy chain very strongly, with a K_d of approximately 10^{-11} M. (The concentration of IgE in the plasma is approximately 10^{-9} M, so even in normal individuals, mast cells are always coated with IgE bound to FcεRI.) The other two chains of the receptor are signaling proteins. The same FcεRI is also present on basophils, which are circulating cells with many of the features of mast cells, but the role of basophils in immediate hypersensitivity is not as well established as the role of mast cells.

When mast cells sensitized by IgE are exposed to the allergen, the cells are activated to secrete their mediators (Fig. 11–4). Mast cell activation results from binding of the allergen to two or more IgE antibodies on the cell. When this happens, the FcεRI molecules

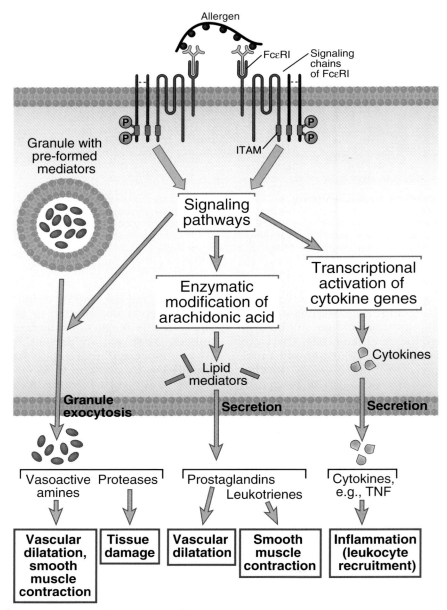

FIGURE 11–4 Production and actions of mast cell mediators. Cross-linking of immunoglobulin E (IgE) on a mast cell by an allergen stimulates phosphorylation of immunoreceptor tyrosine-based activation motifs (ITAMs) in the signaling chains of the IgE Fc receptor (FcεRI), which then initiates multiple signaling pathways. These signaling pathways stimulate the release of mast cell granule contents (amines, proteases), the synthesis of arachidonic acid metabolites (prostaglandins, leukotrienes), and the synthesis of various cytokines. TNF, tumor necrosis factor.

that are carrying the IgE are cross-linked, triggering biochemical signals from the signal-transducing chains of FcεRI. The signals lead to three types of responses in the mast cell: rapid release of granule contents (degranulation), synthesis and secretion of lipid mediators, and synthesis and secretion of cytokines.

The most important mediators produced by mast cells are vasoactive amines and proteases stored in and released from granules, newly generated and secreted products of arachidonic acid metabolism, and cytokines (Fig. 11–4). These mediators have different actions. The major amine, histamine, causes the dilation of small blood vessels, increases vascular permeability, and stimulates the transient contraction of smooth muscles. Proteases may cause damage to local tissues. Arachidonic acid metabolites include prostaglandins, which cause vascular dilation, and leukotrienes, which stimulate prolonged smooth muscle contraction. Cytokines induce local inflammation (the late-phase reaction, described next). Thus, mast cell mediators are responsible for acute vascular and smooth muscle reactions and inflammation, the hallmarks of immediate hypersensitivity.

Cytokines produced by mast cells stimulate the recruitment of leukocytes, which cause the late-phase reaction. The principal leukocytes involved in this reaction are eosinophils, neutrophils, and T$_H$2 cells. Mast cell–derived tumor necrosis factor (TNF) and IL-4 promote neutrophil- and eosinophil-rich inflammation. Chemokines produced by mast cells and by epithelial cells in the tissues also contribute to leukocyte recruitment. Eosinophils and neutrophils liberate proteases, which cause tissue damage, and T$_H$2 cells may exacerbate the reaction by producing more cytokines. Eosinophils are prominent components of many allergic reactions and are an important cause of tissue injury in these reactions. These cells are activated by the cytokine IL-5, which is produced by T$_H$2 cells and mast cells.

Clinical Syndromes and Therapy

Immediate hypersensitivity reactions have diverse clinical and pathologic features, all of which are attributable to mediators produced by mast cells in different amounts and in different tissues (Fig. 11–5). Some mild

Clinical syndrome	Clinical and pathologic manifestations
Allergic rhinitis, sinusitis (hay fever)	Increased mucus secretion; inflammation of upper airways, sinuses
Food allergies	Increased peristalsis due to contraction of intestinal muscles
Bronchial asthma	Airway obstruction caused by bronchial smooth muscle hyperactivity; inflammation and tissue injury caused by late-phase reaction
Anaphylaxis (may be caused by drugs, bee sting, food)	Fall in blood pressure (shock) caused by vascular dilation; airway obstruction due to laryngeal edema

FIGURE 11–5 Clinical manifestations of immediate hypersensitivity reactions. The table lists manifestations of some common immediate hypersensitivity reactions. Immediate hypersensitivity may be manifested in many other ways, as in development of skin lesions (e.g., urticaria, eczema).

manifestations, such as allergic rhinitis and sinusitis, which are common in hay fever, are reactions to inhaled allergens, such as a protein of ragweed pollen. Mast cells in the nasal mucosa produce histamine, and T$_H$2 cells produce IL-13, and these two mediators cause increased production of mucus. Late-phase reactions may lead to more prolonged inflammation. In food allergies, ingested allergens trigger mast cell degranulation, and the released histamine causes increased peristalsis. Bronchial asthma is most often a form of respiratory allergy in which inhaled allergens (often undefined) stimulate bronchial mast cells to release mediators, including leukotrienes, which cause repeated bouts of bronchial constriction and airway obstruction. In chronic asthma, there are large numbers of eosinophils in the bronchial mucosa and excessive secretion of mucus in the airways, and the bronchial smooth muscle becomes hypertrophied and hyperreactive to various stimuli. Some cases of asthma are not associated with IgE production, although all are caused by mast cell activation.

In some patients, asthma may be triggered by cold or exercise; how either of these causes mast cell activation is unknown.

The most severe form of immediate hypersensitivity is **anaphylaxis,** a systemic reaction characterized by edema in many tissues, including the larynx, accompanied by a fall in blood pressure. Some of the most frequent inducers of anaphylaxis include bee stings, injected or ingested penicillin-family antibiotics, and ingested nuts or shellfish. The reaction is caused by widespread mast cell degranulation in response to the systemic distribution of the antigen, and it is life threatening because of the sudden fall in blood pressure and airway obstruction.

The therapy for immediate hypersensitivity diseases is aimed at inhibiting mast cell degranulation, antagonizing the effects of mast cell mediators, and reducing inflammation (Fig. 11–6). Common drugs include antihistamines for hay fever, agents that relax bronchial smooth muscles in asthma, and epinephrine in anaphylaxis. In diseases with inflammation as an important pathologic component, such as asthma, corticosteroids are used to inhibit inflammation. Many patients benefit from repeated administration of small doses of allergens, called desensitization or allergen-specific immunotherapy. This treatment may work by changing the T cell response away from T_H2 dominance, by inducing tolerance in allergen-specific T cells, or by stimulating regulatory T cells (Tregs).

Before concluding the discussion of immediate hypersensitivity, it is important to address the question of why evolution has preserved an IgE antibody–mediated and mast cell–mediated immune response whose major effects are pathologic. There is no definitive answer to this puzzle,

Syndrome	Therapy	Mechanism of action
Anaphylaxis	Epinephrine	Causes vascular smooth muscle contraction and increases cardiac output (to counter shock); relaxes airway muscle; inhibits mast cell degranulation
Bronchial asthma	Corticosteroids	Reduce inflammation
	Leukotriene antagonists	Relax bronchial smooth muscle and reduce inflammation
	Phosphodiesterase inhibitors	Relax bronchial smooth muscle
Various allergic diseases	Desensitization (repeated administration of low doses of allergens)	Unknown; may inhibit IgE production and increase production of other Ig isotypes; may induce T cell tolerance
	Anti-IgE antibody	Neutralize and eliminate IgE
	Antihistamines	Block actions of histamine on vessels and smooth muscles
	Cromolyn	Inhibits mast cell degranulation

FIGURE 11–6 Treatment of immediate hypersensitivity reactions. The table summarizes the principal mechanisms of action of the various drugs used to treat allergic disorders; Ig, immunoglobulin.

but immediate hypersensitivity reactions likely evolved to protect against pathogens or toxins. It is known that IgE antibody and eosinophils are important mechanisms of defense against helminthic infections, and mast cells play a role in innate immunity against some bacteria and in destroying venomous toxins.

DISEASES CAUSED BY ANTIBODIES AND ANTIGEN-ANTIBODY COMPLEXES

Antibodies other than IgE may cause disease by binding to their target antigens in cells and tissues or by forming immune complexes that deposit in blood vessels (Fig. 11–7). Antibody-mediated hypersensitivity reactions have long been recognized and are the basis

of many chronic immunologic diseases in humans. Antibodies against cells or extracellular matrix components may deposit in any tissue that expresses the relevant target antigen. Diseases caused by such antibodies usually are specific for a particular tissue. Immune complexes often deposit in blood vessels, especially vessels through which plasma is filtered at high pressure (e.g., in renal glomeruli and joint synovium). Therefore, immune complex diseases tend to be systemic and often manifest as widespread vasculitis, arthritis, and nephritis.

Etiology of Antibody-Mediated Diseases

The antibodies that cause disease most often are autoantibodies against self antigens and less commonly are specific for

FIGURE 11–7 Types of antibody-mediated diseases. Antibodies (other than IgE) may cause tissue injury and disease by: **A,** binding directly to their target antigens on the surface of cells and in the extracellular matrix (type II hypersensitivity) or **B,** by forming immune complexes that deposit mainly in blood vessels (type III hypersensitivity).

foreign (e.g., microbial) antigens. The production of autoantibodies results from a failure of self-tolerance. In Chapter 9 we discussed the mechanisms by which self-tolerance may fail, but why this happens in any human autoimmune disease is still not understood. Autoantibodies may bind to self antigens in tissues or may form immune complexes with circulating self antigens.

Two of the best-described diseases caused by antibodies produced against microbial antigens are rare, late sequelae of streptococcal infections. After such infections, some individuals produce anti-streptococcal antibodies that cross-react with an antigen in heart tissues. Deposition of these antibodies in the heart triggers an inflammatory disease called rheumatic fever, which can lead to acute heart failure, or slow scarring of valves and late-onset heart failure. Other individuals make anti-streptococcal antibodies that deposit in kidney glomeruli, causing an inflammatory process called post-streptococcal glomerulonephritis that can lead to renal failure. Some immune complex diseases are caused by complexes of antimicrobial antibodies and microbial antigens. This may occur in patients with chronic infections with certain viruses (e.g., the Epstein-Barr virus) or parasites (e.g., malaria).

Mechanisms of Tissue Injury and Disease

Antibodies specific for cell and tissue antigens may deposit in tissues and cause injury by inducing local inflammation, they may bind to and promote the destruction of cells, or they interfere with normal cellular functions (Fig. 11–8). Antibodies against tissue antigens and immune complexes deposited in vessels induce inflammation by attracting and activating leukocytes. IgG antibodies of the IgG1 and IgG3 subclasses bind to neutrophil and macrophage Fc receptors and activate these leukocytes, resulting in inflammation (see Chapter 8). The same antibodies, as well as IgM, activate the complement system by the classical pathway, resulting in the production of complement byproducts that recruit leukocytes and induce inflammation. When leukocytes are activated at sites of antibody deposition, these cells release substances such as reactive oxygen species and lysosomal enzymes that damage the adjacent tissues. If antibodies bind to cells, such as erythrocytes and platelets, the cells are opsonized and may be ingested and destroyed by host phagocytes.

Some antibodies may cause disease without directly inducing tissue injury. For example, antibodies against hormone receptors may inhibit receptor function; in some cases of myasthenia gravis, antibodies against the acetylcholine receptor inhibit neuromuscular transmission, causing paralysis. Other antibodies may directly activate receptors, mimicking their physiologic ligands. In a form of hyperthyroidism called Graves' disease, antibodies against the receptor for thyroid-stimulating hormone stimulate thyroid cells even in the absence of the hormone.

Clinical Syndromes and Therapy

Many chronic hypersensitivity disorders in humans are caused by, or are associated with, anti-tissue antibodies (Fig. 11–9) and immune complexes (Fig. 11–10).

Two experimental models of immune complex diseases have provided valuable information about pathogenic mechanisms. **Serum sickness** is induced by systemic administration of a protein antigen, which elicits an antibody response and leads to the formation of circulating immune complexes. In humans, serum sickness can occur after a person receives injections of serum antibody preparations from other individuals or animals, which are sometimes used for the treatment of snakebite or exposure to rabies virus and for the depletion of T cells in transplant recipients. In all these cases, the recipient makes antibody responses against the injected foreign antibodies and other serum proteins, if present, resulting in the formation of immune complexes. The **Arthus reaction** is induced by subcutaneous administration of a protein antigen to a previously immunized animal; it results in the formation of immune complexes at the site of antigen injection, and a local vasculitis.

Therapy for these diseases is intended mainly to limit inflammation and its injurious consequences, with drugs such as corticosteroids. In severe cases, plasmapheresis is used to reduce levels of circulating antibodies or immune complexes. Some of these diseases respond well to treatment with intravenous IgG (IVIG) pooled from healthy donors. How IVIG works is not known; it may induce the expression of and bind to the inhibitory Fc receptor on myeloid cells and

A **Complement- and Fc receptor–mediated inflammation**

Fc receptors

Neutrophil activation

Complement byproducts (C5a, C3a)

Complement activation

Neutrophil enzymes, reactive oxygen species

Inflammation and tissue injury

B **Opsonization and phagocytosis**

Opsonized cell

Fc receptor

C3b

C3b receptor

Complement activation

Phagocyte

Phagocytosed cell

Phagocytosis

C **Abnormal physiologic responses without cell/tissue injury**

Antibody against TSH receptor

TSH receptor

Thyroid epithelial cell

Thyroid hormones

Antibody stimulates receptor without hormone

Nerve ending

Acetylcholine (ACh)

Antibody to ACh receptor

ACh receptor

Muscle

Antibody inhibits binding of neurotransmitter to receptor

FIGURE 11–8 Effector mechanisms of antibody-mediated diseases. Antibodies cause disease by **A,** inducing inflammation at the site of deposition; **B,** opsonizing cells for phagocytosis; and **C,** interfering with normal cellular functions, such as hormone receptor signaling. All three mechanisms are seen with antibodies that bind directly to their target antigens, but immune complexes cause disease mainly by inducing inflammation (**A**). TSH, Thyroid-stimulating hormone.

B cells (see Chapter 7, Fig. 7–15), or it may reduce the half-life of pathogenic antibodies by competing for binding to the neonatal Fc receptor in endothelial and other cells (see Chapter 8, Fig. 8–2). Treatment of patients with an antibody specific for CD20, a surface protein of mature B cells, results in depletion of the B cells and may be useful for treating some antibody-mediated disorders. Other approaches for inhibiting the production of autoantibodies include treating patients with antagonists that block CD40 ligand and thus inhibit helper T cell–dependent B cell activation, and using antibodies to block cytokines that promote the survival of B cells and plasma cells. There is also interest in inducing tolerance in cases in which the autoantigens are

Antibody-mediated disease	Target antigen	Mechanisms of disease	Clinicopathologic manifestations
Autoimmune hemolytic anemia	Erythrocyte membrane proteins (Rh blood group antigens, I antigen)	Opsonization and phagocytosis of erythrocytes	Hemolysis, anemia
Autoimmune (idiopathic) thrombocytopenic purpura	Platelet membrane proteins (gpIIb/IIIa integrin)	Opsonization and phagocytosis of platelets	Bleeding
Goodpasture's syndrome	Non-collagenous protein in basement membranes of kidney glomeruli and lung alveoli	Complement- and Fc receptor–mediated inflammation	Nephritis, lung hemorrhage
Graves' disease (hyperthyroidism)	Thyroid-stimulating hormone (TSH) receptor	Antibody-mediated stimulation of TSH receptors	Hyperthyroidism
Myasthenia gravis	Acetylcholine receptor	Antibody inhibits acetylcholine binding, down-modulates receptors	Muscle weakness, paralysis
Pemphigus vulgaris	Proteins in intercellular junctions of epidermal cells (epidermal cadherin)	Antibody-mediated activation of proteases, disruption of intercellular adhesions	Skin vesicles (bullae)
Pernicious anemia	Intrinsic factor of gastric parietal cells	Neutralization of intrinsic factor, decreased absorption of vitamin B_{12}	Abnormal erythropoiesis, anemia
Rheumatic fever	Streptococcal cell wall antigen; antibody cross-reacts with myocardial antigen	Inflammation, macrophage activation	Myocarditis, arthritis

FIGURE 11–9 Human antibody-mediated diseases (type II hypersensitivity). The table lists examples of human diseases caused by antibodies. In most of these diseases, the role of antibodies is inferred from the detection of antibodies in the blood or the lesions, and in some cases by similarities with experimental models in which the involvement of antibodies can be formally established by transfer studies.

known. These newer therapies are at the stage of preclinical testing and early clinical trials.

DISEASES CAUSED BY T LYMPHOCYTES

The role of T lymphocytes in human immunologic diseases has been increasingly recognized with improved methods for identifying and isolating these cells from lesions and through animal models of human disease in which a pathogenic role of T cells is established by experiments. In fact, much of the recent interest in the pathogenesis and treatment of human autoimmune diseases has focused on disorders in which tissue injury is caused mainly by T lymphocytes.

Etiology of T Cell–Mediated Diseases

The major causes of T cell–mediated hypersensitivity reactions are autoimmunity and exaggerated or persistent responses to

Immune complex disease	Antibody specificity	Clinicopathologic manifestations
Systemic lupus erythematosus	DNA, nucleoproteins, others	Nephritis, arthritis, vasculitis
Polyarteritis nodosa	Often microbial antigens (e.g., hepatitis B virus surface antigen)	Vasculitis
Post-streptococcal glomerulonephritis	Streptococcal cell wall antigen(s)	Nephritis
Serum sickness (clinical and experimental)	Various protein antigens	Systemic vasculitis, nephritis, arthritis
Arthus reaction (experimental)	Various protein antigens	Cutaneous vasculitis

FIGURE 11–10 Immune complex diseases (type III hypersensitivity). Table lists examples of human diseases caused by the deposition of immune complexes, as well as two experimental models. In the diseases, immune complexes are detected in the blood or in the tissues that are the sites of injury. In all the disorders, injury is caused by complement-mediated and Fc receptor–mediated inflammation.

environmental antigens. The autoimmune reactions usually are directed against cellular antigens with restricted tissue distribution. Therefore, T cell–mediated autoimmune diseases tend to be limited to a few organs and usually are not systemic. Examples of T cell–mediated hypersensitivity reactions against environmental antigens include contact sensitivity to chemicals (e.g., those found in poison ivy). Tissue injury also may accompany T cell responses to microbes. For example, in tuberculosis, a T cell–mediated immune response develops against protein antigens of *Mycobacterium tuberculosis,* and the response becomes chronic because the infection is difficult to eradicate. The resultant granulomatous inflammation causes injury to normal tissues at the site of infection. In hepatitis virus infection, the virus itself may not be highly cytopathic, but the cytotoxic T lymphocyte (CTL) response to infected hepatocytes may cause liver injury. T_H2 cells may also play a role in some inflammatory diseases other than allergies, especially in the late fibrotic stages of inflammation.

Excessive polyclonal T cell activation by certain microbial toxins produced by some bacteria and viruses can lead to production of large amounts of inflammatory cytokines, causing a syndrome similar to septic shock. These toxins are called **superantigens** because they stimulate large numbers of T cells. Superantigens bind to invariant parts of T cell receptors on many different clones of T cells, regardless of antigen specificity, thereby activating these cells.

Mechanisms of Tissue Injury

In different T cell–mediated diseases, tissue injury is caused by inflammation induced by cytokines that are produced mainly by $CD4^+$ T cells or by killing of host cells by $CD8^+$ CTLs (Fig. 11–11). The mechanisms of tissue injury are the same as the mechanisms used by T cells to eliminate cell-associated microbes.

$CD4^+$ T cells may react against cell or tissue antigens and secrete cytokines that induce local inflammation and activate macrophages. Different diseases may be associated with activation of T_H1 and T_H17 cells. T_H1 cells are the source of interferon-γ (IFN-γ), the principal macrophage-activating cytokine, and T_H17 cells are responsible for recruitment of leukocytes, including neutrophils. The actual tissue injury in these diseases is caused mainly by the macrophages and neutrophils. The typical reaction mediated by T cell cytokines is **delayed-type**

FIGURE 11–11 Mechanisms of T cell–mediated tissue injury (type IV hypersensitivity). T cells may cause tissue injury and disease by two mechanisms. **A,** Inflammation may be triggered by cytokines produced mainly by CD4⁺ T cells and in which tissue injury is caused by activated macrophages and inflammatory cells; APC, Antigen-presenting cell. **B,** Direct killing of target cells is mediated by CD8⁺ cytotoxic T lymphocytes (CTLs).

hypersensitivity (DTH), so called because it occurs 24 to 48 hours after an individual previously exposed to a protein antigen is challenged with the antigen (i.e., the reaction is delayed). The delay occurs because it takes several hours for circulating effector T lymphocytes to home to the site of antigen challenge, respond to the antigen at this site, and induce a detectable reaction. DTH reactions are manifested by infiltrates of T cells and blood monocytes in the tissues, edema and fibrin deposition caused by increased vascular permeability in response to cytokines produced by CD4⁺ T cells, and tissue damage induced by leukocyte products, mainly macrophages, activated by the T cells (Fig. 11–12). DTH reactions often are used to determine if people have been previously exposed to and have responded to an antigen. For example, a DTH reaction to a mycobacterial antigen, PPD (purified protein derivative), is an indicator of a T cell response to the mycobacteria. This is the basis for the PPD skin test, used to detect past or active mycobacterial infection.

FIGURE 11–12 Delayed-type hypersensitivity reaction in the skin. A, Perivascular accumulation (cuffing) of mononuclear inflammatory cells (lymphocytes and macrophages), with associated dermal edema and fibrin deposition. **B,** Immunoperoxidase staining reveals a predominantly perivascular cellular infiltrate that marks positively with anti-CD4 antibodies. (B courtesy Dr. Louis Picker, Department of Pathology, Oregon Health Sciences University, Portland.)

CD8+ T cells specific for antigens on host cells may directly kill these cells. CD8+ T cells also produce cytokines that induce inflammation, but they are usually not the major sources of cytokines in immune reactions. In many T cell–mediated autoimmune diseases, both CD4+ T cells and CD8+ T cells specific for self antigens are present, and both contribute to tissue injury.

Clinical Syndromes and Therapy

Many organ-specific autoimmune diseases in humans are believed to be caused by T cells, based on the identification of these cells in lesions and similarities with animal models in which the diseases are known to be T cell mediated (Fig. 11–13). These disorders typically are chronic and progressive, in part because T cell reactions tend to be prolonged and often self-perpetuating, and because the inciting antigens, such as tissue antigens or proteins expressed by resident microbes, are often never cleared. Also, tissue injury causes release and alteration of self proteins, which may result in reactions against these newly encountered proteins. This phenomenon has been called epitope spreading to indicate that the initial immune response against one or a few self antigen epitopes may expand to include responses against many more self antigens. Chronic inflammatory diseases that are initiated by immune reactions are called **immune-mediated inflammatory diseases.**

The therapy for T cell–mediated hypersensitivity disorders is designed to reduce inflammation and to inhibit T cell responses. For many reasons, the mainstay of treatment of such diseases has been the potent anti-inflammatory steroids, but these drugs have significant side effects. The development of more targeted therapies based on understanding of the fundamental mechanisms of these diseases has been one of the most impressive accomplishments of immunology. Antagonists of TNF have proved to be beneficial in patients with rheumatoid arthritis and inflammatory bowel disease by reducing inflammation. Newer agents developed to inhibit T cell responses include drugs that block costimulators such as B7 and antagonists against receptors for cytokines such as IL-1, IL-6, and IL-17. B cell depletion with anti-CD20 has also been effective in rheumatoid arthritis and multiple sclerosis; it is not clear if this is because antibodies contribute to the diseases or because B cells

function as APCs to promote T cell activation. There also is great hope for inducing tolerance in pathogenic T cells, but no successful clinical trials have yet been reported.

SUMMARY

* Immune responses that cause tissue injury are called hypersensitivity reactions, and the diseases caused by these reactions are called hypersensitivity diseases or immune-mediated inflammatory diseases.
* Hypersensitivity reactions may arise from uncontrolled or abnormal responses to foreign antigens or autoimmune responses against self antigens.
* Hypersensitivity reactions are classified according to the mechanism of tissue injury.
* Immediate hypersensitivity (type I, commonly called allergy) is caused by the production of IgE antibody against environmental antigens or drugs (allergens), sensitization of mast cells by the IgE, and degranulation of these mast cells on subsequent encounter with the allergen.
* Clinicopathologic manifestations of immediate hypersensitivity result from the actions of mediators secreted by the mast cells: amines dilate vessels and contract smooth muscles, arachidonic acid metabolites also contract muscles, and cytokines induce inflammation, the hallmark of the late-phase reaction. Treatment of allergies is designed to inhibit the production of mediators, antagonize their actions, and counteract their effects on end organs.
* Antibodies against cell and tissue antigens may cause tissue injury and disease (type II hypersensitivity). IgM and IgG antibodies promote the phagocytosis of cells to which they bind, induce inflammation by complement-mediated and Fc receptor–mediated leukocyte recruitment, and may interfere with the functions of cells by binding to essential molecules and receptors.
* In immune complex diseases (type III hypersensitivity), antibodies may bind to circulating antigens to form immune complexes, which deposit in vessels,

Disease	Specificity of pathogenic T cells	Clinicopathologic manifestations
Multiple sclerosis	Myelin proteins	Demyelination in the central nervous system, sensory and motor dysfunction
Rheumatoid arthritis	Unknown antigens in joint	Inflammation of synovium and erosion of cartilage and bone in joints
Type 1 (insulin-dependent) diabetes mellitus	Pancreatic islet antigens	Impaired glucose metabolism, vascular disease
Crohn's disease	Unknown, ? role of intestinal microbes	Inflammation of the bowel wall; abdominal pain, diarrhea, hemorrhage
Contact sensitivity (e.g., poison ivy reaction)	Modified skin proteins	DTH reaction in skin, rash
Chronic infections (e.g., tuberculosis)	Microbial proteins	Chronic (e.g., granulomatous) inflammation
Viral hepatitis (HBV, HCV)	Virally encoded proteins	CTL-mediated hepatocyte death, liver dysfunction; fibrosis
Superantigen-mediated diseases (toxic shock syndrome)	Polyclonal (microbial superantigens activate many T cells of different specificities)	Fever, shock related to systemic inflammatory cytokine release

FIGURE 11–13 T cell–mediated diseases. The table lists diseases in which T cells play a dominant role in causing tissue injury; antibodies and immune complexes may also contribute. Note that multiple sclerosis, rheumatoid arthritis, and type 1 diabetes are autoimmune disorders. Crohn's disease, an inflammatory bowel disease, is likely caused by reactions against microbes in the intestine and may have a component of autoimmunity. The other diseases are caused by reactions against foreign (microbial or environmental) antigens. In most of these diseases, the role of T cells is inferred from the detection and isolation of T cells reactive with various antigens from the blood or lesions, and from the similarity with experimental models in which the involvement of T cells has been established by a variety of approaches. The specificity of pathogenic T cells has been defined in animal models and in some of the lesions in humans. Viral hepatitis and toxic shock syndrome are clinical examples of disorders in which T cells play an important pathogenic role, but these are not considered examples of hypersensitivity. CTL, Cytotoxic T lymphocyte; DTH, delayed-type hypersensitivity; HBV, hepatitis B virus; HCV, hepatitis C virus.

leading to inflammation in the vessel wall (vasculitis), which secondarily causes tissue injury due to impaired blood flow.

* T cell–mediated diseases (type IV hypersensitivity) result from inflammation caused by cytokines produced by CD4$^+$ T$_H$1 and T$_H$17 cells, or killing of host cells by CD8$^+$ CTLs.

REVIEW QUESTIONS

1. What are the major types of hypersensitivity reactions?
2. What types of antigens may induce immune responses that cause hypersensitivity reactions?
3. What is the sequence of events in a typical immediate hypersensitivity reaction? What is the late-phase reaction, and how is it caused?

4. What are some examples of immediate hypersensitivity disorders, what is their pathogenesis, and how are they treated?
5. How do antibodies cause tissue injury and disease?
6. What are some examples of diseases caused by antibodies specific for cell surface or tissue matrix antigens?
7. How do immune complexes cause disease, and how are the clinical manifestations different from most diseases caused by antibodies specific for cell surface or tissue matrix proteins?
8. What are some examples of diseases caused by T cells, what is their pathogenesis, and what are their principal clinical and pathologic manifestations?

Answers to and discussion of the Review Questions are available at studentconsult.com.

Congenital and Acquired Immunodeficiencies
Diseases Caused by Defective Immune Responses

Defects in the development and functions of the immune system result in increased susceptibility to newly acquired infections; reactivation of latent infections such as cytomegalovirus, Epstein-Barr virus, and tuberculosis, in which the normal immune response keeps the infection in check but does not eradicate it; and increased incidence of certain cancers. These consequences of defective immunity are predictable because, as emphasized throughout this book, the normal function of the immune system is to defend individuals against infections and some cancers. Disorders caused by defective immunity are called **immunodeficiency diseases.** Some of these diseases may result from genetic abnormalities in one or more components of the immune system; these are called **congenital** (or **primary**) **immunodeficiencies.** Other defects in the immune system may result from infections, nutritional abnormalities, or medical treatments that cause loss or inadequate function of various components of the immune system; these are called **acquired** (or **secondary**) **immunodeficiencies.**

In this chapter we describe the causes and pathogenesis of congenital and acquired immunodeficiencies. Among the acquired diseases, we emphasize acquired immunodeficiency syndrome (AIDS), which results from infection by human immunodeficiency virus (HIV) and is one of the most devastating health problems worldwide. We address the following questions:

- What are the mechanisms by which immunity is compromised in the common immunodeficiency diseases?
- How does HIV cause the clinical and pathologic abnormalities of AIDS?
- What approaches are being used to treat immunodeficiency diseases?

Information about the clinical features of these disorders can be found in textbooks of pediatrics and medicine.

CONGENITAL (PRIMARY) IMMUNODEFICIENCIES

Congenital immunodeficiencies are caused by genetic defects that lead to blocks in the maturation or functions of different components of the immune system. It is estimated that as many as 1 in 500 individuals in the United States and Europe suffer from congenital immune deficiencies of varying severity. Congenital immunodeficiencies share several features, the most common being infectious complications (Fig. 12–1). Different congenital immunodeficiency diseases, however, may differ considerably in clinical and pathologic manifestations. Some of these disorders result in greatly increased susceptibility to infections that may manifest early after birth and may be fatal unless the immunologic defects are corrected. Other congenital immunodeficiencies lead to mild infections and may first be detected in adult life.

The following discussion summarizes the pathogenesis of select immunodeficiencies, several of which are mentioned in earlier chapters to illustrate the physiologic importance of various components of the immune system. Congenital deficiencies in molecules involved in self-tolerance are manifested as autoimmune disease, as discussed in Chapter 9.

Defects in Lymphocyte Maturation

Many congenital immunodeficiencies are the result of genetic abnormalities that cause blocks in the maturation of B lymphocytes, T lymphocytes, or both (Figs. 12–2 and 12–3). Disorders manifesting as defects in both the B cell and T cell arms of the adaptive immune system are classified as **severe combined immunodeficiency (SCID)**.

Several different genetic abnormalities may cause SCID. About half of the cases are X-linked, affecting only male children. More than 99% of cases of **X-linked SCID** are caused by mutations in the common γ (γ$_c$) chain signaling subunit of the receptors for several cytokines, including interleukin-2 (IL-2), IL-4, IL-7, IL-9, IL-15, and IL-21. (Because the γ$_c$ chain was first identified as one of the three chains of the IL-2 receptor, it is also called the IL-2Rγ chain.) When the γ$_c$ chain is not functional, immature lymphocytes, especially pro-T cells, cannot proliferate in response to IL-7, which is the major growth factor for these cells. Defective responses to IL-7 result in reduced survival and maturation

Type of immunodeficiency	Histopathology and laboratory abnormalities	Common infectious consequences
B cell deficiencies	Absent or reduced follicles and germinal centers in lymphoid organs Reduced serum Ig levels	Pyogenic bacterial infections, enteric bacterial and viral infections
T cell deficiencies	May be reduced T cell zones in lymphoid organs Reduced DTH reactions to common antigens Defective T cell proliferative responses to mitogens *in vitro*	Viral and other intracellular microbial infections (e.g., *Pneumocystis jiroveci*, atypical mycobacteria, fungi) Virus-associated malignancies (e.g., EBV associated lymphomas)
Innate immune deficiencies	Variable, depending on which component of innate immunity is defective	Variable; pyogenic bacterial and viral infections

FIGURE 12–1 Features of immunodeficiency diseases. The table summarizes important diagnostic features and clinical manifestations of immunodeficiencies affecting different components of the immune system. Within each group, different diseases, and even different patients with the same disease, may show considerable variation. Reduced numbers of circulating B or T cells are often detected in some of these diseases. DTH, Delayed-type hypersensitivity; EBV, Epstein-Barr virus; Ig, immunoglobulin.

FIGURE 12–2 Congenital immunodeficiencies caused by defects in genetic lymphocyte maturation. Lymphocyte maturation pathways are described in Chapter 4. JAK3 (Janus kinase 3) is a kinase involved in signaling by many cytokine receptors; ARTEMIS is a protein involved in antigen receptor gene recombination; BTK (Bruton tyrosine kinase) is a kinase that delivers signals from the pre-B cell receptor (BCR) and BCR; ZAP70 is a kinase involved in TCR signaling; and TAP proteins transport peptides for presentation by class I MHC molecules. ADA, Adenosine deaminase; CLP, common lymphoid progenitor; HSC, hematopoietic stem cell; PNP, purine nucleoside phosphorylase; RAG, recombinase-activating gene.

of lymphocyte precursors. In humans, the defect affects mainly T cell maturation (whereas in mice, B cells are also greatly reduced). The consequence of this block is a profound decrease in the numbers of mature T cells, deficient cell-mediated immunity, and defective humoral immunity because of absent T cell help (even though B cells may mature almost normally). Natural killer (NK) cells also are deficient, because the γ_c chain is part of the receptor for IL-15, the major cytokine involved in NK cell proliferation and maturation.

About half the cases of **autosomal SCID** are caused by mutations in an enzyme called adenosine deaminase (ADA), which is involved in the breakdown of adenosine. Deficiency of ADA leads to the accumulation of toxic purine metabolites in cells that are actively synthesizing DNA, namely, proliferating cells. Lymphocytes are particularly susceptible to injury by purine metabolites because these cells undergo tremendous proliferation during their maturation. ADA deficiency results in a block in T cell maturation more than in B cell maturation; defective humoral immunity is largely a consequence of

the lack of T cell helper function. A similar phenotype is seen in individuals who have a deficiency in purine nucleotide phosphorylase (PNP). Another important cause of autosomal SCID is mutation of the gene encoding a kinase that is involved in signaling by the γ_c cytokine receptor chain. Such mutations result in the same abnormalities as those in X-linked SCID caused by γ_c mutations, described previously. Rare cases of autosomal SCID are caused by mutations in the *RAG1* or *RAG2* gene, which encode the VDJ recombinase that is required for immunoglobulin (Ig) and T cell receptor gene recombination and lymphocyte maturation (see Chapter 4). With increasing application of newborn screening to identify congenital immunodeficiencies, other causes of SCID are being discovered.

The most common clinical syndrome caused by a block in B cell maturation is **X-linked agammaglobulinemia** (first described as Bruton's agammaglobulinemia). In this disorder, B cells in the bone marrow fail to mature beyond the pre-B cell stage, resulting in a marked decrease or absence of mature B lymphocytes

Severe combined immunodeficiency (SCID)

Disease	Functional deficiencies	Mechanism of defect
X-linked SCID	Markedly decreased T cells; normal or increased B cells; reduced serum Ig	Cytokine receptor common γ chain gene mutations, defective T cell maturation due to lack of IL-7 signals
Autosomal recessive SCID due to ADA, PNP deficiency	Progressive decrease in T and B cells (mostly T); reduced serum Ig in ADA deficiency, normal B cells and serum Ig in PNP deficiency	ADA or PNP deficiency leads to accumulation of toxic metabolites in lymphocytes
Autosomal recessive SCID due to other causes	Decreased T and B cells; reduced serum Ig	Defective maturation of T and B cells; may be mutations in *RAG* genes and other genes involved in VDJ recombination or IL-7R signaling

B cell immunodeficiencies

Disease	Functional deficiencies	Mechanism of defect
X-linked agammaglobulinemia	Decrease in all serum Ig isotypes; reduced B cell numbers	Block in maturation beyond pre-B cells, because of mutation in Bruton tyrosine kinase (BTK)
Ig heavy-chain deletions	IgG1, IgG2, or IgG4 absent; sometimes associated with absent IgA or IgE	Chromosomal deletion involving Ig heavy-chain locus at 14q32

T cell immunodeficiencies

Disease	Functional deficiencies	Mechanism of defect
DiGeorge syndrome	Decreased T cells; normal B cells; normal or decreased serum Ig	Anomalous development of 3rd and 4th branchial pouches, leading to thymic hypoplasia

FIGURE 12–3 Features of congenital immunodeficiencies caused by defects in lymphocyte maturation. Table summarizes the most common congenital immunodeficiencies in which the genetic blocks are known, and their principal features. ADA, Adenosine deaminase; Ig, immunoglobulin; IL-7, interleukin-7; PNP, purine nucleoside phosphorylase; RAG, recombinase-activating gene.

and serum immunoglobulins. The disease is caused by mutations in the gene encoding a kinase called Bruton tyrosine kinase (BTK), resulting in defective production or function of the enzyme. The enzyme is activated by the pre-B cell receptor expressed in pre-B cells, and it delivers biochemical signals that promote the survival, proliferation, and maturation of these cells. The gene for this enzyme is located on the X chromosome. Therefore, women who carry a mutant allele of the *BTK* gene on one of their X chromosomes are carriers of the disease, but male offspring who inherit the abnormal X chromosome are affected. In about a fourth of patients with X-linked agammaglobulinemia, autoimmune diseases, notably arthritis, develop as well. A link between an immuno-deficiency and autoimmunity seems paradoxical. One possible explanation for this association is that BTK contributes to BCR signaling and is required for central B cell tolerance, so defective BTK may result in the accumulation of autoreactive B cells.

Selective defects in T cell maturation are quite rare. Of these, **DiGeorge syndrome** is the most common. It results from incomplete development of the thymus (and parathyroid glands) and a failure of T cell maturation. Patients with DiGeorge syndrome tend to improve with age, probably because the small amount of thymic tissue that does develop is able to support some T cell maturation.

Treatment of primary immunodeficiencies that affect lymphocyte maturation varies with the disease. SCID is fatal in early life unless the patient's immune system is reconstituted. The most widely used treatment is hematopoietic stem cell transplantation, with careful matching of donor and recipient to avoid potentially serious graft-versus-host disease. For selective B cell defects, patients may be given pooled immunoglobulin from healthy donors to provide passive immunity. Ig replacement therapy has provided enormous benefit in patients with X-linked agammaglobulinemia. Although the ideal treatment for all congenital immunodeficiencies is to replace the defective gene, this remains a distant goal for most diseases. Successful gene therapy has been reported in patients with X-linked SCID; a normal γ_c gene was introduced into their bone marrow stem cells, which were then transplanted back into the patients. In some of these patients, however, T cell leukemia has subsequently developed, apparently because the introduced γ_c gene was inserted near an oncogene and activated it. In all patients with these diseases, infections are treated with antibiotics as needed.

Defects in Lymphocyte Activation and Function

Better understanding of the molecules involved in lymphocyte activation and function has led to the recognition of mutations and other abnormalities in these molecules that result in immunodeficiency disorders (Fig. 12–4). This section describes some of the diseases in which lymphocytes mature normally but the activation and effector functions of the cells are defective.

The **X-linked hyper-IgM syndrome** is characterized by defective B cell heavy-chain isotype (class) switching, so that IgM is the major serum antibody, and by severe deficiency of cell-mediated immunity against intracellular microbes. The disease is caused by mutations in CD40 ligand (CD40L), the helper T cell protein that binds to CD40 on B cells, dendritic cells, and macrophages and thus mediates T cell–dependent activation of these cells (see Chapters 6 and 7). Failure to express functional CD40L leads to defective T cell–dependent B cell responses, such as isotype switching, in humoral immunity, and to defective T cell–dependent macrophage activation in cell-mediated immunity. Boys with this disease are susceptible to infection by *Pneumocystis jiroveci*, a fungus that survives within phagocytes in the absence of T cell help. A rare autosomal recessive form of hyper-IgM syndrome is seen in subjects with mutations affecting the enzyme activation-induced deaminase (AID), which is involved in isotype switching and somatic hypermutation (see Chapter 7).

Genetic deficiencies in the production of selected Ig isotypes are quite common. IgA deficiency is believed to affect as many as 1 in 700 people but causes no clinical problems in most patients. The defect causing these deficiencies is not known in a majority of cases; rarely, the deficiencies may be caused by mutations of Ig heavy-chain constant (C) region genes. **Common variable immunodeficiency** (CVID) is a heterogeneous group of disorders that represent a common form of primary immunodeficiency. These disorders are characterized by poor antibody responses to infections and reduced serum levels of IgG, IgA, and often IgM. The underlying causes of CVID include defects in various genes involved in B cell maturation and activation. Some patients have mutations in genes encoding receptors for B cell growth factors or costimulators that play a role in T cell–B cell interactions. Patients have recurrent infections, autoimmune disease, and lymphomas.

Defective activation of T lymphocytes may result from deficient expression of major histocompatibility complex (MHC) molecules. The **bare lymphocyte syndrome** is a disease caused by a failure to express class II MHC molecules, as a result of mutations in the transcription factors that normally induce class II MHC expression. Recall that class II MHC molecules display peptide antigens for recognition by CD4$^+$ T cells,

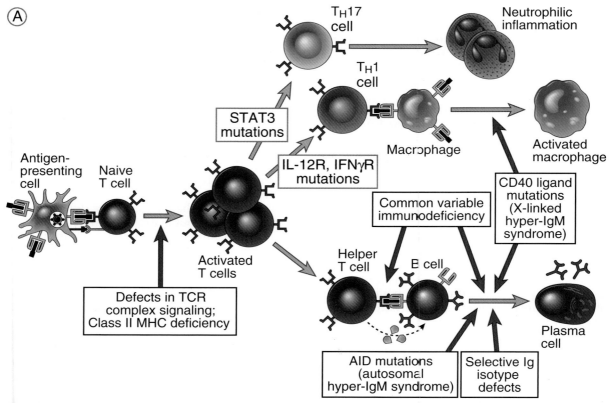

FIGURE 12–4 Congenital immunodeficiencies associated with defects in lymphocyte activation and effector functions. Congenital immunodeficiencies may be caused by genetic defects in the expression of molecules required for antigen presentation to T cells, T or B lymphocyte antigen receptor signaling, helper T cell activation of B cells and macrophages, and differentiation of antibody-producing B cells. **A,** Examples showing the sites at which immune responses may be blocked.

and that this recognition is critical for maturation and activation of the T cells. The disease is manifested by a profound decrease in CD4$^+$ T cells, because of defective maturation of these cells in the thymus and defective activation in peripheral lymphoid organs.

Rare cases of selective T cell deficiency are caused by mutations affecting various signaling pathways or cytokines and receptors involved in differentiation of naive T cells into effector cells. Depending on the mutation and the extent of the defect, affected patients show severe T cell deficiency or deficiency in particular arms of T cell–mediated immunity, such as in T$_H$1 responses (associated with atypical mycobacterial infections) and T$_H$17 responses (associated with fungal and bacterial infections). These defects have revealed the importance of various pathways of T cell activation, but these are rare disorders.

Defects in Innate Immunity

Abnormalities in two components of innate immunity, phagocytes and the complement system, are important causes of immunodeficiency (Fig. 12–5). **Chronic granulomatous disease** is caused by mutations in genes encoding subunits of the enzyme phagocyte oxidase, which catalyzes the production of microbicidal reactive oxygen species in lysosomes (see Chapter 2). As a result, neutrophils and macrophages that phagocytose microbes are unable to kill the microbes. The immune system tries to compensate for this defective microbial killing by calling in more and more macrophages, and by activating T cells, which stimulate recruitment and activation of even more phagocytes. Therefore, collections of phagocytes accumulate around foci of infections by intracellular microbes, but the

B

Disease	Functional Deficiencies	Mechanisms of Defect
X-linked hyper-IgM syndrome	Defects in helper T cell–dependent B cell and macrophage activation	Mutations in CD40 ligand
Common variable immunodeficiency	Reduced or no production of selective isotypes or subtypes of immunoglobulins; susceptibility to bacterial infections or no clinical problems	Mutations in receptor for B cell growth factors, costimulators
Defective class II MHC expression: The bare lymphocyte syndrome	Lack of class II MHC expression and impaired CD4+ T cell activation; defective cell-mediated immunity and T cell–dependent humoral immunity	Mutations in genes encoding transcription factors required for class II MHC gene expression
Defects in T cell receptor complex expression or signaling	Decreased T cells or abnormal ratios of CD4+ and CD8+ subsets; decreased cell-mediated immunity	Rare cases due to mutations or deletions in genes encoding CD3 proteins, ZAP-70
Defects in T_H1 responses	Decreased T cell–mediated macrophage activation; susceptibility to intracellular microbial infection	Rare cases due to mutations encoding the receptors for IL-12 or interferon-γ
Defects in T_H17 responses	Decreased T cell–mediated inflammatory responses; susceptibility to infections with pyogenic bacteria and mucocutaneous candidiasis	Rare cases due to mutations in genes encoding STAT3, IL-17, IL-17R
X-linked lymphoproliferative syndrome	Uncontrolled EBV-induced B cell proliferation, uncontrolled macrophage and CTL activation, defective NK cell and CTL function	Mutations in *SAP*

FIGURE 12–4, cont'd B, Table summarizes the features of select congenital immunodeficiency disorders. Note that abnormalities in class II MHC expression and TCR complex signaling can cause defective T cell maturation (see Fig. 12–2), as well as defective activation of the cells that do mature, as shown here. AID, Activation-induced deaminase; ZAP-70, ζ chain–associated protein of 70 kD.

microbes cannot be destroyed effectively. These collections resemble granulomas, giving rise to the name of this disease. **Leukocyte adhesion deficiency** is caused by mutations in genes encoding integrins, molecules required for the expression of ligands for selectins, or signaling molecules activated by chemokine receptors required to activate integrins. Integrins and selectin ligands are involved in the adhesion of leukocytes to other cells. As a result of these mutations, blood leukocytes do not bind firmly to vascular endothelium and are not recruited normally to sites of infection.

Deficiencies of almost every complement protein, and many complement regulatory proteins, have been described (see Chapter 8). C3 deficiency results in severe infections and usually is fatal. Deficiencies of C2 and C4, two components of the classical pathway of complement activation, result in increased bacterial or viral infection or increased incidence of systemic lupus erythematosus, presumably because of defective clearance of immune complexes. Deficiencies of complement regulatory proteins lead to various syndromes associated with excessive complement activation.

Disease	Functional Deficiencies	Mechanisms of Defect
Chronic granulomatous disease	Defective production of reactive oxygen intermediates by phagocytes	Mutations in genes encoding components of the phagocyte oxidase enzyme, most often cytochrome b558
Leukocyte adhesion deficiency-1	Absent or deficient expression of β2 integrins causing defective leukocyte adhesion–dependent functions	Mutations in gene encoding the β chain (CD18) of β_2 integrins
Leukocyte adhesion deficiency-2	Absent or deficient expression of leukocyte ligands for endothelial E- and P-selectins, causing failure of leukocyte migration into tissues	Mutations in gene encoding a protein required for synthesis of the sialyl-Lewis X component of E- and P-selectin ligands
Complement C3 deficiency	Defect in complement cascade activation	Mutations in the C3 gene
Complement C2, C4 deficiency	Deficient activation of classical pathway of complement leading to susceptibility to infection and development of lupus-like disease	Mutations in C2 or C4 genes
Chédiak-Higashi syndrome	Defective lysosomal function in neutrophils, macrophages and dendritic cells, and defective granule function in natural killer cells	Mutation in a gene encoding a lysosomal trafficking regulatory protein
Herpes simplex virus 1 (HSV-1) encephalitis	Defective antiviral immunity in the CNS	Mutations in gene encoding TLR3
Recurrent bacterial pneumonia	Defective innate immune responses to pyogenic bacteria	Mutations in gene encoding MyD88

FIGURE 12–5 Congenital immunodeficiencies caused by defects in innate immunity. The table lists immunodeficiency diseases caused by defects in various components of the innate immune system.

The **Chédiak-Higashi syndrome** is an immunodeficiency disease in which the lysosomal granules of leukocytes do not function normally. The immune defect is thought to affect phagocytes and NK cells and manifests as increased susceptibility to bacterial infection.

Rare patients have been described with mutations affecting Toll-like receptors (TLRs) or signaling pathways downstream of TLRs, including molecules required for activation of the nuclear factor κB (NF-κB) transcription factor.

Somewhat surprisingly, several of these mutations make patients susceptible to only a limited set of infections. For example, mutations affecting MyD88, an adaptor protein downstream of many TLRs, are associated with severe bacterial (most often pneumococcal) pneumonia, and mutations affecting TLR3 are associated with recurrent herpesvirus encephalitis but apparently not other viral infections. These quite restricted clinical phenotypes suggest considerable redundancy in host defense mechanisms, so

Cause	Mechanism
Human immunodeficiency virus infection	Depletion of CD4$^+$ helper T cells
Irradiation and chemotherapy treatments for cancer	Decreased bone marrow precursors for all leukocytes
Immunosuppression for graft rejection and inflammatory diseases	Depletion or functional impairment of lymphocytes
Involvement of bone marrow by cancers (metastases, leukemias)	Reduced site of leukocyte development
Protein-calorie malnutrition	Metabolic derangements inhibit lymphocyte maturation and function
Removal of spleen	Decreased phagocytosis of microbes

FIGURE 12–6 Acquired (secondary) immunodeficiency. The table lists the most common causes of acquired immunodeficiency diseases and how they lead to defects in immune responses.

that defects in one pathway can be compensated by other pathways, and patients are not susceptible to a wide variety of infections.

Lymphocyte Abnormalities Associated with Other Diseases

Some systemic diseases that involve multiple organ systems, and whose major manifestations are not immunologic, may have a component of immunodeficiency. The **Wiskott-Aldrich syndrome** is characterized by eczema, reduced blood platelets, and immunodeficiency. This X-linked disease is caused by a mutation in a gene that encodes a protein that binds to various adaptor molecules and cytoskeletal components in hematopoietic cells. Because of the absence of this protein, platelets and leukocytes do not develop normally, are small, and fail to migrate normally. **Ataxia-telangiectasia** is characterized by gait abnormalities (ataxia), vascular malformations (telangiectasia), and immunodeficiency. The disease is caused by mutations in a gene whose product is involved in DNA repair. Defects in this protein lead to abnormal DNA repair (e.g., during recombination of antigen

receptor gene segments), resulting in defective lymphocyte maturation.

ACQUIRED (SECONDARY) IMMUNODEFICIENCIES

Deficiencies of the immune system often develop because of abnormalities that are not genetic but are acquired during life (Fig. 12–6). The most serious of these abnormalities worldwide is HIV infection, as described later. The most frequent causes of secondary immunodeficiencies in developed countries are cancers involving the bone marrow and various therapies. Cancer treatment with chemotherapeutic drugs and irradiation may damage proliferating cells, including bone marrow precursors and mature lymphocytes, resulting in immunodeficiency. Immunosuppressive drugs used to prevent graft rejection and drugs for inflammatory diseases, including some of the newer therapies (e.g., TNF antagonists, costimulation blockade), are designed to blunt immune responses. Therefore, immunodeficiency is a complication of such therapies. Protein-calorie malnutrition results in deficiencies of virtually all components of the immune system and is a common cause of immunodeficiency in developing countries.

ACQUIRED IMMUNODEFICIENCY SYNDROME

Although AIDS was first recognized as a distinct entity in the 1980s, it has become one of the most devastating afflictions in history. AIDS is caused by infection with HIV. Of the estimated 34 million HIV-infected people worldwide, about 70% are in Africa and 20% in Asia. More than 30 million deaths are attributable to HIV/AIDS, with about 2 million deaths annually. Effective antiretroviral drugs have been developed, but the infection continues to spread in parts of the world where these therapies are not widely available, and in some African countries, more than 30% of the population has HIV infection. This section describes the important features of HIV, how it infects humans, and the disease it causes, with a brief discussion of the current status of therapy and vaccine development.

Human Immunodeficiency Virus

Human immunodeficiency virus is a retrovirus that infects cells of the immune system, mainly CD4$^+$ T lymphocytes, and causes progressive destruction of these cells. An infectious HIV particle consists of two RNA strands within a protein core, surrounded by a lipid envelope derived from infected host cells but containing viral proteins (Fig. 12–7). The viral RNA encodes structural proteins, various enzymes, and proteins that regulate transcription of viral genes and the viral life cycle.

The life cycle of HIV consists of the following sequential steps: infection of cells, production of viral DNA and its integration into the host genome, expression of viral genes, and production of viral particles (Fig. 12–8). HIV infects cells by virtue of its major envelope glycoprotein, called gp120 (for 120-kD glycoprotein), which binds to CD4 and to particular chemokine receptors on human cells (mainly CXCR4 on T cells and CCR5 on macrophages). The major cell types that may be infected by HIV are CD4$^+$ T lymphocytes, macrophages, and dendritic cells. After binding to cellular receptors, the viral membrane fuses with the host cell membrane, and the virus enters the cell's cytoplasm. Here the virus is uncoated by viral protease, and its RNA is released. A DNA copy of the viral RNA is synthesized by the viral reverse transcriptase enzyme (a process characteristic of all retroviruses), and the DNA integrates into the host cell's DNA by the action of the integrase enzyme. The integrated viral DNA is called a provirus. If the infected T cell, macrophage, or dendritic cell is activated by some extrinsic stimulus, such as another infectious microbe, the cell responds by turning on the transcription of many of its own genes and often by producing cytokines. A negative consequence of this normal protective response is that the cytokines, and the process of cellular activation itself, also may activate the provirus, leading to production of viral RNAs and then proteins. The virus is then able to form a core structure, which migrates to the cell membrane, acquires a lipid envelope from the host, and is shed as an infectious viral particle, ready to infect another cell. The integrated HIV provirus may remain latent within infected cells for months or years, hidden from the patient's immune system (and even from antiviral therapies, discussed later).

Most cases of AIDS are caused by HIV-1 (i.e., HIV type 1). A related virus, HIV-2, causes some cases of the disease.

Pathogenesis of AIDS

AIDS develops over many years as latent HIV becomes activated and destroys cells of the immune system. Virus production leads to death of infected cells, as well as to death of uninfected lymphocytes, subsequent immune deficiencies, and clinical AIDS (Fig. 12–9). HIV infection is acquired by sexual intercourse, sharing contaminated needles used by intravenous drug users, transplacental transfer, or transfusion of infected blood or blood products. After infection there may be a brief, acute viremia, when the virus is detected in the blood, and the host may respond as in any mild viral infection. The virus infects CD4$^+$ T cells, dendritic cells, and macrophages at sites of entry through epithelia, in lymphoid organs such as lymph nodes, and in the circulation. In mucosal tissues at the sites of entry, there may be considerable destruction of infected T cells. Because a large fraction of the body's lymphocytes, and especially memory T cells, reside in these tissues, the result of the local

LTR Long Terminal Repeat: Integration of viral DNA into host genome; binding site for transcription factors

gag Pr55gag: Nuclear import of viral DNA

pol Polymerase: Encodes a variety of viral enzymes

vif Viral infectivity factor (p23): Overcomes inhibitory effects of host cell factors

vpr Viral protein R (p15): Promotes infection of macrophages by regulating nuclear import of HIV pre-integration complex

tat Transcriptional activator (p14): Promotes cell cycle arrest and enhances integrated viral DNA transcription

rev Regulator of viral gene expression (p19): Inhibits viral RNA splicing and promotes export of incompletely spliced viral RNA

vpu Viral protein U: Promotes CD4 degradation and influences virion release

env Envelope protein gp160: Cleaved into gp120, which mediates CD4 and chemokine receptor binding, and gp41, which mediates fusion

nef Negative effector: Promotes down-regulation of surface CD4 and class I MHC expression; blocks apoptosis; enhances virion infectivity

FIGURE 12–7 Structure and genes of the human immunodeficiency virus (HIV). A, An HIV-1 virion is shown next to a T cell surface. HIV-1 consists of two identical strands of RNA (the viral genome) and associated enzymes, including reverse transcriptase, integrase, and protease, packaged in a cone-shaped core composed of the p24 capsid protein with a surrounding p17 protein matrix, all surrounded by a phospholipid membrane envelope derived from the host cell. Virally encoded membrane proteins (gp41 and gp120) are bound to the envelope. CD4 and chemokine receptors on the host cell surface function as the receptors for HIV-1. **B,** The HIV-1 genome consists of genes whose positions are indicated here as differently colored blocks. Some genes contain sequences that overlap with sequences of other genes, as shown by overlapping blocks, but are read differently by host cell RNA polymerase. Similarly shaded blocks separated by lines *(tat, rev)* indicate genes whose coding sequences are separated in the genome and require RNA splicing to produce functional messenger RNA. The major functions of the proteins encoded by different viral genes are listed. MHC, Major histocompatibility complex. *(A adapted from front cover, The New Face of AIDS. Science 272:1841-2102, 1996. © Terese Winslow. B adapted from Greene WC: AIDS and the immune system. © 1993 by Scientific American, Inc. All rights reserved.)*

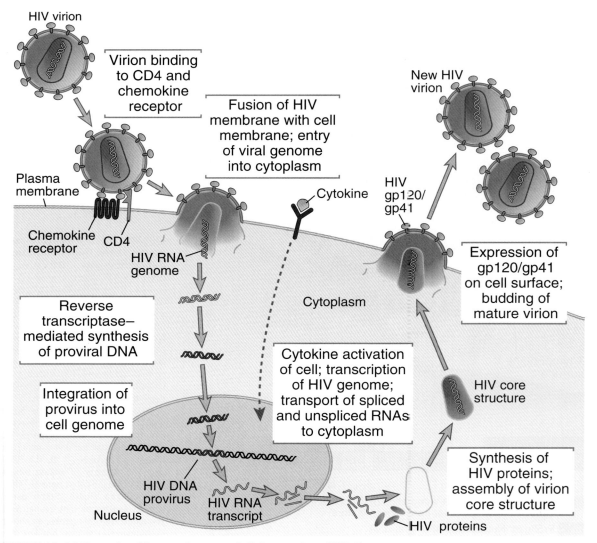

FIGURE 12–8 Life cycle of human immunodeficiency virus (HIV-1). The sequential steps in HIV reproduction are shown, from initial infection of a host cell to release of a new virus particle (virion). For the sake of clarity, the production and release of only one new virion are shown. An infected cell actually produces many virions, each capable of infecting nearby cells, leading to spread of the infection.

destruction may be a significant functional deficit that is not reflected in the presence of infected cells in the blood or the depletion of circulating T cells. Dendritic cells may capture the virus as it enters through mucosal epithelia and transport it to peripheral lymphoid organs, where it infects T cells. Rare individuals with *CCR5* mutations that do not permit HIV entry into macrophages can remain disease free for years after HIV infection, indicating the importance of macrophage

infection in the progression to AIDS. The integrated provirus may be activated in infected cells, as described previously, leading to production of viral particles and spread of the infection. During the course of HIV infection, the major source of infectious viral particles is activated CD4⁺ T cells; dendritic cells and macrophages are reservoirs of infection.

The depletion of CD4⁺ T cells after HIV infection is caused by a cytopathic effect of

the virus, resulting from production of viral particles in infected cells, as well as death of uninfected cells. Active viral gene expression and protein production may interfere with the synthetic machinery of the T cells. Therefore, infected T cells in which the virus is replicating are killed during this process. The number of T cells lost during the progression to AIDS is greater than the number of infected cells. The mechanism of this T cell loss remains poorly defined. One possibility is that T cells are chronically activated, perhaps by infections that are common in these patients, and the chronic stimulation culminates in apoptosis, by the pathway called activation-induced cell death.

Other infected cells, such as dendritic cells and macrophages, may also die, resulting in destruction of the architecture of lymphoid organs. Many studies have suggested that immune deficiency results not only from depletion of T cells but, in addition, from various functional abnormalities in T lymphocytes and other immune cells (dendritic cells and macrophages). The significance of these functional defects has not been established, however, and loss of T cells (followed by a fall in the blood CD4$^+$ T cell count) remains the most reliable indicator of disease progression.

Clinical Features of HIV Infection and AIDS

The clinical course of HIV infection is characterized by several phases, culminating in immune deficiency (Fig. 12–10, A). Early after HIV infection, patients may experience a mild acute illness with fever and malaise, correlating with the initial viremia. This illness subsides within a few days, and the disease enters a period of clinical latency. During this latency, there usually is a progressive loss of CD4$^+$ T cells in lymphoid tissues and destruction of the architecture of the lymphoid tissues. Eventually, the blood CD4$^+$ T

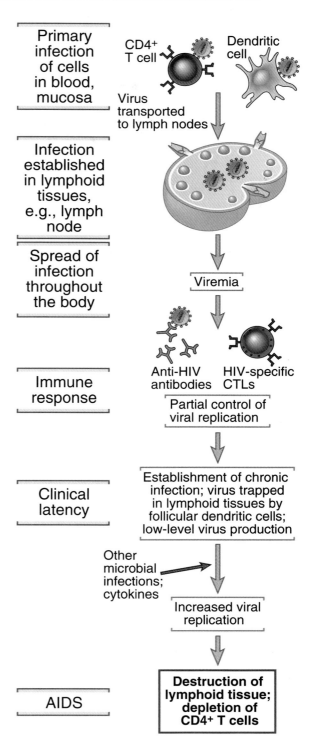

FIGURE 12–9 Pathogenesis of disease caused by human immunodeficiency virus. The stages of HIV disease correlate with spread of HIV from the initial site of infection to lymphoid tissues throughout the body. The immune response of the host temporarily controls acute infection but does not prevent establishment of chronic infection of cells in lymphoid tissues. Cytokines produced in response to HIV and other microbes serve to enhance HIV production and progression to acquired immunodeficiency syndrome (AIDS). CTLs, cytotoxic T lymphocytes.

FIGURE 12–10 Clinical course of HIV disease. A, Blood-borne virus (plasma viremia) is detected early after infection and may be accompanied by systemic symptoms typical of acute HIV syndrome. The virus spreads to lymphoid organs, but plasma viremia falls to very low levels (detectable only by sensitive reverse transcriptase–polymerase chain reaction assays) and stays this way for many years. CD4+ T cell counts steadily decline during this clinical latency period because of active viral replication and T cell destruction in lymphoid tissues. As the level of CD4+ T cells falls, there is increasing risk of infection and other clinical components of acquired immunodeficiency syndrome (AIDS). **B,** Magnitude and kinetics of immune responses, shown in arbitrary relative units. CTLs, Cytotoxic T lymphocytes. *(Reproduced with permission from Pantaleo G, Graziosi C, Fauci A: The immunopathogenesis of human immunodeficiency virus infection. N Engl J Med 328:327-335, 1993.)*

cell count begins to decline, and when the count falls below 200 cells per mm³ (normal level about 1500 cells/mm³), patients become susceptible to infections and are diagnosed as having AIDS.

The clinicopathologic manifestations of full-blown AIDS are primarily the result of increased susceptibility to infections and some cancers, as a consequence of immune deficiency. Patients not given antiretroviral drugs often are infected by intracellular microbes, such as viruses, the fungal pathogen *Pneumocystis jiroveci*, and atypical mycobacteria, all of which normally are combated by T cell–mediated immunity. Many of these microbes are present in the environment, but they do not infect healthy persons with intact immune systems. Because these infections are seen in immunodeficient persons, in whom the microbes have an opportunity to establish infection, these types of infections are said to be opportunistic. Many of the opportunistic infections are caused by viruses, such as cytomegalovirus. Patients with AIDS show defective cytotoxic T lymphocyte (CTL) responses to viruses, even though HIV does not infect CD8+ T cells. The CTL responses are defective probably because CD4+ helper T cells (the main targets of HIV) are required for full CD8+

CTL responses against many viral antigens (see Chapters 5 and 6). AIDS patients are at increased risk for infections by extracellular bacteria, probably because of impaired helper T cell–dependent antibody responses to bacterial antigens. Patients also become susceptible to cancers caused by oncogenic viruses. The two most common types of cancers are B cell lymphomas, caused by the Epstein-Barr virus, and a tumor of small blood vessels called Kaposi's sarcoma, caused by a herpesvirus. Patients with advanced AIDS often have a wasting syndrome with significant loss of body mass, caused by altered metabolism and reduced caloric intake. The dementia that develops in some patients with AIDS is likely caused by infection of macrophages (microglial cells) in the brain.

The clinical course of HIV/AIDS has been dramatically changed by effective antiretroviral drug therapy. With appropriate treatment, patients exhibit much slower progression of the disease, fewer opportunistic infections, and greatly reduced incidence of cancers and dementia.

The immune response to HIV is ineffective in controlling spread of the virus and its pathologic effects. Infected patients produce antibodies and CTLs against viral antigens, and the responses help to limit the early, acute HIV syndrome (Fig. 12–10, *B*). But these immune responses usually do not prevent progression of the disease. Antibodies against envelope glycoproteins, such as gp120, may be ineffective because the virus rapidly mutates the region of gp120 that is the target of most antibodies. CTLs often are ineffective in killing infected cells because the virus inhibits the expression of class I MHC molecules by the infected cells. Immune responses to HIV may paradoxically promote spread of the infection. Antibody-coated viral particles may bind to Fc receptors on macrophages and follicular dendritic cells in lymphoid organs, thus increasing virus entry into these cells and creating additional reservoirs of infection. If CTLs are able to kill infected cells, the dead cells may be cleared by phagocytosis, resulting in spread of the virus to macrophages. By infecting and thus interfering with the function of immune cells, the virus is able to prevent its own eradication.

A small fraction of patients control HIV infection without therapy; these individuals are often referred to as elite controllers or long-term nonprogressors. There has been great interest in defining the genes that may protect these individuals, because elucidation of these genes may suggest therapeutic approaches. Some of these subjects inherit a deletion in the CCR5 chemokine receptor that compromises its ability to function as a coreceptor for viral entry. The presence of certain HLA alleles, such as HLA-B57 and HLA-B27, also seems to be protective, perhaps because these HLA molecules are particularly efficient at presenting HIV peptides to CD8+ T cells.

Therapy and Vaccination Strategies

The current treatment for AIDS is aimed at controlling replication of HIV and the infectious complications of the disease. Combinations of drugs that block the activity of the viral reverse transcriptase, protease, and integrase enzymes are now being administered early in the course of the infection, with considerable benefit. This therapeutic approach is called highly active antiretroviral therapy (HAART) or combination antiretroviral therapy (ART). The virus is capable of mutations that may render it resistant to the drugs used, and reservoirs of latent virus are not eradicated by these drugs. Additional drugs that inhibit fusion of the virus with host cells have been developed.

The development of effective vaccines will likely be a major component of the strategy for control of HIV infection worldwide. A successful vaccine probably needs to induce an innate immune response, high titers of neutralizing antibodies, and a strong T cell response, as well as mucosal immunity. It has proved difficult to achieve all these goals with current vaccination strategies. An additional challenge is the ability to protect against all subtypes of HIV. Early efforts focused on gp120 as an immunogen but were largely unsuccessful because of the high rate of mutations in gp120. More recent attempts have involved combinations of DNA immunization and recombinant poxviruses encoding several different HIV proteins. It will take years to judge the effectiveness of new vaccines in clinical trials.

SUMMARY

- Immunodeficiency diseases are caused by defects in various components of the immune system that result in increased susceptibility to infections and some cancers. Congenital (primary) immunodeficiency diseases are caused by genetic abnormalities. Acquired (secondary) immunodeficiencies are the result of infections, cancers, malnutrition, or treatments for other conditions that adversely affect the cells of the immune system.

- Some congenital immunodeficiency diseases result from mutations that block the maturation of lymphocytes. Severe combined immunodeficiency may be caused by mutations in the cytokine receptor γ_c chain that reduces the IL-7–driven proliferation of immature lymphocytes, by mutations in enzymes involved in purine metabolism, or by other defects in lymphocyte maturation. Selective B cell maturation defects are seen in X-linked agammaglobulinemia, caused by abnormalities in an enzyme involved in B cell maturation (BTK), and selective T cell maturation defects are seen in the DiGeorge syndrome, in which the thymus does not develop normally.

- Some immunodeficiency diseases are caused by defects in lymphocyte activation, despite their normal maturation. The X-linked hyper-IgM syndrome is caused by mutations in the gene encoding CD40 ligand, and helper T cell–dependent B cell responses (e.g., Ig heavy chain class switching) and T cell–dependent macrophage activation are defective. The bare lymphocyte syndrome is caused by defective expression of class II MHC proteins, resulting in defective maturation and activation of CD4$^+$ T cells.
- Acquired immunodeficiency syndrome is caused by the retrovirus HIV, which infects CD4$^+$ T cells, macrophages, and dendritic cells by using an envelope protein (gp120) to bind to CD4 and chemokine receptors. The viral RNA is reverse transcribed and the resulting DNA integrates into the host genome, where it may be activated to produce infectious virus. Infected cells die during this process of virus replication, and death of cells of the immune system is the principal mechanism by which the virus causes immune deficiency.
- The clinical course of HIV infection typically consists of acute viremia, clinical latency with progressive destruction of CD4$^+$ T cells and dissolution of lymphoid tissues, and ultimately AIDS, with severe immunodeficiency resulting in opportunistic infections, some cancers, weight loss, and occasionally dementia. Treatment of HIV infection is designed to interfere with the life cycle of the virus. Vaccine development is ongoing.

REVIEW QUESTIONS

1. What are the most common clinicopathologic manifestations of immunodeficiency diseases?
2. What are some of the proteins affected by mutations that may block the maturation of T and B lymphocytes in human immunodeficiency diseases?
3. What are some of the mutations that may block activation or effector functions of both mature CD4$^+$ T cells and B cells, and what are the clinicopathologic consequences of these mutations?
4. How does HIV infect cells and replicate inside infected cells?
5. What are the principal clinical manifestations of advanced HIV infection, and what is the pathogenesis of these manifestations?

Answers to and discussion of the Review Questions are available at studentconsult.com

Suggested Readings

CHAPTER 1

Bromley SK, Mempel TR, Luster AD: Orchestrating the orchestrators: chemokines in control of T cell traffic. Nature Immunology 9:970-980, 2008.

Burnet FM: A modification of Jerne's theory of antibody production using the concept of clonal selection. Australian Journal of Science 20:67-69, 1957.

Drayton DL, Liao S, Mounzer RW, Ruddle NH: Lymphoid organ development: from ontogeny to neogenesis. Nature Immunology 7:344-353, 2006.

Jerne NK: The natural-selection theory of antibody formation. Proceedings of the National Academy of Sciences of the United States of America 41:849-857, 1955.

Luster AD, Alon R, von Andrian UH: Immune cell migration in inflammation: present and future therapeutic targets. Nature Immunology 6:1182-1190, 2005.

Mebius RE, Kraal G: Structure and function of the spleen. Nature Reviews Immunology 5:606-616, 2005.

Sallusto F, Baggiolini M: Chemokines and leukocyte traffic. Nature Immunology 9:949-952, 2008.

Von Andrian UH, Mempel TR: Homing and cellular traffic in lymph nodes. Nature Reviews Immunology 3:867-878, 2003.

CHAPTER 2

Akira S, Uematsu S, Takeuchi O: Pathogen recognition and innate immunity. Cell 124:783-801, 2006.

Amulic B, Cazalet C, Hayes GL, et al: Neutrophil function: from mechanisms to disease. Annual Review of Immunology 30:459-489, 2012.

Blasius AL, Beutler B: Intracellular Toll-like receptors. Immunity 32:305-315, 2010.

Borregaard N: Neutrophils: from marrow to microbes. Immunity 33:657-670, 2010.

Chen G, Shaw MH, Kim YG, Nuñez G: Nod-like receptors: role in innate immunity and inflammatory disease. Annual Review of Pathology 4:365-398, 2009.

Dale DC, Boxer L, Liles WC: The phagocytes: neutrophils and monocytes. Blood 112:935-945, 2008.

Franchi L, Munoz-Planilla R, Nunez G: Sensing and reacting to microbes through the inflammasomes. Nature Immunology 13:325-332, 2012.

Hotchkiss RS, Karl IE: The pathophysiology and treatment of sepsis. New England Journal of Medicine 348:138-150, 2003.

Janeway C, Medzhitov R: Innate immune recognition. Annual Review of Immunology 20:197-216, 2002.

Kawai T, Akira S: Innate immune recognition of viral infection. Nature Immunology 7:131-137, 2006.

Klotman ME, Chang TL: Defensins in innate antiviral immunity. Nature Reviews Immunology 6:447-456, 2006.

Lanier LL: NK cell recognition. Annual Review of Immunology 23:225-274, 2005.

Ley K, Laudanna C, Cybulsky MI, Nourshargh S: Getting to the site of inflammation: the leukocyte adhesion cascade updated. Nature Reviews Immunology 7:678-689, 2007.

Masters SL, Simon A, Aksentijevich I, Kastner DL: Horror autoinflammaticus: the molecular pathophysiology of autoinflammatory disease. Annual Review of Immunology 27:621-668, 2009.

Pichlmair A, Reis e Sousa C: Innate recognition of viruses. Immunity 27:370-383, 2007.

Rock KL, Latz E, Ontiveros F, Kono H: The sterile inflammatory response. Annual Review of Immunology 28:321-342, 2010.

Schroder K, Tschopp J: The inflammasomes. Cell 140:821-832, 2010.

Selsted ME, Ouellette AJ: Mammalian defensins in the anti-microbial immune response. Nature Immunology 6:551-557, 2005.

Steinman RM: Decisions about dendritic cells: past, present and future. Annual Review of Immunology, 30:1-22, 2012.

Takeuchi O, Akira S: Pattern recognition receptors and inflammation. Cell 140:805-820, 2010.

Underhill DM, Ozinsky A: Phagocytosis of microbes: complexity in action. Annual Review of Immunology 20:825-852, 2002.

Vivier E, Tomasello E, Baratin M, et al: Functions of natural killer cells. Nature Immunology 9:503-510, 2008.

Zlotnik A, Yoshie O: The chemokine superfamily revisited. Immunity 36:705-716, 2012.

CHAPTER 3

Bousso P: T-cell activation by dendritic cells in the lymph node: lessons from the movies. Nature Reviews Immunology 8:675-684, 2008.

Germain RN, Jenkins MK: In vivo antigen presentation. Current Opinion in Immunology 16:120-125, 2004.

Hansen TH, Bouvier M: MHC class I antigen presentation: learning from viral evasion strategies. Nature Reviews Immunology 9:503-513, 2009.

Heath WR, Carbone FR: Dendritic cell subsets in primary and secondary T cell responses at body surfaces. Nature Immunology 10:1237-1244, 2009.

Horton R, Wilming L, Lovering RC, et al: Gene map of the extended human MHC. Nature Reviews Genetics 5:889-899, 2004.

Joffre OP, Segura E, Savina A, Amigorena S: Cross-presentation by dendritic cells. Nature Reviews Immunology 12:557-569, 2012.

Kurts C, Robinson BW, Knolle PA: Cross-priming in health and disease. Nature Reviews Immunology 10:403-414, 2010.

López-Bravo M, Ardavín C: In vivo induction of immune responses to pathogens by conventional dendritic cells. Immunity 29:343-351, 2008.

Neefjes J, Jongsma ML, Paul P, Bakke O: Towards a systems understanding of MHC class I and MHC class II antigen presentation. Nature Review Immunology 11:823-836, 2011.

Ramachandra L, Simmons D, and Harding CV: MHC molecules and microbial antigen processing in phagosomes. Current Opinion in Immunology 21:98-104, 2009.

Segura E, Villadangos JA: Antigen presentation by dendritic cells in vivo. Current Opinion in Immunology 21:105-110, 2009.

Trombetta ES, Mellman I: Cell biology of antigen processing in vitro and in vivo. Annual Review of Immunology 23:975-1028, 2005.

Watts C: The exogenous pathway for antigen presentation on major histocompatibility complex class II and CD1 molecules. Nature Immunology 5:685-692, 2004.

CHAPTER 4

Boehm T: Thymus development and function. Current Opinion in Immunology 20:178-184, 2008.

Davis SJ, Ikemizu S, Evans EJ, et al: The nature of molecular recognition by T cells. Nature Immunology 4:217-224, 2003.

Jung D, Giallourakis C, Mostoslavsky R, Alt FW: Mechanism and control of V(D)J recombination at the immunoglobulin heavy chain locus. Annual Review of Immunology 24:541-570, 2006.

Klein L, Hinterberger M, Wirnsberger G, Kyewski B: Antigen presentation in the thymus for positive selection and central tolerance induction. Nature Reviews Immunology 9:833-844, 2009.

Law M, Hengartner L: Antibodies against viruses: passive and active immunization. Current Opinion in Immunology 20:486-492, 2008.

Matthews AG, Oettinger MA: RAG: a recombinase diversified. Nature Immunology 10:817-821, 2009.

Nemazee D: Receptor selection in B and T lymphocytes. Annual Review of Immunology 18:19-51, 2000.

Pillai S, Cariappa A, Moran ST: Marginal zone B cells. Annual Review of Immunology 23:161-196, 2005.

Rothenberg EV: Cell lineage regulators in B and T cell development. Nature Immunology 8:441-444, 2007.

Rudolph MG, Stanfield RL, Wilson IA: How TCRs bind MHCs, peptides, and coreceptors. Annual Review of Immunology 24:419-466, 2006.

Stritesky GL, Jameson SC, Hogquist K: Selection of self-reactive T cells in the thymus. Annual Review of Immunology 30:95-114, 2012.

Von Boehmer H, Melchers F: Checkpoints in lymphocyte development and autoimmune disease. Nature Immunology 11:14-20, 2010.

CHAPTER 5

Amsen D, Spilanakis CG, Flavell RA: How are T_H1 and T_H2 cells made? Current Opinion in Immunology 21:153-160, 2009.

Boyman O, Sprent J: The role of interleukin-2 during homeostasis and activation of the immune system. Nature Reviews Immunology 12:180-190, 2012.

Dustin ML: A dynamic view of the immunological synapse. Seminars in Immunology 17:400-410, 2005.

Fooksman DR, Varchana S, Vasiliver-Shamis G, et al: Functional anatomy of T cell activation and synapse formation. Annual Review of Immunology 28:79-105, 2010.

Gallo EM, Cante-Barrett K, Crabtree GR: Lymphocyte calcium signaling from membrane to nucleus. Nature Immunology 7:25-32, 2006.

Greenwald RJ, Freeman GJ, Sharpe AH: The B7 family revisited. Annual Review of Immunology 23:515–548, 2005.

Kaech SM, Wherry EJ: Heterogeneity and cell-fate decisions in effector and memory $CD8^+$ T cell differentiation during viral infection. Immunity 27:393-405, 2007.

Krammer PH, Arnold R, Lavrik IN: Life and death in peripheral T cells. Nature Reviews Immunology 7:532-542, 2007.

Vignali DA, Kuchroo VK: IL-12 cytokines: Immunological playmakers. Nature Immunology 13:722-728, 2012.

Zhu J, Yamane H, Paul WE: Differentiation of effector CD4 T cell populations. Annual Review of Immunology 28:445-489, 2010.

CHAPTER 6

Bettelli E, Oukka M, Kuchroo VK: T(H)-17 cells in the circle of immunity and autoimmunity. Nature Immunology 8:345-350, 2007.

Billiau P, Matthys P: Interferon-γ: a historical perspective. Cytokine and Growth Factor Reviews 20:97-113, 2009.

Choi J, Enis DR, Koh KP, et al: T lymphocyte–endothelial cell interactions. Annual Review of Immunology 22: 683-709, 2004.

Gordon S, Martinez FO: Alternative activation of macrophages: mechanisms and functions. Immunity 32:593-604, 2010.

Kapsenberg ML: Dendritic-cell control of pathogen-derived T-cell polarization. Nature Reviews Immunology 3:984-993, 2003.

Lieberman J: The ABCs of granule-mediated cytotoxicity: new weapons in the arsenal Nature Reviews Immunology 3:361-370, 2003.

Littman DR, Rudensky AY: Th17 and regulatory T cells in mediating and restraining inflammation. Cell 140:845-858, 2010.

Pribila JT, Quale AC, Mueller KL, Shimizu Y: Integrins and T cell–mediated immunity. Annual Review of Immunology 22:157-180, 2004.

Reiner SL: Development in motion: helper T cells at work. Cell 129:33-36, 2007.

Reiner SL, Sallusto F, Lanzavecchia A: Division of labor with a workforce of one: challenges in specifying effector and memory T cell fate. Science 317:622-625, 2007.

Sallusto F, Geginat J, Lanzavecchia A: Central memory and effector memory T cell subsets: function, generation, and maintenance. Annual Review of Immunology 22:745-763, 2004.

Schaible UE, Collins HL, Kaufmann SH: Confrontation between intracellular bacteria and the immune system. Advances in Immunology 71:267-377, 1999.

Von Andrian UH, Mackay CR: T-cell function and migration. New England Journal of Medicine 343:1020-1034, 2000.

Wan YY, Flavell RA: How diverse: CD4 effector T cells and their functions. Journal of Molecular and Cell Biology 1:20-36, 2009.

Zhang N, Bevan MJ: CD8(+) T cells: foot soldiers of the immune system. Immunity 35:161-168, 2011.

CHAPTER 7

Allen CD, Okada T, Cyster JG: Germinal-center organization and cellular dynamics Immunity 27:190-202, 2007.

Carroll MC: The complement system in B cell regulation. Molecular Immunology 41:141-146, 2004.

Dorner T, Radbruch A: Antibodies and B cell memory in viral immunity. Immunity 27:384-392, 2007.

Dudley DD, Chaudhuri J, Bassing CH, Alt FW: Mechanism and control of V(D)J recombination versus class switch recombination: Similarities and differences. Advances in Immunology 86:43-112, 2005.

Honjo T, Muramatsu M, Fagarasan S: AID: How does it aid antibody diversity? Immunity 20:659-668, 2004.

Manz RA, Hauser AE, Hiepe F, Radbruch A: Maintenance of serum antibody levels. Annual Review of Immunology 23:367-386, 2005.

Pan-Hammarstrom Q, Zhao Y, Hammarstrom L: Class switch recombination: A comparison between mouse and human. Advances in Immunology 93:1-61, 2007.

Radbruch A, Muehlinghaus G, Luger EO, et al: Competence and competition: The challenge of becoming a long-lived plasma cell. Nature Reviews Immunology 6:741-750, 2006.

Shapiro-Shelef M, Calame K: Regulation of plasma cell development. Nature Reviews Immunology 5:230-242, 2005.

Shlomchik MJ, Weisel F: Germinal center selection and the development of memory B and plasma cells. Immunology Reviews. 247:52-63, 2012.

Victora GD, Nussenzweig MC: Germinal centers. Annual Review of Immunology 30:429-457, 2012.

CHAPTER 8

Baker K, Qiao SW, Kuo T, et al: Immune and non-immune functions of the (not so) neonatal Fc receptor, FcRn. Seminars in Immunopathology 31:223-236, 2009.

Carroll MC: The complement system in regulation of adaptive immunity. Nature Immunology 5:981-986, 2004.

Carroll MV, Sim RB: Complement in health and disease. Advances in Drug Delivery Reviews 63:965-975, 2011.

Fargarsan S, Honjo T: Regulation of IgA synthesis at mucosal surfaces. Current Opinion in Immunology 16:277-283, 2004.

Macpherson AJ, Geuking MB, McCoy KD. Homeland Security: IgA immunity at the frontiers of the body. Trends in Immunology 33:160-167, 2012.

Marshall-Clarke S, Reen D, Tasker L, Hassan J: Neonatal immunity: how well has it grown up? Immunology Today 21:35-41, 2000.

Nimmerjahn F, Ravetch JV: FcγRs in health and disease. Current Topics in Microbiology and Immunology 350:105-125, 2011.

Parren PW, Burton DR: The antiviral activity of antibodies in vitro and in vivo. Advances in Immunology 77:195-262, 2001.

Roozendaal R, Carroll MC: Emerging patterns in complement-mediated pathogen recognition. Cell 125:29-32, 2006.

Ward ES: Acquiring maternal immunoglobulin: different receptors, similar functions. Immunity 20:507-508, 2004.

CHAPTER 9

Cheng MH, Anderson M: Monogenic autoimmunity. Annual Review of Immunology 30:393-427, 2012.

Chervonsky A: Influence of microbial environment on autoimmunity. Nature Immunology 11:28-35, 2010.

Fathman CG, Lineberry NB: Molecular mechanisms of CD4+ T-cell anergy. Nature Reviews Immunology 7:599-609, 2007.

Goodnow CC: Multistep pathogenesis of autoimmune disease. Cell 130:25-35, 2007.

Hogquist KA, Baldwin TA, Jameson SC: Central tolerance: learning self-control in the thymus. Nature Reviews Immunology 5:772-782, 2005.

Josefowicz SZ, Lu LF, Rudensky AY: Regulatory T cells: mechanisms of differentiation and function. Annual Review of Immunology 30:531-564, 2012.

Kyewski B, Klein L: A central role for central tolerance. Annual Review of Immunology 24:571-606, 2006.

Miller SD, Turley DM, Podojil JR: Antigen-specific tolerance strategies for the prevention and treatment of autoimmune disease. Nature Reviews Immunology 7:665-677, 2007.

Mueller DL: Mechanisms maintaining peripheral tolerance. Nature Immunology 11:21-27, 2010.

Nemazee D: Receptor editing in lymphocyte development and central tolerance. Nature Reviews Immunology 6:728-740, 2006.

Parish IA, Heath WR: Too dangerous to ignore: self-tolerance and the control of ignorant autoreactive T cells. Immunology Cell Biology 86:146-152, 2008.

Sakaguchi S, Miyara M, Costantino CM, Hafler DA: FOXP3+ regulatory T cells in the human immune system. Nature Reviews Immunology 10:490-500, 2010.

Sakaguchi S, Yamaguchi T, Nomura T, Ono M: Regulatory T cells and immune tolerance. Cell 133:775-787, 2008.

Singh NJ, Schwartz RH: Primer: mechanisms of immunologic tolerance. Nature Clinical Practice Rheumatology 2:44-52, 2006.

Steinman RM, Hawiger D, Nussenzweig MC: Tolerogenic dendritic cells. Annual Review of Immunology 21:685-711, 2003.

Von Boehmer H, Melchers F: Checkpoints in lymphocyte development and autoimmune disease. Nature Immunology 11:14-20, 2010.

Zenewicz L, Abraham C, Flavell RA, Cho J: Unraveling the genetics of autoimmunity. Cell 140:791-797, 2010.

Zheng Y, Rudensky AY: Foxp3 in control of the regulatory T cell lineage. Nature Immunology 8:457-462, 2007.

CHAPTER 10

Baldwin WM, Valujskikh A, Fairchild RL: Antibody mediated rejection: emergence of animal models to answer clinical questions. American Journal of Transplantation 10:1135-1142, 2010.

Boon T, Coulie PG, van den Eynde BJ, van der Bruggen P: Human T cell responses against melanoma. Annual Review of Immunology 24:175-208, 2006.

Burnet FM: The concept of immunological surveillance. Progress in Experimental Tumor Research 13:1-27, 1970.

Chidgey AP, Layton D, Trounson A, Boyd RL: Tolerance strategies for stem-cell-based therapies. Nature 453:330-377, 2008.

Chinen J, Buckley RH: Transplantation immunology: solid organ and bone marrow. Journal of Allergy and Clinical Immunology 125:S324-S335, 2010.

Clarkson MR, Sayegh MH: T-cell costimulatory pathways in allograft rejection and tolerance. Transplantation 80:555-563, 2005.

Colvin RB, Smith RN: Antibody-mediated organ-allograft rejection. Nature Reviews Immunology 5:807-817, 2005.

Farkas AM, Finn OJ: Vaccines based on abnormal self antigens as tumor-associated antigens: immune regulation. Seminars in Immunology 22:125-131, 2010.

Finn OJ: Cancer immunology. New England Journal of Medicine 358:2704-2715, 2008.

Gibbons C, Sykes M: Manipulating the immune system for anti-tumor responses and transplant tolerance via mixed hematopoietic chimerism. Immunological Reviews 223:33-36, 2008.

Gilboa E: DC-based cancer vaccines. Journal of Clinical Investigation 117:1195-1203, 2007.

Gould DS, Auchincloss H Jr: Direct and indirect recognition: the role of MHC antigens in graft rejection. Immunology Today 20:77-82, 1999.

Grivennikov SI, Greten FR, Karin M: Immunity, inflammation, and cancer. Cell 140:883-899, 2010.

Halloran PF: Immunosuppressive drugs for kidney transplantation. New England Journal of Medicine 351:2715-2729, 2004.

Harris M: Monoclonal antibodies as therapeutic agents for cancer. Lancet Oncology 5:292-302, 2004.

June CH: Principles of adoptive T cell cancer therapy. Journal of Clinical Investigation 117:1204-1212, 2007.

Mantovani A, Allavena P, Sica A, Balkwill F: Cancer-related inflammation. Nature 454:436-444, 2008.

Mellman I, Coukos G, Dranoff G: Cancer immunotherapy comes of age. Nature 480:480-489, 2012.

Nankivell BJ, Alexander SI: Rejection of the kidney allograft. New England Journal of Medicine 363:1451-1462, 2010.

Safinia N, Sagoo P, Lechler R, Lombardi G: Adoptive regulatory T cell therapy: challenges in clinical transplantation. Current Opinions in Organ Transplantation 15:427-434, 2010.

Schreiber RD, Old LJ, Smyth MJ: Cancer immunoediting: integrating immunity's roles in cancer suppression and promotion. Science 331:1565-1570, 2011.

Swann JB, Smyth MJ: Immune surveillance of tumors. Journal of Clinical Investigation 117:1137-1146, 2007.

Weiner LM, Surana R, Wang S: Monoclonal antibodies: versatile platforms for cancer immunotherapy. Nature Reviews Immunology 10:317-327, 2010.

Yang YG, Sykes M: Xenotransplantation: current status and a perspective on the future. Nature Reviews Immunology 7:519-531, 2007.

CHAPTER 11

Bach JF: Infections and autoimmune diseases. Journal of Autoimmunity 25(Suppl 1):74-80, 2005.

Bischoff SC: Role of mast cells in allergic and non-allergic immune responses: comparison of human and murine data. Nature Reviews Immunology 7:93-104, 2007.

Chatenoud L: Immune therapies of autoimmune diseases: are we approaching a real cure? Current Opinion in Immunology 18:710-717, 2006.

Cohn L, Elias JA, Chupp GL: Asthma: mechanisms of disease persistence and progression. Annual Review of Immunology 22:789-815, 2004.

Costa JJ, Weller PF, Galli SJ: The cells of the allergic response. Journal of the American Medical Association 278:1815-1822, 1997.

Davidson A, Diamond B: Autoimmune diseases. New England Journal of Medicine 345:340-350, 2001.

Frohman EM, Racke MK, Raine CS: Multiple sclerosis: the plague and its pathogenesis. New England Journal of Medicine 354:942-955, 2006.

Galli SJ, Kalesnikoff J, Grimbaldeston MA, et al: Mast cells as "tunable" effector and immunoregulatory cells: recent advances. Annual Review of Immunology 23:749-786, 2005.

Goodnow CC: Multistep pathogenesis of autoimmune disease. Cell 130:25-35, 2007.

Gould HJ, Sutton BJ: IgE in allergy and asthma today. Nature Reviews Immunology 8:205-217, 2008.

Gutcher I, Becher B: APC-derived cytokines and T cell polarization in autoimmune inflammation. Journal of Clinical Investigation 117:1119-1127, 2007.

Kay AB: Allergy and allergic diseases. New England Journal of Medicine 344:30-37, 109-113, 2001.

Kim HY, DeKruyff RH, Umetsu DT: The many paths to asthma: phenotype shaped by innate and adaptive immunity. Nature Immunology 11:577-584, 2010.

Marshak-Rothstein A: Toll-like receptors in systemic autoimmune disease. Nature Reviews Immunology 6:823-835, 2006.

McInnes IB, Schett G: The pathogenesis of rheumatoid arthritis. New England Journal of Medicine 365:2205-2219, 2011.

Palmer MT, Weaver CT: Autoimmunity: increasing suspects in the CD4$^+$ T cell lineage. Nature Immunology 11:36-40, 2010.

Rioux JD, Abbas AK: Paths to understanding the genetic basis of autoimmune disease. Nature 435:584-589, 2005.

Stone KD, Prussin C, Metcalfe DD: IgE, mast cells, basophils, and eosinophils. Journal of Allergy and Clinical Immunology 125:S73-S80, 2010.

Strober W, Fuss I, Mannon P: The fundamental basis of inflammatory bowel disease. Journal of Clinical Investigation 117:514-521, 2007.

Tsokos GC: Systemic lupus erythematosus. New England Journal of Medicine 365:2110-2121, 2011.

Wills-Karp M, Ewart SL: Time to draw breath: asthma-susceptibility genes are identified. Nature Reviews Genetics 5:376-387, 2004.

CHAPTER 12

Barouch DH: Challenges in the development of an HIV-1 vaccine. Nature 455:613-619, 2008.

Booth C, Gaspar HB, Thrasher AJ: Gene therapy for primary immunodeficiency. Current Opinion in Pediatrics 23:659-666, 2011.

Buckley RH: Molecular defects in human severe combined immunodeficiency and approaches to immune reconstitution. Annual Review of Immunology 22:625-655, 2004.

Bustamante J, Boisson-Dupuis S, Jouangay E, et al: Novel primary immunodeficiencies revealed by the investigation of paediatric infectious diseases. Current Opinion in Immunology 20:39-48, 2008.

Chen X, Jensen PE: MHC class II antigen presentation and immunological abnormalities due to deficiency of MHC class II and its associated genes. Experimental and Molecular Pathology 85:40-44, 2008.

Cunningham-Rundles C, Ponda PP: Molecular defects in T- and B-cell primary immunodeficiency diseases. Nature Reviews Immunology 5:880-892, 2005.

Ganser-Pornillos BK, Yeager M, Pornillos O: Assembly and architecture of HIV. Advances in Experimental Medicine and Biology 726:441-465, 2012.

Hladik F, McElrath MJ: Setting the stage: host invasion by HIV. Nature Reviews Immunology 8:447-457, 2008.

Holland SM: Chronic granulomatous disease. Clinical Review of Allergy and Immunology 38:3-10, 2010.

Mascola JR, Montefiori DC: The role of antibodies in HIV vaccines. Annual Review of Immunology 28:413-444, 2010.

McMichael AJ, Borrow P, Tomaras GD, et al: The immune response during acute HIV-1 infection: clues for vaccine development. Nature Reviews Immunology 10:11-23, 2010.

Moir S, Chun TW, Fauci AS: Pathogenic mechanisms of HIV disease. Annual Review of Pathololgy 6:223-248, 2011.

Notarangelo LD: Primary immunodeficiencies. Journal of Allergy and Clinical Immunology 125:S182-S194, 2010.

Picker LJ, Hansen SG, Lifson JD: New paradigms for HIV/AIDS vaccine development. Annual Review of Medicine 63:95-111, 2012.

Rezaei N, Hedayat M, Aghamohammadi A, Nichols KE: Primary immunodeficiency diseases associated with increased susceptibility to viral infections and malignancies. Journal of Allergy and Clinical Immunology 127:1329-1341, 2011.

Simon V, Ho DD, Abdool Karim Q: HIV/AIDS epidemiology, pathogenesis, prevention, and treatment. Lancet 368:489-504, 2006.

Sponzilli I, Notarangelo LD: Severe combined immunodeficiency (SCID): from molecular basis to clinical management. Acta Biomedica 82:5-13, 2011.

Volberding PA, Deeks SG: Antiretroviral therapy and management of HIV infection. Lancet 376:49-62, 2010.

Walker BD, Burton DR: Toward an AIDS vaccine. Science 320:760-764, 2008.

Wilen CB, Tilton JC, Doms RW: Molecular mechanisms of HIV entry. Advances in Experimental Medicine and Biology 726:223-242, 2012.

Glossary

αβ T cell receptor (αβ TCR) The most common form of TCR, expressed on both CD4$^+$ and CD8$^+$ T cells. The αβ TCR recognizes peptide antigen bound to an MHC molecule. Both α and β chains contain highly variable (V) regions that together form the antigen-binding site, as well as constant (C) regions. TCR V and C regions are structurally homologous to the V and C regions of immunoglobulin (Ig) molecules.

ABO blood group antigens Carbohydrate antigens attached mainly to cell surface proteins (and a small fraction to lipids) and present on many cell types, including red blood cells. These antigens differ among individuals, depending on inherited alleles encoding the enzymes required for synthesis of the carbohydrate antigens. The ABO antigens act as alloantigens responsible for blood transfusion reactions and hyperacute rejection of allografts.

Acquired immunodeficiency Deficiency in the immune system that is acquired after birth, usually because of infection (e.g., AIDS), and that is not related to a genetic defect; also called secondary immunodeficiency.

Acquired immunodeficiency syndrome (AIDS) Disease caused by human immunodeficiency virus (HIV) infection that is characterized by depletion of CD4$^+$ T cells, leading to a profound defect in cell-mediated immunity. Clinically, AIDS includes opportunistic infections, malignant tumors, wasting, and encephalopathy.

Activation-induced cell death (AICD) Apoptosis of activated lymphocytes, generally used for T cells; considered Fas-mediated apoptosis by some, but this is not the only mechanism of AICD.

Activation-induced (cytidine) deaminase (AID) Enzyme expressed in B cells that catalyzes the conversion of cytidine into uridine in DNA molecules and that is required for somatic hypermutation and Ig class switch recombination.

Activation protein 1 (AP-1) Family of DNA-binding transcription factors composed of dimers of two proteins that bind to one another through a shared structural motif called a leucine zipper. The best-characterized AP-1 factor is composed of the proteins Fos and Jun. AP-1 is involved in transcriptional regulation of many different genes important in the immune system, such as cytokine genes.

Active immunity The form of adaptive immunity that is induced by exposure to a foreign antigen and activation of lymphocytes and in which the immunized individual plays an active role in responding to the antigen. This type contrasts with passive immunity, in which an individual receives antibodies or lymphocytes from another individual who was previously actively immunized.

Acute rejection The form of graft rejection involving vascular and parenchymal injury mediated by T cells, macrophages, and antibodies that usually occurs days or weeks after transplantation but may occur later if immunosuppression becomes inadequate.

Acute-phase reactants Proteins, mostly synthesized in the liver, whose plasma concentrations increase shortly after infection as part of the systemic inflammatory response syndrome. Examples include C-reactive protein, fibrinogen, and serum amyloid A protein. Hepatic synthesis of these molecules is upregulated by inflammatory cytokines, especially IL-6 and TNF. The acute-phase reactants play various roles in the innate immune response to microbes.

Acute-phase response Increase in plasma concentrations of several proteins, called acute-phase reactants, which occurs as part of the early innate immune response to infections.

Adaptive immunity The form of immunity that is mediated by lymphocytes and stimulated by exposure to infectious agents. In contrast to innate immunity, adaptive immunity is characterized by exquisite specificity for distinct macromolecules and memory, which is the ability to respond more vigorously to repeated exposure to the same microbe. Also called specific immunity or acquired immunity.

Adaptor protein Proteins involved in intracellular signal transduction pathways by serving as bridge molecules or scaffolds for the recruitment of other signaling molecules. During lymphocyte antigen receptor or cytokine receptor signaling, adaptor molecules may be phosphorylated on tyrosine residues to enable them to bind other proteins containing Src homology 2 (SH2) domains. Adaptor molecules involved in T cell activation include LAT, SLP-76, and Grb-2.

Adhesion molecule Cell surface molecule whose function is to promote adhesive interactions with other cells or the extracellular matrix. Leukocytes express various types of adhesion molecules, such as selectins, integrins, and members of the Ig superfamily, and these molecules play crucial roles in cell migration and cellular activation in innate and adaptive immune responses.

Adjuvant A substance, distinct from antigen, which enhances T and B cell activation mainly by promoting the accumulation and activation of antigen-presenting cells (APCs) at the site of antigen exposure. Adjuvants stimulate expression of T cell–activating costimulators and cytokines by APCs and may also prolong the expression of peptide-MHC complexes on the surface of APCs.

Adoptive transfer Process of transferring lymphocytes from one, usually immunized individual into another individual. Adoptive transfer is used in research to define the role of a particular cell population (e.g., T cells) in an immune response. Clinically, adoptive transfer of tumor-reactive T lymphocytes is used in experimental cancer therapy.

Affinity Strength of the binding between a single binding site of a molecule (e.g., an antibody) and a ligand (e.g., an antigen). The affinity of a molecule X for a ligand Y is represented by the dissociation constant (K_d), which is the concentration of Y that is required to occupy the combining sites of half the X molecules present in a solution. A smaller K_d indicates a stronger or higher-affinity interaction, and a lower concentration of ligand is needed to occupy the sites.

Affinity maturation Process that leads to increased affinity of antibodies for a particular antigen as a humoral response progresses. Affinity maturation takes place in germinal centers of lymphoid tissues and is the result of somatic mutation of Ig genes, followed by selective survival of the B cells producing the highest-affinity antibodies.

Allele One of different forms of a gene present at a particular chromosomal locus. An individual who is heterozygous at a locus has two different alleles, each on a different member of a pair of chromosomes, one inherited from the mother and one from the father. If a particular gene in a population has many different alleles, the gene or locus is said to be polymorphic. The MHC locus is extremely polymorphic.

Allelic exclusion The exclusive expression of only one of two inherited alleles encoding Ig heavy and light chains and T cell receptor (TCR) β chains. Allelic exclusion occurs when the protein product of one, productively recombined antigen receptor locus on one chromosome blocks rearrangement of the corresponding locus on the other chromosome. This property ensures that each lymphocyte will express a single antigen receptor, and that all the antigen receptors expressed by one clone of lymphocytes will have the identical specificity. Because the TCR α chain locus does not show allelic exclusion, some T cells do express two different types of TCR.

Allergen An antigen that elicits an immediate hypersensitivity (allergic) reaction. Allergens are proteins or chemicals bound to proteins that induce IgE antibody responses in atopic individuals.

Allergy Disorder caused by an immediate hypersensitivity reaction, often referring to the type of antigen that elicits the disease, such as food allergy, bee sting allergy, and penicillin allergy. All these conditions are the result of antigen-induced T_H2 generation and IgE production, and mast cell or basophil activation.

Alloantibody An antibody specific for an alloantigen (i.e., an antigen present in some individuals of a species but not in others).

Alloantigen Cell or tissue antigen that is present in some members of a species but not in others and that is recognized as foreign on an allograft. Alloantigens are usually products of polymorphic genes.

Alloantiserum The alloantibody-containing serum of an individual who has previously been exposed to one or more alloantigens.

Allogeneic graft Organ or tissue graft from a donor who is of the same species but genetically nonidentical to the recipient; also called an allograft.

Alloreactive Reactive to alloantigens; describes T cells or antibodies from one individual that will recognize antigens on cells or tissues of another, genetically nonidentical individual.

Alternative macrophage activation Macrophage activation by IL-4 and IL-13 leading to an antiinflammatory and tissue reparative phenotype, in contrast to classical macrophage activation by interferon-γ and TLR ligands.

Alternative pathway of complement activation Antibody-independent pathway of activation of the complement system that occurs when the C3b protein binds to microbial cell surfaces. The alternative pathway is a component of the innate immune system and mediates inflammatory responses to infection as well as direct lysis of microbes.

Anaphylactic shock Cardiovascular collapse occurring in the setting of a systemic immediate hypersensitivity reaction.

Anaphylatoxins The C5a, C4a, and C3a complement fragments that are generated during complement activation. The anaphylatoxins bind specific cell surface receptors and promote acute inflammation by stimulating neutrophil chemotaxis and activating mast cells.

Anaphylaxis Severe systemic form of immediate hypersensitivity in which mast cell or basophil mediators cause bronchial constriction, tissue edema, and cardiovascular collapse.

Anchor residues Amino acid residues of a peptide whose side chains fit into pockets in the peptide-binding cleft of an MHC molecule. The side chains bind to complementary amino acids in the MHC molecule and therefore serve to anchor the peptide in the cleft of the MHC molecule.

Anergy State of unresponsiveness to antigenic stimulation. Lymphocyte anergy (also called clonal anergy) is the failure of clones of T or B cells to react to antigen and is a mechanism of maintaining immunologic tolerance to self. Clinically, anergy describes the lack of T cell–dependent, cutaneous delayed-type hypersensitivity reactions to common antigens.

Antibody Type of glycoprotein molecule, also called immunoglobulin (Ig), produced by B lymphocytes that binds antigens, often with a high degree of specificity and affinity. The basic structural unit of an antibody is composed of two identical heavy chains and two identical light chains. N-terminal variable regions of the heavy and light chains form the antigen-binding sites, whereas the C-terminal constant regions of the heavy chains functionally interact with other molecules in the immune system. Every individual has millions of different antibodies, each with a unique antigen-binding site. Secreted antibodies perform various effector functions, including neutralizing antigens, activating complement, and promoting leukocyte-dependent destruction of microbes.

Antibody-dependent cell-mediated cytotoxicity (ADCC) Process by which NK cells are targeted to IgG-coated cells, resulting in lysis of the antibody-coated cells. A specific receptor for the constant region of IgG, called FcγRIII (CD16), is expressed on the NK cell membrane and mediates binding to the IgG.

Antibody feedback Downregulation of antibody production by secreted IgG antibodies that occurs when antigen-antibody complexes simultaneously engage B cell membrane Ig and Fcγ receptors (FcγRII). Under these conditions, the cytoplasmic tails of the Fcγ receptors transduce inhibitory signals inside the B cell.

Antibody repertoire Collection of different antibody specificities expressed in an individual.

Antibody-secreting cell B lymphocyte that has undergone differentiation and produces the secretory form of Ig. Antibody-secreting cells are produced in response to antigen and reside in the spleen and lymph nodes as well as in the bone marrow. Often used synonymously with plasma cells.

Antigen A molecule that binds to an antibody or a T cell receptor (TCR). Antigens that bind to antibodies include all classes of molecules. TCRs bind only peptide fragments of proteins complexed with MHC molecules; both the peptide ligand and the native protein from which it is derived are called T cell antigens.

Antigen presentation The display of peptides bound by MHC molecules on the surface of an APC that permits specific recognition by TCRs and activation of T cells.

Antigen-presenting cell (APC) A cell that displays peptide fragments of protein antigens, in association with MHC molecules, on its surface and activates antigen-specific T cells. APCs also express costimulatory molecules to activate T lymphocytes optimally.

Antigen processing Intracellular conversion of protein antigens derived from the extracellular space or the cytosol into peptides and loading of these peptides onto MHC molecules for display to T lymphocytes.

Antiretroviral therapy (ART) Combination chemotherapy for HIV infection consisting of reverse-transcriptase inhibitors and a viral protease inhibitor. ART can reduce plasma virus titers to below detectable levels for more than 1 year and slow the progression of HIV disease. Also called highly active antiretroviral therapy (HAART).

Antiserum Serum from an individual previously immunized with an antigen that contains antibody specific for that antigen.

Apoptosis Process of cell death characterized by DNA cleavage, nuclear condensation and fragmentation, and plasma membrane blebbing that leads to phagocytosis of cell fragments without inducing an inflammatory response. This type of cell death is important in lymphocyte development, regulation of lymphocyte responses to foreign antigens, and maintenance of tolerance to self antigens.

Arthus reaction Localized form of experimental immune complex–mediated vasculitis induced by injection of an antigen subcutaneously into a previously immunized animal or into an animal that has been given intravenous antibody specific for the antigen. Circulating antibodies bind to the injected antigen and form immune complexes that are deposited in the walls of small arteries at the injection site and give rise to a local cutaneous vasculitis with necrosis.

Atopy Propensity of an individual to produce IgE antibodies in response to various environmental antigens and to develop strong immediate hypersensitivity (allergic) responses. People who have allergies to environmental antigens, such as pollen or house dust, are said to be atopic.

Autoantibody Antibody produced in an individual that is specific for a self antigen. Autoantibodies can cause damage to cells and tissues and are produced in excess in systemic autoimmune diseases, such as systemic lupus erythematosus.

Autocrine factor Molecule that acts on the same cell that produces the factor. For example, IL-2 is an autocrine T cell growth factor that stimulates mitotic activity of the T cell that produces it.

Autoimmune disease Disorder caused by a breakdown of self-tolerance such that the adaptive immune system responds to self antigens and mediates cell and tissue damage. Autoimmune diseases can be organ specific (e.g., thyroiditis or diabetes) or systemic (e.g., systemic lupus erythematosus).

Autoimmune regulator (AIRE) Protein that functions to stimulate expression of peripheral tissue protein antigens in thymic epithelial cells. Mutations in the *AIRE* gene in humans and mice lead to tissue-specific autoimmune disease, because of defective expression of tissue antigens in the thymus and failure to delete T cells specific for these antigens.

Autoimmunity The state of adaptive immune system responsiveness to self antigens that occurs when mechanisms of self-tolerance fail.

Autologous graft Tissue or organ graft in which the donor and recipient are the same individual. Autologous bone marrow and skin grafts are performed in clinical medicine.

Autophagy Process by which a cell degrades its own components by lysosomal catabolism. Polymorphisms of genes that regulate autophagy are linked to risk for some autoimmune diseases.

Avidity Overall strength of interaction between two molecules, such as an antibody and antigen. Avidity depends on both the affinity and the valency of interactions. Therefore, the avidity of a pentameric IgM antibody, with 10 antigen-binding sites, for a multivalent antigen may be much greater than the avidity of a dimeric IgG molecule for the same antigen. Avidity can be used to describe the strength of cell-cell interactions, which are mediated by many binding interactions between cell surface molecules.

B-1 B lymphocytes Subset of B lymphocytes that develop earlier during ontogeny than do conventional B cells, express a limited repertoire of V genes with little junctional diversity, and secrete IgM antibodies that bind T-independent antigens. Many B-1 cells express the CD5 (Ly-1) molecule.

B cell receptor (BCR) The cell surface antigen receptor on B lymphocytes, which is a membrane-bound immunoglobulin molecule.

B cell receptor (BCR) complex Multiprotein complex expressed on the surface of B lymphocytes that recognizes antigen and transduces activating signals into the cell. The BCR complex includes membrane Ig, which is responsible for binding antigen, and Igα and Igβ proteins, which initiate signaling events.

B lymphocyte The only cell type capable of producing antibody molecules and therefore the mediator of humoral immune responses. B lymphocytes, or B cells, develop in the bone marrow, and mature B cells are found mainly in lymphoid follicles in secondary lymphoid tissues, in bone marrow, and in low numbers in the circulation.

Bare lymphocyte syndrome Immunodeficiency disease characterized by a lack of class II MHC molecule expression that leads to defects in antigen presentation and cell-mediated immunity. The disease is caused by mutations in genes encoding factors that regulate class II MHC gene transcription.

Basophil Type of bone marrow–derived circulating granulocyte with structural and functional similarities to mast cells that has granules containing many of the same inflammatory mediators as mast cells and expresses a high-affinity Fc receptor for IgE. Basophils that are recruited into tissue sites where antigen is present may contribute to immediate hypersensitivity reactions.

Bcl-2 family proteins Family of partially homologous cytoplasmic and mitochondrial membrane proteins that regulate apoptosis by influencing mitochondrial outer membrane permeability. Members of this family can be proapoptotic (Bax, Bad, and Bak) or antiapoptotic (Bcl-2 and Bcl-X_L).

BCR See *B cell receptor.*

Biogenic amines Low-molecular-weight, non-lipid compounds, such as histamine, that share the structural feature of an amine group, are stored in and released from the cytoplasmic granules of mast cells, and mediate many of the biologic effects of immediate hypersensitivity (allergic) reactions. (Biogenic amines are sometimes called vasoactive amines.)

Biologic response modifiers Molecules, such as cytokines, used clinically as modulators of inflammation, immunity, and hematopoiesis.

Bone marrow Central cavity of bone that is the site of generation of all circulating blood cells in adults, including immature lymphocytes, and the site of B cell maturation.

Bone marrow transplantation The transplantation of bone marrow–derived hematopoietic including stem cells that give rise to all mature blood cells and lymphocytes. It is performed clinically to treat hematopoietic or lymphopoietic disorders and malignant diseases and is also used in various immunologic experiments in animals. Used synonymously with *hematopoietic stem cell transplantation.*

Bronchial asthma Inflammatory disease usually caused by repeated immediate hypersensitivity reactions in the lung that leads to intermittent and reversible airway obstruction, chronic bronchial inflammation with eosinophils, and bronchial smooth muscle cell hypertrophy and hyperreactivity.

Bruton's tyrosine kinase (BTK) Tyrosine kinase of the Tec family that plays an essential role in B cell maturation. Mutations in the gene encoding BTK cause X-linked agammaglobulinemia, a disease characterized by failure of B cells to mature beyond the pre-B cell stage.

Burkitt's lymphoma Malignant B cell tumor that is defined by histologic features but almost always carries a reciprocal chromosomal translocation involving Ig gene loci and the cellular *MYC* gene on chromosome 8. Many cases of Burkitt's lymphoma in Africa are associated with Epstein-Barr virus infection.

C (constant region) gene segments The DNA sequences in the Ig and TCR gene loci that encode the nonvariable portions of Ig heavy and light chains and TCR α, β, γ, and δ chains.

C1 A serum complement system protein composed of several polypeptide chains that initiates the classical pathway of complement activation by attaching to the Fc portions of IgG or IgM antibody that has bound antigen.

C1 inhibitor (C1 INH) A plasma protein inhibitor of the classical pathway of complement activation. C1 INH is a serine protease inhibitor (serpin) that mimics the normal substrates of the C1r and C1s components of C1. A genetic deficiency in

C1 INH causes the disease hereditary angioneurotic edema.

C3 The central and most abundant complement system protein; it is involved in both the classical and alternative pathway cascades. C3 is proteolytically cleaved during complement activation to generate a **C3b** fragment, which covalently attaches to cell or microbial surfaces, and a **C3a** fragment, which has various proinflammatory activities.

C3 convertase Multiprotein enzyme complex generated by the early steps of either the classical or the alternative pathway of complement activation. C3 convertase cleaves C3, which gives rise to two proteolytic products called C3a and C3b.

C5 convertase Multiprotein enzyme complex generated by C3b binding to C3 convertase. C5 convertase cleaves C5 and initiates the late steps of complement activation, leading to formation of the membrane attack complex and lysis of cells.

C-reactive protein (CRP) Member of the pentraxin family of plasma proteins involved in innate immune responses to bacterial infections. CRP is an acute-phase reactant, and it binds to the capsule of pneumococcal bacteria. CRP also binds to C1q and may thereby activate complement or act as an opsonin by interacting with phagocyte C1q receptors.

Calcineurin Cytoplasmic serine/threonine phosphatase that dephosphorylates and thereby activates the transcription factor NFAT. Calcineurin is activated by calcium signals generated through TCR signaling in response to antigen recognition, and the immunosuppressive drugs cyclosporine and FK506 work by blocking calcineurin activity.

Caspases Intracellular proteases with cysteines in their active sites that cleave substrates at the C-terminal sides of aspartic acid residues. Most are components of enzymatic cascades that cause apoptosis of cells, but some, such as **caspase-1,** drive inflammation.

Cathelicidins Polypeptides produced by neutrophils and various barrier epithelia that serve various functions in innate immunity, including direct toxicity to microorganisms, activation of leukocytes, and neutralization of lipopolysaccharide.

Cathepsins Thiol and aspartyl proteases with broad substrate specificities. The most abundant proteases of endosomes in APCs, cathepsins play an important role in generating peptide fragments from exogenous protein antigens that bind to class II MHC molecules.

CD molecules Cell surface molecules expressed on various cell types in the immune system that are designated by the "cluster of differentiation" or CD number. (See Appendix III.)

Cell-mediated immunity (CMI) The form of adaptive immunity that is mediated by T lymphocytes and serves as the defense mechanism against microbes that survive within phagocytes or infect nonphagocytic cells. CMI responses include CD4+ T cell–mediated activation of macrophages that have phagocytosed microbes and CD8+ CTL–mediated killing of infected cells.

Central tolerance A form of self-tolerance induced in generative (central) lymphoid organs as a consequence of immature self-reactive lymphocytes recognizing self antigens and subsequently leading to their death or inactivation. Central tolerance prevents the emergence of lymphocytes with high-affinity receptors for the self antigens that are expressed in the bone marrow or thymus.

Chédiak-Higashi syndrome Rare autosomal recessive immunodeficiency disease caused by a defect in the cytoplasmic granules of various cell types that affects the lysosomes of neutrophils and macrophages as well as the granules of CTLs and NK cells. Patients show reduced resistance to infection with pyogenic bacteria.

Chemokine receptors Cell surface receptors for chemokines that transduce signals stimulating the migration of leukocytes. These receptors are members of the seven-transmembrane α-helical, G protein–coupled receptor family.

Chemokines Large family of structurally homologous, low-molecular-weight cytokines that stimulate leukocyte movement and regulate the migration of leukocytes from the blood to tissues.

Chemotaxis Movement of a cell directed by a chemical concentration gradient. The movement of lymphocytes, polymorphonuclear leukocytes, monocytes, and other leukocytes into various tissues is often directed by gradients of low-molecular-weight cytokines called chemokines.

Chronic granulomatous disease (CGD) Rare inherited immunodeficiency disease caused by a defect in the gene encoding a component of the phagocyte oxidase enzyme that is needed for microbial killing by polymorphonuclear leukocytes and macrophages. CGD is characterized by recurrent intracellular bacterial and fungal infections, often accompanied by chronic cell-mediated immune responses and the formation of granulomas.

Chronic rejection A form of allograft rejection characterized by fibrosis with loss of normal organ structures occurring during a prolonged period. In many cases, the major pathologic event in chronic rejection is graft arterial occlusion, which is caused by proliferation of intimal smooth muscle cells and is called graft arteriosclerosis.

c-Kit ligand (stem cell factor) Protein required for hematopoiesis, early steps in T cell development in the thymus, and mast cell development. c-Kit ligand is produced in membrane-bound and soluble forms by stromal cells in the bone marrow and thymus and binds to the c-Kit tyrosine kinase membrane receptor on pluripotent stem cells.

Class I major histocompatibility complex (MHC) molecule One of two forms of polymorphic, heterodimeric membrane proteins that bind and display peptide fragments of protein antigens on the surface of APCs for recognition by T lymphocytes. Class I MHC molecules usually display peptides derived from the cytoplasm of the cell.

Class II–associated invariant chain peptide (CLIP) Peptide remnant of the invariant chain that sits in the class II MHC peptide-binding cleft and is removed by action of the HLA-DM molecule before the cleft becomes accessible to peptides produced from extracellular protein antigens.

Class II major histocompatibility complex (MHC) molecule One of two major classes of polymorphic, heterodimeric membrane proteins that bind and display peptide fragments of protein antigens on the surface of APCs for recognition by T lymphocytes. Class II MHC molecules usually display peptides derived from extracellular proteins that are internalized into phagocytic or endocytic vesicles.

Classical macrophage activation Macrophage activation by interferon-γ, T_H1 cells, and TLR ligands, leading to a proinflammatory and microbicidal phenotype. "Classically activated" macrophages are also called M1 macrophages.

Classical pathway of complement activation The pathway of activation of the complement system that is initiated by binding of antigen-antibody complexes to the C1 molecule and induces a proteolytic cascade involving multiple other complement proteins. The classical pathway is an effector arm of the humoral immune system that generates inflammatory mediators, opsonins for phagocytosis of antigens, and lytic complexes that destroy cells.

Clonal anergy State of antigen unresponsiveness of a clone of T lymphocytes experimentally induced by recognition of antigen in the absence of additional signals (costimulatory signals) required for functional activation. Clonal anergy is considered a model for one mechanism of tolerance to self antigens and may be applicable to B lymphocytes as well.

Clonal deletion Mechanism of lymphocyte tolerance in which an immature T cell in the thymus or an immature B cell in the bone marrow undergoes apoptotic death as a consequence of recognizing an abundant antigen in the generative organ.

Clonal expansion Increase in number of lymphocytes specific for an antigen that results from antigen stimulation and proliferation of naive T cells. Clonal expansion occurs in lymphoid tissues and is required to generate enough antigen-specific effector lymphocytes from rare naive precursors to eradicate infections.

Clonal ignorance A form of lymphocyte unresponsiveness in which self antigens are ignored by the immune system even though lymphocytes specific for those antigens remain viable and functional.

Clonal selection hypothesis Fundamental tenet of the immune system (no longer a hypothesis) stating that every individual possesses numerous clonally derived lymphocytes, each clone having arisen from a single precursor, expresseing one antigen receptor, and capable of recognizing and responding to a distinct antigenic determinant. When an antigen enters, it selects a specific pre-existing clone and activates it.

Clone Population of lymphocytes with identical antigen receptors and specificities.

Collectins Family of proteins, including mannose-binding lectin, characterized by a collagen-like domain and a lectin (i.e., carbohydrate-binding) domain. Collectins play a role in the innate immune system by acting as microbial pattern recognition receptors, and they may activate the complement system by binding to C1q.

Colony-stimulating factors (CSFs) Cytokines that promote the expansion and differentiation of bone marrow progenitor cells. CSFs are essential for the maturation of red blood cells, granulocytes, monocytes, and lymphocytes. Examples of CSFs include granulocyte-monocyte colony-stimulating factor (GM-CSF), granulocyte colony-stimulating factor (G-CSF), and IL-3.

Combinatorial diversity Combinatorial diversity describes the many different combinations of variable, diversity, and joining segments that are possible as a result of somatic recombination of DNA in the Ig and TCR loci during B cell or T cell development. Combinatorial diversity is one mechanism for the generation of large numbers of different antigen receptor genes from a limited number of DNA gene segments.

Complement System of serum and cell surface proteins that interact with one another and with other molecules of the immune system to generate important effectors of innate and adaptive immune responses. The classical, alternative, and lectin pathways of the complement system are activated by antigen-antibody complexes, microbial surfaces, and plasma lectins binding to microbes, respectively, and consist of a cascade of proteolytic enzymes that generate inflammatory mediators and opsonins. All three pathways lead to the formation of a common terminal cell lytic complex that is inserted in cell membranes.

Complement receptor type 1 (CR1) High-affinity receptor for the C3b and C4b fragments of complement. Phagocytes use CR1 to mediate internalization of C3b- or C4b-coated particles. CR1 on erythrocytes serves in the clearance of immune complexes from the circulation. CR1 is also a regulator of complement activation.

Complement receptor type 2 (CR2) Receptor expressed on B cells and follicular dendritic cells that binds proteolytic fragments of the C3 complement protein, including C3d, C3dg, and iC3b. CR2 functions to stimulate humoral immune responses by enhancing B cell activation by antigen and by promoting the trapping of antigen-antibody complexes in germinal centers. CR2 is also the receptor for Epstein-Barr virus.

Complementarity-determining region (CDR) Short segments of Ig and TCR proteins that contain most of the sequence differences among different antibodies or TCRs and that make contact with antigen; also called hypervariable regions. Three CDRs are present in the variable domain of each antigen receptor polypeptide chain and six CDRs in an intact Ig or TCR molecule. These hypervariable segments assume

loop structures that together form a surface complementary to the three-dimensional structure of the bound antigen.

Congenic mouse strains Inbred mouse strains that are identical to one another at every genetic locus except the one for which they are selected to differ; such strains are created by repetitive back-crossbreeding and selection for a particular trait. Congenic strains that differ from one another only at a particular MHC allele have been useful in defining the function of MHC molecules.

Congenital immunodeficiency Genetic defect in which an inherited deficiency in some aspect of the innate or adaptive immune system leads to an increased susceptibility to infections. Congenital immunodeficiency is frequently manifested early in infancy and childhood but is sometimes clinically detected later in life; also called primary immunodeficiency.

Conjugate vaccine Polysaccharide coupled to a carrier protein, inducing effective responses against the polysaccharide; useful for inducing protective immunity against bacteria such as *Haemophilus influenzae*, especially in infants.

Constant (C) region Portion of Ig or TCR polypeptide chains that does not vary in sequence among different clones and is not involved in antigen binding.

Contact sensitivity Propensity for a T cell–mediated, delayed-type hypersensitivity reaction to develop in the skin on contact with a particular chemical agent. Chemicals that elicit contact hypersensitivity bind to and modify self proteins or molecules on the surfaces of APCs, which are then recognized by CD4+ or CD8+ T cells.

Co-receptor Lymphocyte surface receptor that binds to an antigen complex at the same time that membrane Ig or TCR binds the antigen and delivers signals required for optimal lymphocyte activation. CD4 and CD8 are T cell co-receptors that bind nonpolymorphic parts of an MHC molecule concurrently with the TCR binding to polymorphic residues and the bound peptide. CR2 is a co-receptor on B cells that binds to complement-opsonized antigens at the same time that membrane Ig binds another part of the antigen.

Costimulator Molecule on the surface of or secreted by an antigen-presenting cell that provides a stimulus (or second signal) required for the activation of naive T cells, in addition to antigen. The best-defined costimulators are the

B7 molecules (CD80 and CD86) on APCs that bind to the CD28 molecule on T cells.

CpG nucleotides Unmethylated cytidine-guanine sequences found in microbial DNA that stimulate innate immune responses. CpG nucleotides are recognized by TLR-9, have adjuvant properties in the mammalian immune system, and may be important to the efficacy of DNA vaccines.

Crossmatching Screening test performed to minimize the chance of graft rejection in which a patient in need of an allograft is tested for the presence of preformed antibodies against donor cell surface antigens (usually MHC antigens). The test involves mixing the recipient serum with leukocytes from potential donors, adding complement, and observing whether cell lysis occurs.

Cross-presentation Mechanism by which a dendritic cell activates (or primes) a naive CD8⁺ CTL specific for the antigens of a third cell (e.g., a virus-infected or tumor cell); also called cross-priming. Cross-presentation occurs, for example, when an infected (often apoptotic) cell is ingested by a dendritic cell and the microbial antigens are processed and presented in association with class I MHC molecules, unlike the general rule for phagocytosed antigens, which are presented in association with class II MHC molecules. The dendritic cell also provides costimulation for the T cells.

C-type lectin Member of a large family of calcium-dependent carbohydrate-binding proteins, many of which play important roles in innate and adaptive immunity. For example, soluble C-type lectins bind to microbial carbohydrate structures and mediate phagocytosis or complement activation (e.g., mannose-binding lectin, dectins, collectins, ficolins).

Cutaneous immune system Components of the innate and adaptive immune system found in the skin that function together in a specialized way to detect and respond to environmental antigens. Components of the cutaneous immune system include keratinocytes, Langerhans cells, intraepithelial lymphocytes, and dermal lymphocytes.

Cyclosporine Immunosuppressive drug used to prevent allograft rejection that functions by blocking T cell cytokine gene transcription. Cyclosporine (also called cyclosporin A) binds to a cytosolic protein called cyclophilin, and cyclosporine-cyclophilin complexes bind to and inhibit calcineurin, thereby inhibiting activation

and nuclear translocation of the transcription factor NFAT.

Cytokines Proteins produced by many different cell types that mediate inflammatory and immune reactions. Cytokines are principal mediators of communication between cells of the immune system. (See Appendix II.)

Cytotoxic (or cytolytic) T lymphocyte (CTL) Type of T lymphocyte whose major effector function is to recognize and kill host cells infected with viruses or other intracellular microbes. CTLs usually express CD8 and recognize microbial peptides displayed by class I MHC molecules. CTL killing of infected cells involves the release of cytoplasmic granules whose contents include enzymes that initiate apoptosis of the infected cell and proteins that facilitate entry of these enzymes into the target cells.

Damage-associated molecular patterns (DAMPs) Endogenous molecules produced by or released from damaged and dying cells that bind to pattern recognition receptors and stimulate innate immune responses. Examples include high-mobility group box 1 (HMGB1) protein, extracellular ATP, and uric acid. DAMPs are sometimes called alarmins.

Dectins Pattern recognition receptors expressed on dendritic cells that recognize fungal cell wall carbohydrates and induce signaling events that promote inflammation and enhance adaptive immune responses.

Defensins Cysteine-rich peptides produced by epithelial barrier cells in the skin, gut, lung, and other tissues and in neutrophil granules that act as broad-spectrum antibiotics to kill a wide variety of bacteria and fungi. The synthesis of defensins is increased in response to stimulation of innate immune system receptors such as Toll-like receptors and inflammatory cytokines such as IL-1 and TNF.

Delayed-type hypersensitivity (DTH) Immune reaction in which T cell–dependent macrophage activation and inflammation cause tissue injury. A DTH reaction to the subcutaneous injection of antigen is often used as an assay for cell-mediated immunity (e.g., the purified protein derivative skin test for immunity to *Mycobacterium tuberculosis*).

Dendritic cells (DCs) Bone marrow–derived cells found in epithelial and lymphoid tissues that are morphologically characterized by thin, membranous projections. Many subsets of DCs exist with diverse functions. Activated (mature) DCs function as APCs for naive T lymphocytes and are important for initiation of adaptive immune responses to protein antigen. Immature (resting) DCs are important for induction of tolerance to self antigens.

Desensitization Method of treating immediate hypersensitivity disease (allergies) that involves repetitive administration of low doses of an antigen to which individuals are allergic. This process often prevents severe allergic reactions on subsequent environmental exposure to the antigen, but the mechanisms are not well understood. Also called allergen-specific immunotherapy.

Determinant Specific portion of a macromolecular antigen to which an antibody binds. In the case of a protein antigen recognized by a T cell, the determinant is the peptide portion that binds to an MHC molecule for recognition by the TCR. Also called epitope.

Diacylglycerol (DAG) Signaling molecule generated by phospholipase C (PLCγ1)–mediated hydrolysis of the plasma membrane phospholipid phosphatidylinositol 4,5-bisphosphate (PIP2) during antigen activation of lymphocytes. The main function of DAG is to activate an enzyme called protein kinase C that participates in the generation of active transcription factors.

DiGeorge syndrome Selective T cell deficiency caused by a congenital malformation that results in defective development of the thymus, parathyroid glands, and other structures that arise from the third and fourth pharyngeal pouches.

Direct antigen presentation Presentation of cell surface allogeneic MHC molecules by graft APCs to a graft recipient's T cells that leads to activation of the alloreactive T cells. In direct recognition of foreign MHC molecules, a TCR that was selected to recognize a self MHC molecule plus foreign peptide cross-reacts with an allogeneic MHC molecule plus peptide. Direct presentation is partly responsible for strong T cell responses to allografts. Also called direct allorecognition.

Diversity The existence of a large number of lymphocytes with different antigenic specificities in any individual. Diversity is a fundamental property of the adaptive immune system and is the result of variability in the structures of the antigen-binding sites of lymphocyte receptors for antigens (antibodies and TCRs).

Diversity (D) segments Short coding sequences between the variable (V) and constant (C) gene segments in the Ig heavy chain and TCR β and γ loci that together with J segments are somatically recombined with V segments during lymphocyte development. The resulting recombined VDJ DNA codes for the carboxyl-terminal ends of the antigen receptor V regions, including the third hypervariable (CDR) regions. Random use of D segments contributes to the diversity of the antigen receptor repertoire.

DNA vaccine A vaccine composed of a bacterial plasmid containing a complementary DNA encoding a protein antigen. DNA vaccines presumably work because professional APCs are transfected in vivo by the plasmid and express immunogenic peptides that elicit specific responses. Furthermore, the plasmid DNA contains CpG nucleotides that act as potent adjuvants.

Double-negative thymocyte Subset of developing T cells in the thymus (thymocytes) that express neither CD4 nor CD8. Most double-negative thymocytes are at an early developmental stage and do not express antigen receptors. They will later express both CD4 and CD8 during the intermediate double-positive stage before further maturation to single-positive T cells expressing only CD4 or CD8. Also called double-negative T cell.

Double-positive thymocyte Subset of developing T cells in the thymus (thymocytes) that express both CD4 and CD8 and are at an intermediate developmental stage. Double-positive thymocytes also express TCRs and are subject to selection processes, and they mature to single-positive T cells expressing only CD4 or CD8. Also called double-positive T cell.

Effector cells The cells that perform effector functions during an immune response, such as secreting cytokines (e.g., helper T cells), killing microbes (e.g., macrophages), killing microbe-infected host cells (e.g., CTLs), or secreting antibodies (e.g., differentiated B cells).

Effector phase Phase of an immune response in which a foreign antigen is destroyed or inactivated. For example, in a humoral immune response, the effector phase may be characterized by antibody-dependent complement activation and phagocytosis of antibody- and complement-opsonized bacteria.

Endosome Intracellular membrane-bound vesicle into which extracellular proteins are internalized during antigen processing. Endosomes have an acidic pH and contain proteolytic enzymes that degrade proteins into peptides that bind to class II MHC molecules. A subset of class II MHC–rich endosomes. called MIIC, play a special role in antigen processing and presentation by the class II pathway.

Endotoxin Component of the cell wall of gram-negative bacteria that is released from dying bacteria and stimulates many innate immune responses, including the secretion of cytokines, induction of microbicidal activities of macrophages, and expression of leukocyte adhesion molecules on endothelium. Endotoxin contains both lipid components and carbohydrate (poly-saccharide) moieties. Also called lipopolysaccharide (LPS).

Enhancer Regulatory nucleotide sequence in a gene that is located either upstream or downstream of the promoter, binds transcription factors, and increases the activity of the promoter. In cells of the immune system, enhancers are responsible for integrating cell surface signals that lead to induced transcription of genes encoding many of the effector proteins of an immune response, such as cytokines.

Enzyme-linked immunosorbent assay (ELISA) Method of quantifying an antigen immobilized on a solid surface by use of a specific antibody with a covalently coupled enzyme. The amount of antibody that binds the antigen is proportional to the amount of antigen present and is determined by spectrophotometrically measuring the conversion of a clear substrate to a colored product by the coupled enzyme. (See Appendix IV.)

Eosinophil A bone marrow–derived granulocyte that is abundant in the inflammatory infiltrates of immediate hypersensitivity late-phase reactions and that contributes to many of the pathologic processes in allergic diseases. Eosinophils are important in defense against extracellular parasites, including helminths.

Epitope The specific portion of a macromolecular antigen to which an antibody binds. In the case of a protein antigen recognized by a T cell, an epitope is the peptide portion that binds to an MHC molecule for recognition by the TCR. Also called determinant.

Epstein-Barr virus (EBV) Double-stranded DNA virus of the herpesvirus family that is the etiologic agent of infectious mononucleosis and is associated with some B cell malignant tumors and nasopharyngeal carcinoma. EBV infects B lymphocytes and some epithelial cells by specifically binding to CR2 (CD21).

Experimental autoimmune encephalomyelitis (EAE) Animal model of multiple sclerosis, an autoimmune demyelinating disease of the central nervous system. EAE is induced in rodents by immunization with components of the myelin sheath (e.g., myelin basic protein) of nerves, mixed with an adjuvant. The disease is mediated in large part by cytokine-secreting $CD4^+$ T cells specific for the myelin sheath proteins.

Fab (fragment, antigen-binding) Proteolytic fragment of an IgG antibody molecule that includes one complete light chain paired with one heavy-chain fragment containing the variable domain and only the first constant domain. Fab fragment retains the ability to monovalently bind an antigen but cannot interact with IgG Fc receptors on cells or with complement. Therefore, Fab preparations are used in research and therapeutic applications when antigen binding is desired without activation of effector functions. (The Fab' fragment retains the hinge region of the heavy chain.)

F(ab')2 fragment Proteolytic fragment of an IgG molecule that includes two complete light chains but only the variable domain, first constant domain, and hinge region of the two heavy-chains. $F(ab')_2$ fragments retain the entire bivalent antigen-binding region of an intact IgG molecule but cannot bind complement or IgG Fc receptors. They are used in research and therapeutic applications when antigen binding is desired without antibody effector functions.

Fas (CD95) Death receptor of the TNF receptor family that is expressed on the surface of T cells and many other cell types and initiates a signaling cascade leading to apoptosis of the cell. The death pathway is initiated when Fas binds to Fas ligand expressed on activated T cells. Fas-mediated killing of lymphocytes is important for the maintenance of self-tolerance. Mutations in the *FAS* gene cause systemic autoimmune disease.

Fas ligand (CD95 ligand) Membrane protein that is a member of the TNF family of proteins expressed on activated T cells. Fas ligand binds to Fas, thereby stimulating a signaling pathway leading to apoptotic cell death of the Fas-expressing cell. Mutations in the Fas ligand gene cause systemic autoimmune disease in mice.

Fc (fragment, crystalline) Proteolytic fragment of IgG that contains only the disulfide-linked carboxyl-terminal regions of the two heavy chains. Fc is also used to describe the corresponding region of an intact Ig molecule that mediates effector functions by binding to cell surface receptors or the C1q complement protein. (Fc fragments are so named because they tend to crystallize out of solution.)

Fc receptor Cell surface receptor specific for the carboxyl-terminal constant region of an Ig molecule. Fc receptors are typically multichain protein complexes that include signaling components and Ig-binding components. Several types of Fc receptors exist, including those specific for different IgG isotypes, IgE, and IgA. Fc receptors mediate many of the cell-dependent effector functions of antibodies, including phagocytosis of antibody-bound antigens, antigen-induced activation of mast cells, and targeting and activation of NK cells.

FcεRI High-affinity receptor for the carboxyl-terminal constant region of IgE molecules that is expressed on mast cells, basophils, and eosinophils. FcεRI molecules on mast cells are usually occupied by IgE, and antigen-induced cross-linking of these IgE-FcεRI complexes activates the mast cell and initiates immediate hypersensitivity reactions.

Fcγ receptor (FcγR) Specific cell surface receptor for the carboxyl-terminal constant region of IgG molecules. There are several different types of Fcγ receptors, including a high-affinity FcγRI that mediates phagocytosis by macrophages and neutrophils, a low-affinity FcγRIIB that transduces inhibitory signals in B cells, and a low-affinity FcγRIIIA that mediates targeting and activation of NK cells.

Ficolins Pentameric innate immune system plasma proteins, containing collagen-like domains and fibrinogen-like carbohydrate-recognizing domains, which bind to cell wall components of gram-positive bacteria, opsonizing them and activating complement.

First-set rejection Allograft rejection in an individual who has not previously received a graft or otherwise been exposed to tissue alloantigens from the same donor. First-set rejection usually takes about 7 to 14 days.

Flow cytometry Method of analysis of the phenotype of cell populations requiring a specialized instrument (flow cytometer) that can detect fluorescence on individual cells in a suspension and thereby determine the number of cells expressing the molecule to which a fluorescent probe binds. Suspensions of cells are incubated with fluorescently labeled antibodies or other probes, and the amount of probe bound by each cell in the population is measured by passing the cells one at a time through a fluorimeter with a laser-generated incident beam.

Fluorescence-activated cell sorter (FACS) Adaptation of the flow cytometer that is used for the purification of cells from a mixed population according to which and how much fluorescent probe the cells bind. Cells are first stained with fluorescently labeled probe, such as an antibody specific for a surface antigen of a cell population. The cells are then passed one at a time through a fluorimeter with a laser-generated incident beam and are differentially deflected by electromagnetic fields whose strength and direction are varied according to the measured intensity of the fluorescence signal.

Follicle See *Lymphoid follicle.*

Follicular dendritic cells (FDCs) Cells found in lymphoid follicles that express complement receptors, Fc receptors, and CD40 ligand and have long cytoplasmic processes that form a meshwork integral to the architecture of a lymphoid follicle. FDCs display antigens on their surface for B cell recognition and are involved in the activation and selection of B cells expressing high-affinity membrane Ig during the process of affinity maturation.

Follicular helper T cell (T$_{FH}$) See *T follicular helper (T$_{FH}$) cells.*

N-Formylmethionine Amino acid that initiates all bacterial proteins and no mammalian proteins (except those synthesized within mitochondria) and serves as a signal to the innate immune system of infection. Specific receptors for N-formylmethionine–containing peptides are expressed on neutrophils and mediate activation of the neutrophils.

FoxP3 A forkhead family transcription factor expressed by and required for the development of CD4$^+$ regulatory T cells. Mutations in FoxP3 in mice and humans result in an absence of CD25$^+$ regulatory T cells and multisystem autoimmune disease.

γδ T cell receptor (γδ TCR) A form of TCR that is distinct from the more common αβ TCR and is expressed on a subset of T cells found mostly in epithelial barrier tissues. Although the γδ TCR is structurally similar to the αβ TCR, the forms of antigen recognized by γδ TCRs are poorly understood; they do not recognize peptide complexes bound to polymorphic MHC molecules.

G protein–coupled receptor family Diverse family of receptors for hormones, lipid inflammatory mediators, and chemokines that use associated trimeric G proteins for intracellular signaling.

G proteins Proteins that bind guanyl nucleotides and act as exchange molecules by catalyzing the replacement of bound guanosine diphosphate (GDP) by guanosine triphosphate (GTP). G proteins with bound GTP can activate a variety of cellular enzymes in different signaling cascades. Trimeric GTP-binding proteins are associated with the cytoplasmic portions of many cell surface receptors, such as chemokine receptors. Other small, soluble G proteins, such as Ras and Rac, are recruited into signaling pathways by adaptor proteins.

GATA-3 Transcription factor that promotes the differentiation of T_H2 cells from naive T cells.

Generative lymphoid organ An organ in which lymphocytes develop from immature precursors. The bone marrow and thymus are the major generative lymphoid organs in which B cells and T cells develop, respectively.

Germinal center Specialized structure in lymphoid organs generated during T-dependent humoral immune responses, where extensive B cell proliferation, isotype switching, somatic mutation, affinity maturation, memory B cell generation, and induction of long-lived plasma cells take place. Germinal centers appear as lightly staining regions within a lymphoid follicle in spleen, lymph node, and mucosal lymphoid tissue.

Germinal center reaction In this reaction, high-affinity B cells selected in the germinal center result in the production of high-affinity antibodies and the generation of long-lived plasma cells and memory B cells.

Germline organization The inherited arrangement of variable, diversity, joining, and constant region gene segments of the antigen receptor loci in nonlymphoid cells or in immature lymphocytes. In developing B or T lymphocytes, the germline organization is modified by somatic recombination to form functional Ig or TCR genes.

Glomerulonephritis Inflammation of the renal glomeruli, often initiated by immunopathologic mechanisms such as deposition of circulating antigen-antibody complexes in the glomerular basement membrane or binding of antibodies to antigens expressed in the glomerulus. The antibodies can activate complement and phagocytes, and the resulting inflammatory response can lead to renal failure.

Graft A tissue or organ that is removed from one site and placed in another site, usually in a different individual.

Graft arteriosclerosis Occlusion of graft arteries caused by proliferation of intimal smooth muscle cells. This process is evident within 6 months to a year after transplantation and is responsible for chronic rejection of vascularized organ grafts. The mechanism is likely to be a chronic immune response to vessel wall alloantigens. Also called accelerated arteriosclerosis.

Graft rejection Specific immune response to an organ or tissue graft that leads to inflammation, damage, and possibly graft failure.

Graft-versus-host disease (GVHD) Disorder occurring in bone marrow transplant recipients caused by the reaction of mature T cells in the marrow graft with alloantigens on host cells. GVHD most often affects the skin, liver, and intestines.

Granulocyte colony-stimulating factor (G-CSF) Cytokine made by activated T cells, macrophages, and endothelial cells at sites of infection that acts on bone marrow to increase the production of and mobilize neutrophils to replace those consumed in inflammatory reactions.

Granulocyte-monocyte colony-stimulating factor (GM-CSF) Cytokine made by activated T cells, macrophages, endothelial cells, and stromal fibroblasts that acts on bone marrow to increase the production of neutrophils and monocytes. GM-CSF is also a macrophage-activating factor and promotes the differentiation of Langerhans cells into mature dendritic cells.

Granuloma Nodule of inflammatory tissue composed of clusters of activated macrophages and T lymphocytes, often with associated necrosis and fibrosis. Granulomatous inflammation is a form of chronic delayed-type hypersensitivity, often in response to persistent microbes, such as *Mycobacterium tuberculosis* and some fungi, or in response to particulate antigens that are not readily phagocytosed.

Granzyme Serine-protease enzyme found in the granules of CTLs and NK cells that is released by exocytosis, enters target cells, and proteolytically cleaves and activates caspases, which in turn cleave several substrates and induce target cell apoptosis.

Gut-associated lymphoid tissue (GALT) Collections of lymphocytes and APCs within the mucosa of the gastrointestinal tract where adaptive immune responses to intestinal microbial flora and ingested antigens are initiated; see also *Mucosa-associated lymphoid tissues.*

H-2 molecule An MHC molecule in the mouse. The mouse MHC was originally called the H-2 locus.

Haplotype The set of MHC alleles inherited from one parent and therefore on one chromosome.

Hapten Small chemical that can bind to an antibody but must be attached to a macromolecule (carrier) to stimulate an adaptive immune response specific for that chemical. For example, immunization with dinitrophenol (DNP) alone will not stimulate an anti-DNP antibody response, but immunization with a protein with covalently bonded DNP hapten will.

Heavy-chain class (isotype) switching Process by which a B lymphocyte changes the class, or isotype, of the antibodies that it produces, from IgM to IgG, IgE, or IgA, without changing the antigen specificity of the antibody. Heavy-chain class switching is regulated by helper T cell cytokines and CD40 ligand and involves recombination of B cell VDJ segments with downstream heavy-chain gene segments.

Helminth Parasitic worm. Helminthic infections often elicit T_H2-dependent immune responses characterized by eosinophil-rich inflammatory infiltrates and IgE production.

Helper T cells The class of T lymphocytes whose main functions are to activate macrophages in cell-mediated immune responses and to promote B cell antibody production in humoral immune responses. These functions are mediated by secreted cytokines and by T cell CD40 ligand binding to macrophage or B cell CD40. Most helper T cells express the CD4 molecule.

Hematopoiesis Development of mature blood cells, including erythrocytes, leukocytes, and platelets, from pluripotent stem cells in the bone marrow and fetal liver. Hematopoiesis is regulated by several different cytokine growth factors produced by bone marrow stromal cells, T cells, and other cell types.

Hematopoietic stem cell Undifferentiated bone marrow cell that divides continuously and gives rise to additional stem cells and cells of multiple different lineages. A hematopoietic stem cell in the bone marrow will give rise to cells of the lymphoid, myeloid, and erythrocytic lineage.

Hematopoietic stem cell transplantation See *Bone marrow transplantation.*

High endothelial venules (HEVs) Specialized venules that are the sites of lymphocyte migration from the blood into the stroma of a peripheral lymph node or mucosal lymphoid tissue. HEVs are lined by plump endothelial cells that protrude into the vessel lumen and express unique adhesion molecules involved in binding naive T cells.

Hinge region Region of Ig heavy chains between the first two constant domains that can assume multiple conformations, thereby imparting flexibility in the orientation of the two antigen-binding sites. Because of the hinge region, an antibody molecule can simultaneously bind two epitopes that are anywhere within a range of distances from one another.

Histamine Biogenic amine stored in the granules of mast cells that is one of the important mediators of immediate hypersensitivity. Histamine binds to specific receptors in various tissues and causes increased vascular permeability and contraction of bronchial and intestinal smooth muscle.

HLA See *Human leukocyte antigens.*

HLA-DM Peptide exchange molecule that plays a critical role in the class II MHC pathway of antigen presentation. HLA-DM is found in the specialized MIIC endosomal compartment and facilitates removal of the invariant chain–derived CLIP peptide and the binding of other peptides to class II MHC molecules. HLA-DM is encoded by a gene in the MHC and is structurally similar to class II MHC molecules, but it is not polymorphic.

Homeostasis In the adaptive immune system, the maintenance of a constant number and diverse repertoire of lymphocytes, despite the emergence of new lymphocytes and tremendous expansion of individual clones that may occur during responses to immunogenic antigens. Homeostasis is achieved by several regulated pathways of lymphocyte death and inactivation.

Homing receptor Adhesion molecules expressed on the surface of lymphocytes that are responsible for the different pathways of lymphocyte recirculation and tissue homing. Homing receptors bind to ligands (addressins) expressed on endothelial cells in particular vascular beds.

Human immunodeficiency virus (HIV) The etiologic agent of AIDS. HIV is a retrovirus that infects a variety of cell types, including CD4-expressing helper T cells, macrophages, and dendritic cells, and causes chronic progressive destruction of the immune system.

Human leukocyte antigens (HLA) MHC molecules expressed on the surface of human cells. Human MHC molecules were first identified as alloantigens on the surface of white blood cells (leukocytes) that bound serum antibodies from individuals previously exposed to other individuals' cells (e.g., mothers or transfusion recipients).

Humanized antibody Monoclonal antibody encoded by a recombinant hybrid gene and composed of the antigen-binding sites from a murine monoclonal antibody and the constant region of a human antibody. Humanized antibodies are less likely than mouse monoclonal antibodies to induce an anti-antibody response in humans; they are used clinically in the treatment of inflammatory diseases, tumors, and transplant rejection.

Humoral immunity The type of adaptive immune response mediated by antibodies produced by B lymphocytes. Humoral immunity is the principal defense mechanism against extracellular microbes and their toxins.

Hybridoma Cell line derived by fusion, or somatic cell hybridization, between a normal lymphocyte and an immortalized lymphocyte tumor line. B cell hybridomas created by fusion of normal B cells of defined antigen specificity with a myeloma cell line are used to produce monoclonal antibodies. T cell hybridomas created by fusion of a normal T cell of defined specificity with a T cell tumor line are commonly used in research.

Hyperacute rejection The form of allograft or xenograft rejection that begins within minutes to hours after transplantation and that is characterized by thrombotic occlusion of the graft vessels. Hyperacute rejection is mediated by pre-existing antibodies in the host circulation that bind to donor endothelial antigens, such as blood group antigens or MHC molecules, and activate the complement system.

Hypersensitivity diseases Disorders caused by immune responses. Hypersensitivity diseases include autoimmune diseases, in which immune responses are directed against self antigens, and diseases that result from uncontrolled or excessive responses against foreign antigens, such as microbes and allergens. The tissue damage that occurs in hypersensitivity diseases is caused by the same effector mechanisms used by the immune system to protect against microbes.

Hypervariable loop (hypervariable region) Short segments of about 10 amino acid residues within the variable regions of antibody or T cell receptor (TCR) proteins that form loop structures that contact antigen. Three hypervariable loops, also called complementarity-determining regions (CDRs), are present in each antibody heavy chain and light chain and in each TCR chain. Most of the variability between different antibodies or TCRs is located within these loops.

Idiotype Property of a group of antibodies or TCRs defined by their sharing a particular idiotope; that is, antibodies that share a particular idiotope belong to the same idiotype. Idiotype is also used to describe the collection of idiotopes expressed by an Ig molecule, and it is often used synonymously with *idiotope*.

Igα and Igβ Proteins required for surface expression and signaling functions of membrane Ig on B cells. Igα and Igβ pairs are disulfide linked to one another, noncovalently associated with the cytoplasmic tail of membrane Ig, and form the BCR complex. The cytoplasmic domains of Igα and Igβ contain ITAMs that are involved in early signaling events during antigen-induced B cell activation.

IL-1 receptor antagonist (IL-1Ra) Natural inhibitor of IL-1 produced by mononuclear phagocytes that is structurally homologous to IL-1 and binds to the same receptors but is biologically inactive. Recombinant IL-1Ra is an approved drug used to reduce inflammation in diseases such as rheumatoid arthritis.

Immature B lymphocyte Membrane IgM+, IgD− B cell, recently derived from marrow precursors, that does not proliferate or differentiate in response to antigens but rather may undergo apoptotic death or become functionally unresponsive. This property is important for the negative selection of B cells that are specific for self antigens present in the bone marrow.

Immediate hypersensitivity The type of immune reaction responsible for allergic diseases and dependent on IgE plus antigen-mediated stimulation of tissue mast cells and basophils. The mast cells and basophils release mediators that cause increased vascular permeability, vasodilation, bronchial and visceral smooth muscle contraction, and local inflammation.

Immune complex Multimolecular complex of antibody molecules with bound antigen. Because each antibody molecule has a minimum of two antigen-binding sites and many antigens are multivalent, immune complexes can vary greatly in size. Immune complexes activate effector mechanisms of humoral immunity, such as the classical complement pathway and Fc receptor–mediated phagocyte activation. Deposition of circulating immune complexes in blood vessel walls or renal glomeruli can lead to inflammation and disease.

Immune complex disease Inflammatory disease caused by the deposition of antigen-antibody complexes in blood vessel walls, resulting in local complement activation and phagocyte recruitment. Immune complexes may form because of overproduction of antibodies against microbial antigens or as a result of autoantibody production in the setting of an autoimmune disease such as systemic lupus erythematosus. Immune complex deposition in the specialized capillary basement membranes of renal glomeruli can cause glomerulonephritis and impair renal function. Systemic deposition of immune complexes in arterial walls can cause vasculitis, with thrombosis and ischemic damage to various organs.

Immune deviation Conversion of a T cell response associated with one set of cytokines, such as T_H1 cytokines that stimulate cell-mediated immunity, to a response associated with other cytokines, such as T_H2 cytokines that stimulate the production of selected antibody isotypes.

Immune inflammation Inflammation that is a result of an adaptive immune response to antigen. The cellular infiltrate at the inflammatory site may include cells of the innate immune system such as neutrophils and macrophages, which are recruited as a result of the actions of T cell cytokines.

Immune-mediated inflammatory disease Broad group of disorders in which immune responses, either to self or foreign antigens, and chronic inflammation are major components.

Immune response Collective and coordinated response to the introduction of foreign substances in an individual mediated by the cells and molecules of the immune system.

Immune response (Ir) genes Originally defined as genes in inbred strains of rodents that were inherited in a dominant mendelian manner and that controlled the ability of the animals to make antibodies against simple synthetic polypeptides. We now know that Ir genes are polymorphic genes that encode MHC molecules, which display peptides to T lymphocytes and are therefore required for T cell activation and helper T cell–dependent B cell (antibody) responses to protein antigens.

Immune surveillance The concept that a physiologic function of the immune system is to recognize and destroy clones of transformed cells before they grow into tumors and to kill tumors after they are formed. The term immune surveillance is sometimes used in a general sense to describe the function of T lymphocytes to detect and destroy any cell, not necessarily a tumor cell, that is expressing foreign (e.g., microbial) antigens.

Immune system The molecules, cells, tissues, and organs that collectively function to provide immunity, or protection, against foreign organisms.

Immunity Protection against disease, usually infectious disease, mediated by the cells and tissues that are collectively called the immune system. In a broader sense, immunity refers to the ability to respond to foreign substances, including microbes and noninfectious molecules.

Immunoblot Analytical technique in which antibodies are used to detect the presence of an antigen bound to (i.e., blotted on) a solid matrix such as filter paper; also known as *Western blot.*

Immunodeficiency See *Acquired immunodeficiency* and *Congenital immunodeficiency.*

Immunodominant epitope The epitope of a protein antigen that elicits most of the response in an individual immunized with the native protein. Immunodominant epitopes correspond to the peptides of the protein that are proteolytically generated within APCs and bind most avidly to MHC molecules, and are most likely to stimulate T cells.

Immunofluorescence Technique in which a molecule is detected by use of an antibody labeled with a fluorescent probe. For example, in immunofluorescence microscopy, cells that express a particular surface antigen can be stained with a fluorescein-conjugated antibody specific for the antigen and then visualized with a fluorescent microscope.

Immunogen An antigen that induces an immune response. Not all antigens are immunogens. For example, small-molecular-weight compounds (haptens) can bind to antibodies but will not stimulate an immune response unless they are linked to macromolecules (carriers).

Immunoglobulin (Ig) Synonymous with antibody; see *Antibody.*

Immunoglobulin domain Three-dimensional globular structural motif found in many proteins in the immune system, including Igs, TCRs, and MHC molecules. Ig domains are about 110 amino acid residues in length, include an internal disulfide bond, and contain two layers of β-pleated sheets, each layer composed of three to five strands of antiparallel polypeptide chain. Ig domains are classified as V-like or C-like on the basis of closest homology to either the Ig V or C domains.

Immunoglobulin heavy chain One of two types of polypeptide chains in an antibody molecule. The basic structural unit of an antibody includes two identical, disulfide-linked heavy chains and two identical light chains. Each heavy chain is composed of a variable (V) Ig domain and three or four constant (C) Ig domains. The different antibody isotypes, including IgM, IgD, IgG, IgA, and IgE, are distinguished by structural differences in their heavy-chain constant regions. The heavy-chain constant regions also mediate effector functions, such as complement activation or engagement of phagocytes.

Immunoglobulin light chain One of two types of polypeptide chains in an antibody molecule. The basic structural unit of an antibody includes two identical light chains, each disulfide linked to one of two identical heavy chains. Each light chain is composed of one variable (V) Ig domain and one constant (C) Ig domain. There are two light chain isotypes, called κ and λ, both functionally identical. About 60% of human antibodies have κ light chains and 40% have λ light chains.

Immunoglobulin superfamily Large family of proteins that contain a globular structural motif called an Ig domain, or Ig fold, originally described in antibodies. Many proteins of importance in the immune system, including antibodies, TCRs, MHC molecules, CD4, and CD8, are members of this superfamily.

Immunohistochemistry Technique to detect the presence of an antigen in histologic tissue sections by use of an enzyme-coupled antibody that is specific for the antigen. The enzyme converts a colorless substrate to a colored insoluble substance that precipitates at the site where the antibody and thus the antigen are localized. The position of the colored precipitate, and therefore the antigen, in the tissue section is observed by conventional light microscopy. Immunohistochemistry is a routine technique in diagnostic pathology and various fields of research.

Immunologic memory See *Memory.*

Immunologic tolerance See *Tolerance.*

Immunologically privileged site A site in the body that is inaccessible to or constitutively suppresses immune responses. The anterior chamber of the eye, the testes, and the brain are examples of immunologically privileged sites.

Immunology The study of the immune system.

Immunoperoxidase technique Common immunohistochemical technique in which a horseradish peroxidase–coupled antibody is used to identify the presence of an antigen in a tissue section. The peroxidase enzyme converts a colorless substrate to an insoluble brown product that is observable by light microscopy.

Immunoprecipitation Technique for the isolation of a molecule from a solution by binding it to an antibody and then rendering the antigen-antibody complex insoluble, either by precipitation with a second antibody or by coupling the first antibody to an insoluble particle or bead.

Immunoreceptor tyrosine-based activation motif (ITAM) Conserved motif composed of two copies of the sequence tyrosine-x-x-leucine (where x is an unspecified amino acid) found in the cytoplasmic tails of various membrane proteins in the immune system that are involved in signal transduction. ITAMs are present in the ζ and CD3 proteins of the TCR complex, in Igα and Igβ proteins in the BCR complex, and in several Ig Fc receptors. When these receptors bind their ligands, the tyrosine residues of the ITAMs become phosphorylated and form docking sites for other molecules involved in propagating cell-activating signal transduction pathways.

Immunoreceptor tyrosine-based inhibition motif (ITIM) Six–amino acid (isoleucine-x-tyrosine-x-x-leucine) motif found in the cytoplasmic tails of various inhibitory receptors in the immune system, including FcγRIIB on B cells and killer cell Ig-like receptors (KIRs) on NK cells. When these receptors bind their ligands, the ITIMs become phosphorylated on their tyrosine residues and form a docking site for protein tyrosine phosphatases, which in turn function to inhibit other signal transduction pathways.

Immunosuppression Inhibition of one or more components of the adaptive or innate immune system as a result of an underlying disease or intentionally induced by drugs for the purpose of preventing or treating graft rejection or auto-immune disease. A commonly used immuno-suppressive drug is cyclosporine, which blocks T cell cytokine production.

Immunotherapy Treatment of a disease with therapeutic agents that promote or inhibit immune responses. Cancer immunotherapy, for example, involves promotion of active immune responses to tumor antigens or administration of antitumor antibodies or T cells to establish passive immunity.

Inbred mouse strain A strain of mice created by repetitive mating of siblings that is characterized by homozygosity at every genetic locus. Every mouse of an inbred strain is genetically identical (syngeneic) to every other mouse of the same strain.

Indirect antigen presentation In transplantation immunology, a pathway of presentation of donor (allogeneic) MHC molecules by recipient APCs that involves the same mechanisms used to present microbial proteins. The allogeneic MHC proteins are processed by recipient professional APCs, and peptides derived from the allogeneic MHC molecules are presented, in association with recipient (self) MHC molecules, to host T cells. In contrast to indirect antigen presentation, direct antigen presentation involves recipient T cell recognition of unprocessed allogeneic MHC molecules on the surface of graft cells. Also called indirect allorecognition.

Inducible nitric oxide synthase (iNOS) See *Nitric oxide synthase.*

Inflammasome Multiprotein complex in the cytosol of mononuclear phagocytes, dendritic cells, and other cell types that proteolytically generates the active form of IL-1 from an inactive precursor. The formation of the inflammasome complex, which includes NLRP-3 (a NOD-like pattern recognition receptor) and caspase-1, is stimulated by a variety of microbial products, cell damage–associated molecules, and crystals.

Inflammation Complex reaction of vascularized tissue to infection, toxin exposure, or cell injury that involves extravascular accumulation of plasma proteins and leukocytes. Acute inflammation is a common result of innate immune responses, and local adaptive immune responses can also promote inflammation. Although inflammation serves a protective function in controlling infections and promoting tissue repair, it can also cause tissue damage and disease.

Inflammatory bowel disease (IBD) Group of disorders, including ulcerative colitis and Crohn's disease, characterized by chronic inflammation in the gastrointestinal tract. The etiology of IBD is not known, but some evidence indicates that it is caused by inadequate regulation of T cell responses, probably against intestinal commensal bacteria. IBD develops in gene knockout mice lacking IL-2, IL-10, or the TCR α chain.

Innate immunity Protection against infection that relies on mechanisms that exist before infection, are capable of a rapid response to microbes, and react in essentially the same way to repeated infections. The innate immune system includes epithelial barriers, phagocytic cells (neutrophils, macrophages), NK cells, the complement system, and cytokines, largely made by dendritic cells and mononuclear phagocytes, that regulate and coordinate many of the activities of the cells of innate immunity.

Inositol 1,4,5-trisphosphate (IP-3) Cytoplasmic signaling molecule generated by phospholipase C (PLCγ1)–mediated hydrolysis of the plasma membrane phospholipid PIP-2 during antigen activation of lymphocytes. The main function of IP-3 is to stimulate the release of intra-cellular stores of calcium from membrane-bound compartments such as the endoplasmic reticulum.

Integrins Heterodimeric cell surface proteins whose major functions are to mediate the adhesion of leukocytes to other leukocytes, endothelial cells, and extracellular matrix proteins. Integrins are important for T cell interactions with APCs and for migration of leukocytes from blood into tissues. The ligand-binding affinity of the integrins can be regulated by various stimuli, and the cytoplasmic domains of integrins bind to the cytoskeleton. There are two main subfamilies of integrins; the members of each family express a conserved β chain (β_1, or CD29, and β_2, or CD18) associated with different β chains. VLA-4 (very late antigen 4) is a β_1 integrin and LFA-1 (leukocyte function–associated antigen 1) is a β_2 integrin expressed on T cells and other leukocytes.

Interferon regulatory factors (IRFs) Family of inducibly activated transcription factors that are important in expression of inflammatory and antiviral genes. For example, IRF-3 is activated by TLR signals and regulates expression of type I interferons, which are cytokines that protect cells from viral infection.

Interferons (IFNs) Named for ability of these cytokines to interfere with viral infection, blocking viral replication within host cells. IFN-γ activates macrophages to become more effective at killing phagocytosed microbes. Type I IFNs induce resistance to viral infection and replication (antiviral state) and include several forms of IFN-α and one IFN-β.

Interleukins Any of a large number of cytokines named with a numeric suffix roughly sequentially in order of discovery or molecular characterization (e.g., interleukin-1, interleukin-2). Some cytokines were originally named for their biologic activities and do not have an interleukin designation. (See Appendix II.)

Intracellular bacterium A bacterium that survives or replicates within cells, usually in endosomes. The principal defense against intracellular bacteria, such as *Mycobacterium tuberculosis,* is cell-mediated immunity.

Intraepidermal lymphocytes T lymphocytes found within the epidermal layer of the skin. In the mouse, most of the intraepidermal T cells express the γδ form of TCR; see *Intraepithelial T lymphocytes.*

Intraepithelial T lymphocytes T lymphocytes present in the epidermis of the skin and in mucosal epithelia that typically express a limited diversity of antigen receptors. Some of these lymphocytes may recognize microbial products, such as glycolipids, associated with nonpolymorphic class I MHC–like molecules. Intraepithelial T lymphocytes may be considered effector cells of innate immunity and function in host defense by secreting cytokines and activating phagocytes and by killing infected cells.

Invariant chain (I_i) Nonpolymorphic protein that binds to newly synthesized class II MHC molecules in the endoplasmic reticulum. The invariant chain prevents loading of the class II MHC peptide-binding cleft with peptides present in the endoplasmic reticulum, and such peptides are left to associate with class I molecules. The invariant chain also promotes folding and assembly of class II molecules and directs newly formed class II molecules to the specialized endosomal MIIC compartment, where peptide loading takes place.

Isotype One of five types of antibodies, determined by which of five different forms of heavy chain is present. Antibody isotypes include IgM, IgD, IgG, IgA, and IgE, and each isotype performs a different set of effector functions. Additional structural variations characterize distinct subtypes of IgG and IgA.

J chain See *Joining (J) chain.*

JAK-STAT signaling pathway A signaling pathway initiated by cytokine binding to type I and type II cytokine receptors. This pathway sequentially involves activation of receptor-associated Janus kinase (JAK) tyrosine kinases, JAK-mediated tyrosine phosphorylation of the cytoplasmic tails of cytokine receptors, docking of signal transducers and activators of transcription (STATs) to the phosphorylated receptor chains, JAK-mediated tyrosine phosphorylation of the associated STATs, dimerization and nuclear translocation of the STATs, and STAT binding to regulatory regions of target genes, causing transcriptional activation of those genes.

Joining (J) chain Polypeptide that links IgA or IgM molecules to form multimers (e.g., dimeric IgA and pentameric IgM).

Joining (J) segments Short coding sequences, between the variable (V) and constant (C) gene segments in all the Ig and TCR loci, which together with D segments are somatically recombined with V segments during lymphocyte development. The resulting recombined VDJ DNA codes for the carboxyl-terminal ends of the antigen receptor V regions, including the third hypervariable (CDR) regions. Random use of different J segments contributes to the diversity of the antigen receptor repertoire.

Junctional diversity The diversity in antibody and TCR repertoires that is attributed to the random addition or removal of nucleotide sequences at junctions among V, D, and J gene segments.

Kaposi's sarcoma Malignant tumor of vascular cells that frequently arises in patients with AIDS. Kaposi's sarcoma is associated with infection by the Kaposi's sarcoma–associated herpesvirus (human herpesvirus 8).

Killer immunoglobulin-like receptors (KIRs) Ig superfamily receptors expressed by NK cells that recognize different alleles of HLA-A, HLA-B, and HLA-C molecules. Some KIRs have signaling components with ITIMs in their cytoplasmic tails, and these deliver inhibitory signals to inactivate the NK cells. Some members of the KIR family have short cytoplasmic tails without ITIMs but associate with other ITAM-containing polypeptides and function as activating receptors.

Knockout mouse A mouse with a targeted disruption of one or more genes that is created by homologous recombination techniques. Knockout mice lacking functional genes encoding cytokines, cell surface receptors, signaling molecules, and transcription factors have provided extensive information about the roles of these molecules in the immune system.

Lamina propria Layer of loose connective tissue underlying epithelium in mucosal tissues such as the intestines and airways, where dendritic cells, mast cells, lymphocytes, and macrophages mediate immune responses to invading pathogens.

Langerhans cells Immature dendritic cells found as a meshwork in the epidermal layer of the skin whose major function is to trap microbes and antigens that enter through the skin and transport the antigens to draining lymph nodes. During their migration to the lymph nodes, Langerhans cells mature into lymph node dendritic cells, which can efficiently present antigen to naive T cells.

Large granular lymphocyte Another name for an NK cell based on the morphologic appearance of this cell type in the blood.

Late-phase reaction Component of the immediate hypersensitivity reaction that ensues 2 to 4 hours after mast cell degranulation and that is characterized by an inflammatory infiltrate of eosinophils, basophils, neutrophils, and lymphocytes. Repeated bouts of this late-phase inflammatory reaction can cause tissue damage.

Lck Src family nonreceptor tyrosine kinase that noncovalently associates with the cytoplasmic tails of CD4 and CD8 molecules in T cells and is involved in the early signaling events of antigen-induced T cell activation. Lck mediates tyrosine phosphorylation of the cytoplasmic tails of CD3 and ζ proteins of the TCR complex.

Lectin pathway of complement activation A pathway of complement activation triggered, in the absence of antibody, by the binding of microbial polysaccharides to circulating lectins such as mannose-binding protein (MBL). MBL is structurally similar to C1q and activates the C1r-C1s enzyme complex (like C1q) or activates another serine esterase, called MBL-associated serine esterase. The remaining steps of the lectin pathway, beginning with cleavage of C4, are the same as the classical pathway.

Leishmania Obligate intracellular protozoan parasite that infects macrophages and can cause a chronic inflammatory disease involving many tissues. *Leishmania* infection in mice has served as a model system for study of the effector functions of several cytokines and the helper T cell subsets that produce them. T_H1 responses to *Leishmania major* and associated IFN-γ production control infection, whereas T_H2 responses with IL-4 production lead to disseminated lethal disease.

Leukemia Malignant disease of bone marrow precursors of blood cells in which large numbers of leukemic cells usually occupy the bone marrow and often circulate in the bloodstream. Lymphocytic leukemias are derived from B or T cell precursors, myelogenous leukemias are derived from granulocyte or monocyte precursors, and erythroid leukemias are derived from red blood cell precursors.

Leukocyte adhesion deficiency (LAD) One of a rare group of immunodeficiency diseases with infectious complications that is caused by defective expression of the leukocyte adhesion molecules required for tissue recruitment of phagocytes and lymphocytes. LAD-1 is caused by mutations in the gene encoding the CD18 protein, which is part of β_2 integrins. LAD-2 is caused by mutations in a gene that encodes a fucose transporter involved in the synthesis of leukocyte ligands for endothelial selectins.

Leukotrienes Class of arachidonic acid–derived lipid inflammatory mediators produced by the lipoxygenase pathway in many cell types. Mast cells make abundant leukotriene C4 (LTC_4) and its degradation products LTD_4 and LTE_4, which bind to specific receptors on smooth muscle cells and cause prolonged bronchoconstriction. Leukotrienes contribute to the pathologic processes of bronchial asthma. Collectively, LTC_4, LTD_4, and LTE_4 constitute what was once called slow-reacting substance of anaphylaxis.

Lipopolysaccharide (LPS) See *Endotoxin*.

Live virus vaccine A vaccine composed of a live but nonpathogenic (attenuated) form of a virus. Attenuated viruses carry mutations that interfere with the viral life cycle or pathogenesis. Because live virus vaccines actually infect the recipient cells, they can effectively stimulate immune responses, such as the CTL response, that are optimal for protecting against wild-type viral infection. A common live virus vaccine is the Sabin poliovirus vaccine.

Lymph Fluid within lymphatic vessels, derived from interstitial tissue fluid, which transports soluble molecules, particles, and dendritic cells to lymph nodes. Lymph is returned to the blood circulation through the thoracic and right lymphatic ducts.

Lymph node Small, nodular, encapsulated aggregates of lymphocyte-rich tissue situated along lymphatic channels throughout the body where adaptive immune responses to lymph-borne antigens are initiated.

Lymphatic system A system of vessels throughout the body that collects tissue fluid called lymph, originally derived from the blood, and returns it, through the thoracic duct, to the circulation. Lymph nodes are interspersed along these vessels and trap and retain antigens present in the lymph.

Lymphocyte homing Directed migration of subsets of circulating lymphocytes into particular tissue sites. Lymphocyte homing is regulated by the selective expression of endothelial adhesion molecules and chemokines, in different tissues. For example, some lymphocytes preferentially home to the intestinal mucosa, and this directed migration is regulated by the chemokine CCL25 and the endothelial adhesion molecule MadCAM, both expressed in the gut, which bind respectively to the CCR9 chemokine receptor and the $\alpha_4\beta_1$ integrin on gut-homing lymphocytes.

Lymphocyte maturation Process by which pluripotent bone marrow stem cells develop into mature, antigen receptor–expressing naive B or T lymphocytes that populate peripheral lymphoid tissues. This process takes place in the specialized environments of the bone marrow (for B cells) and the thymus (for T cells).

Lymphocyte migration Movement of lymphocytes from the bloodstream into peripheral tissues.

Lymphocyte recirculation Continuous movement of lymphocytes through the bloodstream and lymphatics, between the lymph nodes or spleen and, if activated, peripheral inflammatory sites.

Lymphocyte repertoire Complete collection of antigen receptors and therefore antigen specificities expressed by the B and T lymphocytes of an individual.

Lymphocytes Specialized cells that capture and display microbial antigens.

Lymphoid follicle B cell–rich region of a lymph node or the spleen that is the site of antigen-induced B cell proliferation and differentiation. In T cell–dependent B cell responses to protein antigens, a germinal center forms within the follicles.

Lymphoid tissue inducer cells Hematopoietically derived cells with phenotypic features of both lymphocytes and natural killer cells that stimulate the development of lymph nodes and other secondary lymphoid organs, in part through production of the cytokines lymphotoxin-α (LTα) and lymphotoxin-β (LTβ).

Lymphokine Previous name for a cytokine (soluble protein mediator of immune responses) produced by lymphocytes.

Lymphokine-activated killer (LAK) cells NK cells with enhanced cytolytic activity for tumor cells as a result of exposure to high doses of IL-2. LAK cells generated in vitro have been adoptively transferred back into patients with cancer to treat their tumors.

Lymphoma Malignant tumor of B or T lymphocytes usually arising in and spreading between lymphoid tissues but that may spread to other tissues. Lymphomas often express phenotypic characteristics of the normal lymphocytes from which they were derived.

Lymphotoxin (LT, TNF-β) Cytokine produced by T cells that is homologous to and binds to the same receptors as TNF. As with TNF, LT has proinflammatory effects, including endothelial and neutrophil activation. LT is also critical for the normal development of lymphoid organs.

Lysosome Membrane-bound, acidic organelle abundant in phagocytic cells that contains proteolytic enzymes that degrade proteins derived both from the extracellular environment and from within the cell. Lysosomes are involved in the class II MHC pathway of antigen processing.

M cells Specialized epithelial cells overlying Peyer's patches in the gut that play a role in delivery of antigens to Peyer's patches.

M1 macrophages See *Classical macrophage activation.*

M2 macrophages See *Alternative macrophage activation.*

Macrophage Tissue-based phagocytic cell derived from blood monocytes that plays important roles in innate and adaptive immune responses. Macrophages are activated by microbial products such as endotoxin and by T cell cytokines such as IFN-γ. Activated macrophages phagocytose and kill microorganisms, secrete proinflammatory cytokines, and present antigens to helper T cells. Macrophages may assume different morphologic forms in different tissues, including the microglia of the central nervous system, Kupffer cells in the liver, alveolar macrophages in the lung, and osteoclasts in bone.

Major histocompatibility complex (MHC) Large genetic locus (on human chromosome 6 and mouse chromosome 17) that includes the highly polymorphic genes encoding the peptide-binding molecules recognized by T lymphocytes. The MHC locus also includes genes encoding cytokines, molecules involved in antigen processing, and complement proteins.

Major histocompatibility complex (MHC) molecule Heterodimeric membrane protein encoded in the MHC locus that serves as a peptide display molecule for recognition by T lymphocytes. Two structurally distinct types of MHC molecules exist. Class I MHC molecules are present on most nucleated cells, bind peptides derived from cytosolic proteins, and are recognized by CD8$^+$ T cells. Class II MHC molecules are restricted largely to dendritic cells, macrophages, and B lymphocytes; bind peptides derived from endocytosed proteins; and are recognized by CD4$^+$ T cells.

Mannose-binding lectin (MBL) Plasma protein that binds to mannose residues on bacterial cell walls and acts as an opsonin by promoting phagocytosis of the bacterium by macrophages. Macrophages express a surface receptor for C1q that can also bind MBL and mediate uptake of the opsonized organisms.

Mannose receptor Carbohydrate-binding receptor (lectin) expressed by macrophages that binds mannose and fucose residues on microbial cell walls and mediates phagocytosis of the organisms.

Marginal zone A peripheral region of splenic lymphoid follicles containing macrophages that are particularly efficient at trapping polysaccharide antigens. Such antigens may persist for prolonged periods on the surfaces of marginal-zone macrophages, where they are recognized by specific B cells, or they may be transported into follicles.

Marginal-zone B lymphocytes Subset of B lymphocytes, found exclusively in the marginal zone of the spleen, that respond rapidly to blood-borne microbial antigens by producing IgM antibodies with limited diversity.

Mast cell Major effector cell of immediate hypersensitivity (allergic) reactions. Mast cells are derived from the marrow, reside in most tissues adjacent to blood vessels, express a high-affinity Fc receptor for IgE, and contain numerous mediator-filled granules. Antigen-induced cross-linking of IgE bound to the mast cell Fc receptors causes release of their granule contents as well as new synthesis and secretion of other mediators, leading to an immediate hypersensitivity reaction.

Mature B cell IgM- and IgD-expressing, functionally competent naive B cells that represent the final stage of B cell maturation in the bone marrow and that populate peripheral lymphoid organs.

Membrane attack complex (MAC) Lytic complex of the terminal components of the complement cascade, including multiple copies of C9, which forms in the membranes of target cells. The MAC causes lethal ionic and osmotic changes in cells.

Memory Property of the adaptive immune system to respond more rapidly, with greater magnitude, and more effectively to a repeated exposure to an antigen compared with the response to the first exposure.

Memory cells See *Memory lymphocytes.*

Memory lymphocytes Memory B and T cells are produced by antigen stimulation of naive lymphocytes and survive in a functionally quiescent state for many years after the antigen is eliminated. Memory lymphocytes mediate rapid and enhanced (i.e., memory or recall) responses to second and subsequent exposures to antigens.

MHC restriction The characteristic of T lymphocytes that they recognize a foreign peptide antigen only when it is bound to a particular allelic form of an MHC molecule.

MHC tetramer Reagent used to identify and enumerate T cells that specifically recognize a particular MHC-peptide complex. The reagent consists of four recombinant, biotinylated MHC molecules (usually class I) bound to a fluorochrome-labeled avidin molecule and loaded with a peptide. T cells that bind the MHC tetramer can be detected by flow cytometry.

β$_2$-Microglobulin Light chain of a class I MHC molecule. β$_2$-Microglobulin is an extracellular protein encoded by a nonpolymorphic gene outside the MHC, is structurally homologous to an Ig domain, and is invariant among all class I molecules.

Mitogen-activated protein (MAP) kinase cascade Signal transduction cascade initiated by the active form of the Ras protein and involving the sequential activation of three serine/threonine kinases, the last one being MAP kinase. MAP kinase in turn phosphorylates and activates other enzymes and transcription factors. The MAP kinase pathway is one of several signal pathways activated by antigen binding to the TCR and BCR.

Mixed leukocyte reaction (MLR) In vitro reaction of alloreactive T cells from one individual against MHC antigens on blood cells from another individual. The MLR involves proliferation of and cytokine secretion by both $CD4^+$ and $CD8^+$ T cells.

Molecular mimicry Postulated mechanism of autoimmunity triggered by infection with a microbe containing antigens that cross-react with self antigens. Immune responses to the microbe result in reactions against self tissues.

Monoclonal antibody An antibody that is specific for one antigen and is produced by a B cell hybridoma (a cell line derived by the fusion of a single normal B cell and an immortal B cell tumor line). Monoclonal antibodies are widely used in research and clinical diagnosis and therapy.

Monocyte Type of bone marrow–derived circulating blood cell that is the precursor of tissue macrophages. Monocytes are actively recruited into inflammatory sites, where they differentiate into macrophages.

Monocyte colony-stimulating factor (M-CSF) Cytokine made by activated T cells, macrophages, endothelial cells, and stromal fibroblasts that stimulates the production of monocytes from bone marrow precursor cells.

Mononuclear phagocytes Cells with a common bone marrow lineage whose primary function is phagocytosis. These cells function as accessory cells in the recognition and activation phases of adaptive immune responses and as effector cells in innate and adaptive immunity. Mononuclear phagocytes circulate in the blood in an incompletely differentiated form called monocytes, and once they settle in tissues, they mature into macrophages; called the mononuclear phagocyte system.

Mucosa-associated lymphoid tissue (MALT) Collections of lymphocytes, dendritic cells, and other cell types within the mucosa of the gastrointestinal and respiratory tracts that are sites of adaptive immune responses to antigens. Mucosa-associated lymphoid tissues contain intraepithelial lymphocytes, mainly T cells, and organized collections of lymphocytes, often rich in B cells, below mucosal epithelia, such as Peyer's patches in the gut or pharyngeal tonsils.

Mucosal immune system Part of the immune system that responds to and protects against microbes that enter the body through mucosal surfaces, such as the gastrointestinal and respiratory tracts, but also maintains tolerance to commensal organisms that live on the outside of the mucosal epithelium. The mucosal immune system is composed of organized mucosa-associated lymphoid tissues, such as Peyer's patches, as well as diffusely distributed cells within the lamina propria.

Multiple myeloma Malignant tumor of antibody-producing B cells that often secretes Igs or parts of Ig molecules. The monoclonal antibodies produced by multiple myelomas were critical for early biochemical analyses of antibody structure.

Multivalency See *Polyvalency.*

Mycobacterium Genus of aerobic bacteria, many species of which can survive within phagocytes and cause disease. The principal host defense against mycobacteria such as *Mycobacterium tuberculosis* is cell-mediated immunity.

N nucleotides Name given to nucleotides randomly added to the junctions between V, D, and J gene segments in Ig or TCR genes during lymphocyte development. The addition of up to 20 of these nucleotides, which is mediated by the enzyme terminal deoxyribonucleotidyl transferase, contributes to the diversity of the antibody and TCR repertoires.

Naive lymphocyte Mature B or T lymphocyte that has not previously encountered antigen. When naive lymphocytes are stimulated by antigen, they differentiate into effector lymphocytes, such as antibody-secreting B cells or helper T cells and CTLs. Naive lymphocytes have surface markers and recirculation patterns that are distinct from those of previously activated lymphocytes. ("Naive" also refers to an unimmunized individual.)

Natural antibodies IgM antibodies, largely produced by B-1 cells, specific for bacteria that are common in the environment and gastrointestinal tract. Normal individuals contain natural antibodies without any evidence of infection, and these antibodies serve as a preformed defense mechanism against microbes that succeed in penetrating epithelial barriers. Some of these antibodies cross-react with ABO blood group antigens and are responsible for transfusion reactions.

Natural killer (NK) cells Subset of bone marrow–derived lymphocytes, distinct from B or T cells, which function in innate immune responses to kill microbe-infected cells by direct lytic mechanisms and by secreting IFN-γ. NK cells do not express clonally distributed antigen receptors like Ig receptors or TCRs, and their activation is regulated by a combination of cell surface stimulatory and inhibitory receptors, the latter recognizing self MHC molecules.

Natural killer T cells (NK-T cells) Numerically small subset of lymphocytes that express T cell receptors and some surface molecules characteristic of NK cells. Some NK-T cells, called invariant (iNK-T), express αβ T cell antigen receptors with mimimal diversity, recognize lipid antigens presented by CD1 molecules, and perform various effector functions typical of helper T cells.

Negative selection Process by which developing lymphocytes that express self-reactive antigen receptors are eliminated, thereby contributing to the maintenance of self-tolerance. Negative selection of developing T lymphocytes (thymocytes) is best understood and involves high-avidity binding of a thymocyte to self MHC molecules with bound peptides on thymic APCs, leading to apoptotic death of the thymocyte.

Neonatal Fc receptor (FcRn) An IgG-specific Fc receptor that mediates the transport of maternal IgG across the placenta and the neonatal intestinal epithelium. FcRn resembles a class I MHC molecule. An adult form of this receptor functions to protect plasma IgG antibodies from catabolism.

Neonatal immunity Passive humoral immunity to infections in mammals in the first months of life, before full development of the immune system. Neonatal immunity is mediated by maternally produced antibodies transported across the placenta into the fetal circulation before birth or derived from ingested milk and transported across the gut epithelium.

Neutrophil Phagocytic cell characterized by a segmented lobular nucleus and cytoplasmic granules filled with degradative enzymes. PMNs are the most abundant type of circulating white blood cells and are the major cell type mediating acute inflammatory responses to bacterial infections. Also called polymorphonuclear leukocyte (PMN).

Nitric oxide Biologic effector molecule with a broad range of activities that in macrophages functions as a potent microbicidal agent to kill ingested organisms.

Nitric oxide synthase (NOS) Member of a family of enzymes that synthesize the vasoactive and microbicidal compound nitric oxide from L-arginine. Macrophages express an inducible form of this enzyme (iNOS) on activation by various microbial or cytokine stimuli.

NOD-like receptors (NLRs) Family of cytosolic multidomain proteins that sense cytoplasmic PAMPs and DAMPs and recruit other proteins to form signaling complexes that promote inflammation; NOD, nucleotide oligomerization domain.

Nuclear factor κB (NF-κB) Family of transcription factors composed of homodimers or heterodimers of proteins homologous to the c-Rel protein. NF-κB proteins are required for the inducible transcription of many genes important in both innate and adaptive immune responses.

Nuclear factor of activated T cells (NFAT) Transcription factor required for the expression of IL-2, IL-4, TNF, and other cytokine genes. The four different NFATs are each encoded by separate genes; NFATp and NFATc are found in T cells. Cytoplasmic NFAT is activated by calcium/calmodulin-dependent, calcineurin-mediated dephosphorylation that permits NFAT to translocate into the nucleus and bind to consensus binding sequences in the regulatory regions of IL-2, IL-4, and other cytokine genes, usually in association with other transcription factors such as AP-1.

Nude mouse Strain of mice that lack development of the thymus, and therefore T lymphocytes, as well as hair follicles. Nude mice have been used experimentally to define the role of T lymphocytes in immunity and disease.

Oncofetal antigen Proteins that are expressed at high levels on some types of cancer cells and in normal developing (fetal) but not adult tissues. Antibodies specific for these proteins are often used in histopathologic identification of tumors or to monitor the progression of tumor growth in patients. CEA (CD66) and α-fetoprotein are two oncofetal antigens commonly expressed by certain carcinomas.

Opsonin Macromolecule that becomes attached to the surface of a microbe and can be recognized by surface receptors of neutrophils and macrophages and that increases the efficiency of phagocytosis of the microbe. Opsonins include IgG antibodies, which are recognized by the Fcγ receptor on phagocytes, and fragments of complement proteins, which are recognized by CR1 (CD35) and by the leukocyte integrin Mac-1.

Opsonization Process of attaching opsonins, such as IgG or complement fragments, to microbial surfaces to target the microbes for phagocytosis.

Oral tolerance Suppression of systemic humoral and cell-mediated immune responses to an antigen after the oral administration of that antigen as a result of anergy of antigen-specific T cells or the production of immunosuppressive cytokines (e.g., TGF-β). Oral tolerance is a possible mechanism for prevention of immune responses to food antigens and to bacteria that normally reside as commensals in the intestinal lumen.

P nucleotides Short, inverted repeat nucleotide sequences in the VDJ junctions of rearranged Ig and TCR genes that are generated by RAG-1– and RAG-2–mediated asymmetric cleavage of hairpin DNA intermediates during somatic recombination events. P nucleotides contribute to the junctional diversity of antigen receptors.

Paracrine factor Molecule that acts on cells in proximity to the cell that produces the factor. Most cytokines act in a paracrine fashion.

Passive immunity The form of immunity to an antigen that is established in one individual by transfer of antibodies or lymphocytes from another individual who is immune to that antigen. The recipient of such a transfer can become immune to the antigen without ever having been exposed to or having responded to the antigen. An example of passive immunity is the transfer of human sera containing antibodies specific for certain microbial toxins or snake venom to a previously unimmunized individual.

Pathogen-associated molecular patterns (PAMPs) Structures produced by microorganisms but not mammalian (host) cells, which are recognized by and stimulate the innate immune system. Examples include bacterial lipopolysaccharide and viral double-stranded RNA.

Pathogenicity Ability of a microorganism to cause disease. Multiple mechanisms may contribute to pathogenicity, including production of toxins, stimulation of host inflammatory responses, and perturbation of host cell metabolism.

Pattern recognition receptors Signaling receptors of the innate immune system that recognize PAMPs and DAMPs and thereby activate innate immune responses. Examples include Toll-like receptors (TLRs) and NOD-like receptors (NLRs).

Pentraxins Family of plasma proteins that contain five identical globular subunits; includes the acute-phase reactant C-reactive protein.

Peptide-binding cleft Portion of an MHC molecule that binds peptides for display to T cells. The cleft is composed of paired α helices resting on a floor made up of an eight-stranded β-pleated sheet. The polymorphic residues, which are the amino acids that vary among different MHC alleles, are located in and around this cleft.

Perforin Protein that is homologous to the C9 complement protein and is present in the granules of CTLs and NK cells. When perforin is released from the granules of activated CTLs or NK cells, it promotes entry of granzymes into the target cell, leading to apoptotic death of the cell.

Periarteriolar lymphoid sheath (PALS) A cuff of lymphocytes surrounding small arterioles in the spleen, adjacent to lymphoid follicles. A PALS contains mainly T lymphocytes, about two thirds of which are CD4+ and one third CD8+. In humoral immune responses to protein antigens, B lymphocytes are activated at the interface between the PALS and follicles and then migrate into the follicles to form germinal centers.

Peripheral lymphoid organs and tissues Organized collections of lymphocytes and accessory cells, including the spleen, lymph nodes, and mucosa-associated lymphoid tissues, in which adaptive immune responses are initiated; also called secondary lymphoid organs.

Peripheral tolerance Unresponsiveness to self antigens that are present in peripheral tissues and not usually in the generative lymphoid organs. Peripheral tolerance is induced by the recognition of antigens without adequate levels of the costimulators required for lymphocyte activation or by persistent and repeated stimulation by these self antigens.

Peyer's patches Organized lymphoid tissue in the lamina propria of the small intestine in which immune responses to ingested antigens may be initiated. Peyer's patches are composed mostly of B cells, with smaller numbers of T cells and accessory cells, all arranged in follicles similar to those found in lymph nodes, often with germinal centers.

Phagocytosis The process by which certain cells of the innate immune system, including macrophages and neutrophils, engulf large particles (>0.5 μm in diameter) such as intact microbes. The cell surrounds the particle with extensions of its plasma membrane by an energy- and cytoskeleton-dependent process; this process results in the formation of an intracellular vesicle called a phagosome, which contains the ingested particle.

Phagosome Membrane-bound intracellular vesicle that contains microbes or particulate material from the extracellular environment. Phagosomes are formed during phagocytosis and fuse with other vesicular structures, such as with lysosomes to form phagolysosomes, leading to enzymatic degradation of the ingested material.

Phosphatase (protein phosphatase) Enzyme that removes phosphate groups from the side chains of certain amino acid residues of proteins. Protein phosphatases in lymphocytes, such as CD45 or calcineurin, regulate the activity of various signal transduction molecules and transcription factors. Some protein phosphatases may be specific for phosphotyrosine residues and others for phosphoserine and phosphothreonine residues.

Phospholipase Cγ (PLCγ) Enzyme that catalyzes hydrolysis of the plasma membrane phospholipid PIP-2 to generate two signaling molecules, IP-3 and DAG. PLCγ becomes activated in lymphocytes by antigen binding to the antigen receptor.

Phytohemagglutinin (PHA) Carbohydrate-binding protein, or lectin, produced by plants that cross-links human T cell surface molecules, including the T cell receptor, thereby inducing polyclonal activation and agglutination of T cells. PHA is frequently used in experimental immunology to study T cell activation. In clinical medicine, PHA is used to assess whether a patient's T cells are functional or to induce T cell mitosis for the purpose of generating karyotypic data.

Plasma cell Terminally differentiated, antibody-secreting B lymphocyte with a characteristic histologic appearance, including an oval shape, eccentric nucleus, and perinuclear halo.

Plasmablast Circulating antibody-secreting cells that may be precursors of the plasma cells that reside in the bone marrow and other tissues.

Polyclonal activators Agents capable of activating many clones of lymphocytes, regardless of their antigen specificities. Examples of polyclonal activators include anti-IgM antibodies for B cells and anti-CD3 antibodies, bacterial superantigens, and PHA for T cells.

Poly-Ig receptor An Fc receptor expressed by mucosal epithelial cells that mediates the transport of IgA and IgM through the epithelial cells into the intestinal lumen.

Polymerase chain reaction (PCR) Rapid method of copying and amplifying specific DNA sequences up to about 1 kb in length that is widely used as a preparative and analytical technique in all branches of molecular biology. The method relies on the use of short oligonucleotide primers complementary to the sequences at the ends of the DNA to be amplified and involves repetitive cycles of melting, annealing, and synthesis of DNA.

Polymorphism Existence of two or more alternative forms, or variants, of a gene that are present at stable frequencies in a population. Each common variant of a polymorphic gene is called an allele, and one individual may carry two different alleles of a gene, each inherited from a different parent. The MHC genes are the most polymorphic genes in the mammalian genome.

Polymorphonuclear leukocyte (PMN) See *Neutrophil.*

Polyvalency Presence of multiple identical copies of an epitope on a single antigen molecule, cell surface, or particle. Polyvalent antigens, such as bacterial capsular polysaccharides, are often capable of activating B lymphocytes independent of helper T cells. Used synonymously with *multivalency.*

Positive selection Process by which developing T cells in the thymus (thymocytes) whose TCRs bind to self MHC molecules are rescued from programmed cell death, whereas thymocytes whose receptors do not recognize self MHC molecules die by default. Positive selection ensures that mature T cells are self MHC restricted and that CD8+ T cells are specific for complexes of peptides with class I MHC molecules and CD4+ T cells for complexes of peptides with class II MHC molecules.

Pre-B cell Developing B cell present only in hematopoietic tissues that is at a maturational stage characterized by expression of cytoplasmic Ig μ heavy chains and surrogate light chains but not Ig light chains. Pre-B cell receptors composed of μ chains and surrogate light chains deliver signals that stimulate further maturation of the pre-B cell into an immature B cell.

Pre-B cell receptor A receptor expressed on developing B lymphocytes at the pre-B cell stage that is composed of an Ig μ heavy chain and an invariant surrogate light chain. The surrogate light chain is composed of two proteins, including the λ5 protein, which is homologous to the λ light chain C domain, and the V pre-B protein, which is homologous to a V domain. The pre-B cell receptor associates with the Igα and Igβ signal transduction proteins to form the pre-B cell receptor complex. Pre-B cell receptors are required for stimulating the proliferation and continued maturation of the developing B cell. It is not known whether the pre-B cell receptor binds a specific ligand.

Pre-T cell Developing T lymphocyte in the thymus at a maturational stage characterized by expression of the TCR β chain but not the α chain or CD4 or CD8. In pre-T cells, the TCR β chain is found on the cell surface as part of the pre-T cell receptor.

Pre-T cell receptor A receptor expressed on the surface of pre-T cells that is composed of the TCR β chain and an invariant pre-Tα protein. This receptor associates with CD3 and ζ molecules to form the pre-T cell receptor complex. The function of this complex is similar to that of the pre-B cell receptor in B cell development, namely, the delivery of signals that stimulate further proliferation, antigen receptor gene rearrangements, and other maturational events. It is not known whether the pre-T cell receptor binds a specific ligand.

Pre-Tα Invariant transmembrane protein with a single extracellular Ig-like domain that associates with the TCR β chain in pre-T cells to form the pre-T cell receptor.

Primary immune response Adaptive immune response that occurs after the first exposure of an individual to a foreign antigen. Primary responses are characterized by relatively slow kinetics and small magnitude compared with the responses after a second or subsequent exposure.

Primary immunodeficiency See *Congenital immunodeficiency.*

Pro-B cell Developing B cell in the bone marrow that is the earliest cell committed to the B lymphocyte lineage. Pro-B cells do not produce Ig, but they can be distinguished from other immature cells by the expression of B lineage–restricted surface molecules such as CD19 and CD10.

Pro-T cell Developing T cell in the thymic cortex that is a recent arrival from the bone marrow and does not express TCRs, CD3, ζ chains, or CD4 or CD8 molecules. Pro-T cells are also called double-negative thymocytes.

Professional antigen-presenting cells (professional APCs) Term sometimes used to refer to APCs that activate T lymphocytes; includes dendritic cells, mononuclear phagocytes, and B lymphocytes, all of which are capable of expressing class II MHC molecules and costimulators. The most important professional APCs for initiation of primary T cell responses are dendritic cells.

Programmed cell death A pathway of cell death by apoptosis that occurs in lymphocytes deprived of necessary survival stimuli, such as growth factors or costimulators. Programmed cell death is caused by the release of mitochondrial cytochrome *c* into the cytoplasm, activation of caspase-9, and initiation of the apoptotic pathway.

Promoter DNA sequence immediately 5′ to the transcription start site of a gene where the proteins that initiate transcription bind. The term promoter is often used to mean the entire 5′ regulatory region of a gene, including enhancers, which are additional sequences that bind transcription factors and interact with the basal transcription complex to increase the rate of transcriptional initiation. Other enhancers may be located at a significant distance from the promoter, either 5′ of the gene, in introns, or 3′ of the gene.

Prostaglandins Class of lipid inflammatory mediators derived from arachidonic acid in many cell types through the cyclooxygenase pathway, which have vasodilator, bronchoconstrictor, and chemotactic activities. Prostaglandins made by mast cells are important mediators of allergic reactions.

Proteasome Large multiprotein enzyme complex with a broad range of proteolytic activity that is found in the cytoplasm of most cells and generates from cytosolic proteins the peptides that bind to class I MHC molecules. Proteins are targeted for proteasomal degradation by covalent linkage of ubiquitin molecules.

Protein kinase C (PKC) Any of several isoforms of an enzyme that mediates the phosphorylation of serine and threonine residues in many different protein substrates and thereby serves to propagate various signal transduction pathways leading to transcription factor activation. In T and B lymphocytes, PKC is activated by DAG, which is generated in response to antigen receptor ligation.

Protein tyrosine kinases (PTKs) Enzymes that mediate the phosphorylation of tyrosine residues in proteins and thereby promote phosphotyrosine-dependent protein-protein interactions. PTKs are involved in numerous signal transduction pathways in cells of the immune system.

Protozoa Single-celled eukaryotic organisms, many of which are human parasites and cause diseases. Examples of pathogenic protozoa include *Entamoeba histolytica,* which causes amebic dysentery; *Plasmodium,* which causes malaria; and *Leishmania,* which causes leishmaniasis. Protozoa stimulate both innate and adaptive immune responses. It has proved difficult to develop effective vaccines against many of these organisms.

Provirus DNA copy of the genome of a retrovirus that is integrated into the host cell genome and from which viral genes are transcribed and the viral genome is reproduced. HIV proviruses can remain inactive for long periods and thereby represent a latent form of HIV infection that is not accessible to immune defense.

Purified antigen (subunit) vaccine A vaccine composed of purified antigens or subunits of microbes. Examples of this type of vaccine include diphtheria and tetanus toxoids, pneumococcus and *Haemophilus influenzae* polysaccharide vaccines, and purified polypeptide vaccines against hepatitis B and influenza virus. Purified antigen vaccines may stimulate antibody and helper T cell responses, but they typically do not generate CTL responses.

Pyogenic bacteria Bacteria, such as the gram-positive staphylococci and streptococci, which induce inflammatory responses rich in polymorphonuclear leukocytes (giving rise to pus). Antibody responses to these bacteria greatly enhance the efficacy of innate immune effector mechanisms to clear infections.

Rac Small, guanine nucleotide–binding protein that is activated by the GDP-GTP exchange factor Vav during the early events of T cell activation. GTP·Rac triggers a three-step protein kinase cascade that culminates in activation of the stress-activated protein (SAP) kinase, c-Jun

N-terminal kinase (JNK), and p38 kinase, which are similar to the MAP kinases.

Radioimmunoassay Highly sensitive and specific immunologic method of quantifying the concentration of an antigen in a solution that relies on a radioactively labeled antibody specific for the antigen. Usually, two antibodies specific for the antigen are used. The first antibody is unlabeled but attached to a solid support, where it binds and immobilizes the antigen whose concentration is being determined. The amount of the second, labeled antibody that binds to the immobilized antigen, as determined by radioactive decay detectors, is proportional to the concentration of antigen in the test solution.

Rapamycin Immunosuppressive drug (also called sirolimus) used clinically to prevent allograft rejection. Rapamycin inhibits the activation of a protein called molecular target of rapamycin (mTOR), which is a key signaling molecule in a variety of metabolic and cell growth pathways including the pathway required for interleukin-2–mediated T cell proliferation.

Ras Member of a family of 21-kD guanine nucleotide–binding proteins with intrinsic GTPase activity that are involved in many different signal transduction pathways in diverse cell types. Mutated *RAS* genes are associated with neoplastic transformation. In T cell activation, Ras is recruited to the plasma membrane by tyrosine-phosphorylated adaptor proteins, where it is activated by GDP-GTP exchange factors. GTP·Ras then initiates the MAP kinase cascade, which leads to expression of the *FOS* gene and assembly of the AP-1 transcription factor.

Reactive oxygen species (ROS) Highly reactive metabolites of oxygen, including superoxide anion, hydroxyl radical, and hydrogen peroxide, that are produced by activated phagocytes. Reactive oxygen species are used by the phagocytes to form oxyhalides that damage ingested bacteria. They may also be released from cells and promote inflammatory responses or cause tissue damage.

Reagin IgE antibody that mediates an immediate hypersensitivity reaction.

Receptor editing Process by which some immature B cells that recognize self antigens in the bone marrow may be induced to change their Ig specificities. Receptor editing involves reactivation of the *RAG* genes, additional light chain VJ recombinations, and new Ig light chain production, which allows the cell to express a different Ig receptor that is not self-reactive.

Recombinase-activating genes 1 and 2 (*RAG1* and *RAG2*) The genes encoding RAG-1 and RAG-2 proteins, which make up the V(D)J recombinase and are expressed in developing B and T cells. RAG proteins bind to recombination signal sequences and are critical for DNA recombination events that form functional Ig and TCR genes. Therefore, RAG proteins are required for expression of antigen receptors and for the maturation of B and T lymphocytes.

Recombination signal sequences Specific DNA sequences found adjacent to the V, D, and J segments in the antigen receptor loci and recognized by the RAG-1/RAG-2 complex during VDJ recombination. The recognition sequences consist of a highly conserved stretch of 7 nucleotides, called the heptamer, located adjacent to the V, D, or J coding sequence, followed by a spacer of exactly 12 or 23 nonconserved nucleotides and a highly conserved stretch of 9 nucleotides, called the nonamer.

Red pulp Anatomic and functional compartment of the spleen composed of vascular sinusoids, scattered among which are large numbers of erythrocytes, macrophages, dendritic cells, sparse lymphocytes, and plasma cells. Red pulp macrophages clear the blood of microbes, other foreign particles, and damaged red blood cells.

Regulatory T cells Population of T cells that regulates the activation of other T cells and is necessary to maintain peripheral tolerance to self antigens. Most regulatory T cells are CD4+ and constitutively express CD25, the α chain of the IL-2 receptor, and the transcription factor FoxP3.

Respiratory burst Process by which reactive oxygen intermediates such as superoxide anion, hydroxyl radical, and hydrogen peroxide are produced in macrophages and polymorphonuclear leukocytes. The respiratory burst is mediated by the enzyme phagocyte oxidase and is usually triggered by inflammatory mediators, such as LTB$_4$, PAF, and TNF, or by bacterial products, such as *N*-formylmethionyl peptides.

Reverse transcriptase Enzyme encoded by retroviruses, such as HIV, that synthesizes a DNA copy of the viral genome from the RNA genomic template. Purified reverse transcriptase is used widely in molecular biology research for purposes of cloning complementary DNAs encoding a gene of interest from messenger RNA. Reverse-transcriptase inhibitors are used as drugs to treat HIV-1 infection.

Rh blood group antigens Complex system of protein alloantigens expressed on red blood cell membranes that are the cause of transfusion reactions and hemolytic disease of the newborn. The most clinically important Rh antigen is designated D.

Rheumatoid arthritis Autoimmune disease characterized primarily by inflammatory damage to joints and sometimes inflammation of blood vessels, lungs, and other tissues. CD4+ T cells, activated B lymphocytes, and plasma cells are found in the inflamed joint lining (synovium), and numerous proinflammatory cytokines, including IL-1 and TNF, are present in the synovial (joint) fluid.

RIG-like receptors (RLRs) Cytosolic receptors of the innate immune system that recognize viral RNA and induce production of type I interferons. The two best characterized RLRs are RIG-I (retinoic acid–inducible gene I) and MDA5 (melanoma differentiation-associated gene 5).

RORγT (retinoid-related orphan receptor γ T) Transcription factor expressed in and required for differentiation of T$_H$17 cells and lymphoid tissue inducer (LTi) cells.

Scavenger receptors Family of cell surface receptors expressed on macrophages, originally defined as receptors that mediate endocytosis of oxidized or acetylated low-density lipoprotein particles, but that also bind and mediate the phagocytosis of a variety of microbes.

SCID mouse A mouse strain in which B and T cells are absent because of an early block in maturation from bone marrow precursors. SCID mice carry a mutation in a component of the enzyme DNA-dependent protein kinase, which is required for double-stranded DNA break repair. Deficiency of this enzyme results in abnormal joining of Ig and TCR gene segments during recombination and therefore failure to express antigen receptors.

Second-set rejection Allograft rejection in an individual who has previously been sensitized to the donor's tissue alloantigens by having received another graft or transfusion from that donor. In contrast to first-set rejection, which occurs in an individual who has not previously been sensitized to the donor alloantigens, second-set rejection is rapid and occurs in 3 to 7 days as a result of immunologic memory.

Secondary immune response Adaptive immune response that occurs on second exposure to an antigen. A secondary response is characterized by more rapid kinetics and greater magnitude relative to the primary immune response, which occurs on first exposure.

Secondary immunodeficiency See *Acquired immunodeficiency.*

Secretory component Proteolytically cleaved portion of the extracellular domain of the poly-Ig receptor that remains bound to an IgA molecule in mucosal secretions.

Selectin Any one of three separate but closely related carbohydrate-binding proteins that mediate adhesion of leukocytes to endothelial cells. Each of the selectin molecules is a single-chain transmembrane glycoprotein with a similar modular structure, including an extracellular calcium-dependent lectin domain. The selectins include L-selectin (CD62L), expressed on leukocytes; P-selectin (CD62P), expressed on platelets and activated endothelium; and E-selectin (CD62E), expressed on activated endothelium.

Selective immunoglobulin deficiency Immunodeficiencies characterized by a lack of only one or a few Ig classes or subclasses. IgA deficiency is the most common selective Ig deficiency, followed by IgG3 and IgG2 deficiencies. Patients with these disorders may be at increased risk for bacterial infections, but many are normal.

Self MHC restriction Limitation (or restriction) of T cells to recognize antigens displayed by MHC molecules that the T cell encountered during maturation in the thymus (and thus sees as self).

Self-tolerance Unresponsiveness of the adaptive immune system to self antigens, largely as a result of inactivation or death of self-reactive lymphocytes induced by exposure to these antigens. Self-tolerance is a cardinal feature of the normal immune system, and failure of self-tolerance leads to autoimmune diseases.

Septic shock Severe complication of bacterial infections that spread to the bloodstream (sepsis), and is characterized by vascular collapse, disseminated intravascular coagulation, and metabolic disturbances. This syndrome is due to the effects of bacterial cell wall components, such as LPS or peptidoglycan, which bind to TLRs on various cell types and induce expression of inflammatory cytokines, including TNF and IL-12.

Seroconversion Production of detectable antibodies in the serum specific for a microorganism during the course of an infection or in response to immunization.

Serology The study of blood (serum) antibodies and their reactions with antigens. The term serology is often used to refer to the diagnosis of infectious diseases by detection of microbe-specific antibodies in the serum.

Serotype Antigenically distinct subset of a species of an infectious organism that is distinguished from other subsets by serologic (i.e., serum antibody) tests. Humoral immune responses to one serotype of microbes (e.g., influenza virus) may not be protective against another serotype.

Serum The cell-free fluid that remains when blood or plasma forms a clot. Blood antibodies are found in the serum fraction.

Serum amyloid A (SAA) Acute-phase protein whose serum concentration rises significantly in the setting of infection and inflammation, mainly because of IL-1– and TNF-induced synthesis by the liver. SAA activates leukocyte chemotaxis, phagocytosis, and adhesion to endothelial cells.

Serum sickness Disease caused by the injection of large doses of a protein antigen into the blood and characterized by the deposition of antigen-antibody (immune) complexes in blood vessel walls, especially in the kidneys and joints. Immune complex deposition leads to complement fixation and leukocyte recruitment and subsequently to glomerulonephritis and arthritis. Serum sickness was originally described as a disorder that occurred in patients receiving injections of serum containing antitoxin antibodies to prevent diphtheria.

Severe combined immunodeficiency (SCID) Immunodeficiency diseases in which both B and T lymphocytes do not develop or do not function properly, and therefore both humoral immunity and cell-mediated immunity are impaired. Children with SCID usually have infections during the first year of life and succumb to these infections unless the immunodeficiency is treated. SCID has several different genetic causes.

Shwartzman reaction Experimental model of the pathologic effects of bacterial LPS and TNF in which two intravenous injections of LPS are administered to a rabbit 24 hours apart. After the second injection, the rabbit suffers disseminated intravascular coagulation and neutrophil and platelet plugging of small blood vessels.

Signal transducer and activator of transcription (STAT) Member of a family of proteins that function as signaling molecules and transcription factors in response to binding of cytokines to type I and type II cytokine receptors. STATs are present as inactive monomers in the cytoplasm of cells and are recruited to the cytoplasmic tails of cross-linked cytokine receptors, where they are tyrosine phosphorylated by JAKs. The phosphorylated STAT proteins dimerize and move to the nucleus, where they bind to specific sequences in the promoter regions of various genes and stimulate their transcription. Different STATs are activated by different cytokines.

Single-positive thymocyte Maturing T cell precursor in the thymus that expresses CD4 or CD8 molecules but not both. Single-positive thymocytes are found mainly in the medulla and have matured from the double-positive stage, during which thymocytes express both CD4 and CD8 molecules. Also called single-positive T cell.

Smallpox Disease caused by variola virus. Smallpox was the first infectious disease shown to be preventable by vaccination and the first disease to be completely eradicated by a worldwide vaccination program.

Somatic hypermutation High-frequency point mutations in Ig heavy and light chains that occur in germinal center B cells. Mutations that result in increased affinity of antibodies for antigen impart a selective survival advantage to the B cells producing those antibodies and lead to affinity maturation of a humoral immune response.

Somatic recombination Process of DNA recombination by which the functional genes encoding the variable regions of antigen receptors are formed during lymphocyte development. A relatively limited set of inherited, or germline, DNA sequences that are initially separated from one another are brought together by enzymatic deletion of intervening sequences and re-ligation. This process occurs only in developing B or T lymphocytes. Also called somatic rearrangement.

Specificity Cardinal feature of the adaptive immune system, namely, that immune responses are directed toward and able to distinguish between distinct antigens or small parts of macromolecular antigens. This fine specificity is attributed to lymphocyte antigen receptors that may bind to one molecule but not to another, even closely related, molecule.

Spleen Secondary lymphoid organ in the left upper quadrant of the abdomen. The spleen is the major site of adaptive immune responses to blood-borne antigens. The red pulp of the spleen is composed of blood-filled vascular sinusoids lined by active phagocytes that ingest opsonized antigens and damaged red blood cells. The white pulp of the spleen contains lymphocytes and lymphoid follicles where B cells are activated.

Src homology domains Three-dimensional domain structures present in many signaling proteins that permit specific noncovalent interactions with other proteins. Several proteins involved in early signaling events in T and B lymphocytes interact with one another through SH2 and SH3 domains.

Stem cell Undifferentiated cell that divides continuously and gives rise to additional stem cells and to cells of multiple different lineages. For example, all blood cells arise from a common hematopoietic stem cell.

Superantigens Proteins that bind to and activate all the T cells in an individual that express a particular set or family of V_β TCR genes. Superantigens are presented to T cells by binding to nonpolymorphic regions of class II MHC molecules on APCs, and they interact with conserved regions of TCR V_β domains. Several staphylococcal enterotoxins are superantigens. Their importance lies in their ability to activate many T cells, which results in large amounts of cytokine production and a clinical syndrome that is similar to septic shock.

Suppressor T cells T cells that block the activation and function of other T lymphocytes. Clearly identifying suppressor T cells has been difficult, and the term is not widely used now. The better-defined T cells that function to control immune responses are regulatory T cells.

Surrogate light chain A complex of two nonvariable proteins that associate with Ig μ heavy chains in pre-B cells to form the pre-B cell receptor. The two surrogate light-chain proteins include V pre-B protein, which is homologous to a light-chain V domain, and λ5, which is covalently attached to the μ heavy chain by a disulfide bond.

Switch recombination Molecular mechanism underlying Ig isotype switching in which a rearranged VDJ gene segment in an antibody-producing B cell recombines with a downstream C gene and the intervening C gene or genes are deleted. DNA recombination events in switch recombination are triggered by CD40 and cytokines and involve nucleotide sequences called **switch regions** located in the introns at the 5' end of each C_H locus.

Syk Cytoplasmic protein tyrosine kinase, similar to ZAP-70 in T cells, that is critical for early signaling steps in antigen-induced B cell activation. Syk binds to phosphorylated tyrosines in the cytoplasmic tails of the Igα and Igβ chains of the BCR complex and in turn phosphorylates adaptor proteins that recruit other components of the signaling cascade.

Syngeneic Genetically identical. All animals of an inbred strain and monozygotic twins are syngeneic.

Syngeneic graft A graft from a donor who is genetically identical to the recipient. Syngeneic grafts are not rejected.

Synthetic vaccine Vaccines composed of recombinant DNA–derived antigens. Synthetic vaccines for hepatitis B virus and herpes simplex virus are now in use.

Systemic lupus erythematosus (SLE) Chronic systemic autoimmune disease that affects predominantly women and is characterized by rashes, arthritis, glomerulonephritis, hemolytic anemia, thrombocytopenia, and central nervous system involvement. Many different autoantibodies are found in patients with SLE, particularly anti-DNA antibodies. Many of the manifestations of SLE are caused by the formation of immune complexes composed of autoantibodies and their specific antigens, with deposition of these complexes in small blood vessels in various tissues. The underlying mechanism for the breakdown of self-tolerance in SLE is not understood.

Tacrolimus Immunosuppressive drug (also known as FK506) used to prevent allograft rejection that functions by blocking T cell cytokine gene transcription, similar to cyclosporine. Tacrolimus binds to a cytosolic protein called FK506-binding protein, and the resulting complex binds to calcineurin, thereby inhibiting activation and nuclear translocation of the transcription factor NFAT.

T cell receptor (TCR) The clonally distributed antigen receptor on CD4+ and CD8+ T lymphocytes that recognizes complexes of foreign peptides bound to self MHC molecules on the surface of APCs. The most common form of TCR is composed of a heterodimer of two disulfide-linked transmembrane polypeptide chains, designated α and β, each containing one N-terminal Ig-like variable (V) domain, one Ig-like constant (C) domain, a hydrophobic transmembrane region, and a short cytoplasmic region. (Another, less common type of TCR, composed of γ and δ chains, is found on a small subset of T cells and recognizes different forms of antigen.)

T cell receptor (TCR) transgenic mouse A mouse in a genetically engineered strain that expresses transgenically encoded functional TCR α and β genes encoding a TCR of a single defined specificity. Because of allelic exclusion of endogenous TCR genes, most or all of the T cells in a TCR transgenic mouse have the same antigen specificity, which is a useful property for various research purposes.

T follicular helper (T_{FH}) cells Heterogeneous subset of CD4+ helper T cells present within lymphoid follicles that are critical in providing signals to B cells in the germinal center reaction. T_{FH} cells express CXCR5, ICOS, IL-21, and Bcl-6.

T lymphocyte The key component of cell-mediated immune responses in the adaptive immune system. T lymphocytes mature in the thymus, circulate in the blood, populate secondary lymphoid tissues, and are recruited to peripheral sites of antigen exposure. They express antigen receptors (TCRs) that recognize peptide fragments of foreign proteins bound to self MHC molecules. Functional subsets of T lymphocytes include CD4+ helper T cells and CD8+ CTLs.

T-bet A T-box family transcription factor that promotes the differentiation of T_H1 cells from naive T cells.

T-dependent antigen An antigen that requires both B cells and helper T cells to stimulate an antibody response. T-dependent antigens are protein antigens that contain some epitopes recognized by T cells and other epitopes recognized by B cells. Helper T cells produce cytokines and cell surface molecules that stimulate B cell growth and differentiation into antibody-secreting cells. Humoral immune responses to T-dependent antigens are characterized by isotype switching, affinity maturation, and memory.

Tertiary lymphoid organ Collection of lymphocytes and antigen-presenting cells organized into B cell follicles and T cell zones that develop in sites of chronic immune-mediated inflammation, such as the joint synovium of rheumatoid arthritis patients.

T-independent antigen Nonprotein antigens, such as polysaccharides and lipids, which can stimulate antibody responses without a requirement for antigen-specific helper T lymphocytes. T-independent antigens usually contain multiple identical epitopes that can cross-link membrane Ig on B cells and thereby activate the cells. Humoral immune responses to T-independent antigens show relatively little heavy-chain isotype switching or affinity maturation, two processes that require signals from helper T cells.

T_H1 cells Subset of CD4$^+$ helper T cells that secrete a particular set of cytokines, including IFN-γ, and whose principal function is to stimulate phagocyte-mediated defense against infections, especially with intracellular microbes.

T_H2 cells Functional subset of CD4$^+$ helper T cells that secrete a particular set of cytokines, including IL-4, IL-5, and IL-3 and whose principal function is to stimulate IgE and eosinophil/mast cell–mediated immune reactions.

T_H17 cells Functional subset of CD4$^+$ helper T cells that secrete a particular set of inflammatory cytokines, including IL-17, which are protective against bacterial and fungal infections and also mediate inflammatory reactions in autoimmune and other inflammatory diseases.

Thymic epithelial cells Epithelial cells abundant in the cortical and medullary stroma of the thymus that play a critical role in T cell development. In the process of positive selection, maturing T cells that weakly recognize self peptides bound to MHC molecules on the surface of thymic epithelial cells are rescued from programmed cell death.

Thymocyte Precursor of a mature T lymphocyte present in the thymus.

Thymus Bilobed organ situated in the anterior mediastinum that is the site of maturation of T lymphocytes from bone marrow–derived precursors. Thymic tissue is divided into an outer cortex and an inner medulla and contains stromal thymic epithelial cells, macrophages, dendritic cells, and numerous T cell precursors (thymocytes) at various stages of maturation.

Tissue typing Determination of the particular MHC alleles expressed by an individual for the purpose of matching allograft donors and recipients. Tissue typing, also called HLA typing, is usually done by molecular (PCR-based) sequencing of HLA alleles, or by serologic methods (lysis of individual's cells by panels of anti-HLA antibodies).

TNF receptor–associated factors (TRAFs) Family of adaptor molecules that interact with the cytoplasmic domains of various receptors in the TNF receptor family, including TNF-RII, lymphotoxin (LT)-β receptor, and CD40. Each of these receptors contains a cytoplasmic motif that binds different TRAFs, which in turn engage other signaling molecules leading to activation of the transcription factors AP-1 and NF-κB.

Tolerance Unresponsiveness of the adaptive immune system to antigens, as a result of inactivation or death of antigen-specific lymphocytes, induced by exposure to the antigens. Tolerance to self antigens is a normal feature of the adaptive immune system, but tolerance to foreign antigens may be induced under certain conditions of antigen exposure.

Tolerogen An antigen that induces immunologic tolerance, in contrast to an immunogen, which induces an immune response. Many antigens can be either tolerogens or immunogens, depending on how they are administered. **Tolerogenic** forms of antigens include large doses of the proteins administered without adjuvants and orally administered antigens.

Toll-like receptors (TLRs) Family of pattern recognition receptors of the innate immune system expressed on the surface and in endosomes of many cell types. TLRs recognize microbial structures such as endotoxin and viral RNA and transduce signals that lead to the expression of inflammatory and antiviral genes.

Toxic shock syndrome Acute illness characterized by shock, skin exfoliation, conjunctivitis, and diarrhea that is associated with tampon use and caused by a *Staphylococcus aureus* superantigen.

Transfusion Transplantation of circulating blood cells, platelets, or plasma from one individual to another. Transfusions are performed to treat blood loss from hemorrhage or to treat a deficiency in one or more blood cell types resulting from inadequate production or excess destruction.

Transfusion reactions Immunologic reaction against transfused blood products, usually mediated by preformed antibodies in the recipient that bind to donor blood cell antigens, such as ABO blood group antigens or histocompatibility antigens. Transfusion reactions can lead to intravascular lysis of red blood cells and, in severe cases, kidney damage, fever, shock, and disseminated intravascular coagulation.

Transgenic mouse A mouse that expresses an exogenous gene that has been introduced into the genome by injection of a specific DNA sequence into the pronuclei of fertilized mouse eggs. Transgenes insert randomly at chromosomal break points and are subsequently inherited as simple mendelian traits. By the design of transgenes with tissue-specific regulatory sequences, mice can be produced that express a particular gene only in certain tissues. Transgenic mice are used extensively in immunology research to study the functions of various cytokines, cell surface molecules, and intracellular signaling molecules.

Transplantation Process of transferring cells, tissues, or organs (i.e., grafts) from one individual to another or from one site to another in the same individual. Transplantation is used to treat a variety of diseases in which there is a functional disorder of a tissue or organ. The major barrier to successful transplantation between individuals is immunologic reaction (rejection) to the transplanted graft.

Transporter associated with antigen processing (TAP) Adenosine triphosphate (ATP)–dependent peptide transporter that mediates the active transport of peptides from the cytosol to the site of assembly of class I MHC molecules inside the endoplasmic reticulum. TAP is a heterodimeric molecule composed of TAP-1 and TAP-2 polypeptides, both encoded by genes in the MHC. Because peptides are required for stable assembly of class I MHC molecules, TAP-deficient animals express few cell surface class I MHC molecules, which results in diminished development and activation of CD8$^+$ T cells.

Tumor immunity Protection against the development of tumors by the immune system. Although immune responses to naturally occurring tumors can frequently be demonstrated, true immunity may occur only in the case of a subset of these tumors that express immunogenic antigens (e.g., tumors that are caused by oncogenic viruses and therefore express viral antigens). Research efforts are under way to enhance weak immune responses to other tumors by a variety of approaches.

Tumor-infiltrating lymphocytes (TILs) Lymphocytes isolated from the inflammatory infiltrates present in and around surgical resection samples of solid tumors that are enriched with tumor-specific CTLs and NK cells. In an experimental mode of cancer treatment, TILs are grown in vitro in the presence of high doses of IL-2 and are then adoptively transferred back into patients with the tumor.

Tumor necrosis factor receptor superfamily (TNFRSF) Large family of structurally homologous transmembrane proteins that bind TNFSF proteins and generate signals that regulate proliferation, differentiation, apoptosis, and inflammatory gene expression. (See Appendix II.)

Tumor necrosis factor superfamily (TNFSF) Large family of structurally homologous transmembrane proteins that regulate diverse functions in responding cells, including proliferation, differentiation, apoptosis, and inflammatory gene expression. TNFSF members typically form homotrimers, either within the plasma membrane or after proteolytic release from the membrane, and bind to homotrimeric TNF receptor superfamily (TNFRSF) molecules, which then initiate a variety of signaling pathways. (See Appendix II.)

Tumor-specific antigen An antigen whose expression is restricted to a particular tumor and is not expressed by normal cells. Tumor-specific antigens may serve as target antigens for antitumor immune responses.

Tumor-specific transplantation antigen (TSTA) An antigen expressed on experimental animal tumor cells that can be detected by induction of immunologic rejection of tumor transplants. TSTAs were originally defined on chemically induced rodent sarcomas and shown to stimulate CTL-mediated rejection of transplanted tumors.

Two-signal hypothesis A now-proven hypothesis that states that the activation of lymphocytes requires two distinct signals, the first being antigen and the second either microbial products or components of innate immune responses to microbes. The requirement for antigen (so-called signal 1) ensures that the ensuing immune response is specific. The requirement for additional stimuli triggered by microbes or innate immune reactions (signal 2) ensures that immune responses are induced when they are needed, that is, against microbes and other noxious substances and not against harmless substances, including self antigens. Signal 2 is referred to as costimulation and is often mediated by membrane molecules on professional APCs, such as B7 proteins.

Type 1 diabetes mellitus Disease characterized by a lack of insulin that leads to various metabolic and vascular abnormalities. The insulin deficiency results from autoimmune destruction of the insulin-producing β cells of the islets of

Langerhans in the pancreas, usually during childhood. CD4$^+$ and CD8$^+$ T cells, antibodies, and cytokines have been implicated in the islet cell damage. Also called insulin-dependent diabetes mellitus.

Ubiquitination Covalent linkage of one or several copies of a small polypeptide called ubiquitin to a protein. Ubiquitination frequently serves to target proteins for proteolytic degradation by proteasomes, a critical step in the class I MHC pathway of antigen processing and presentation.

Urticaria Localized transient swelling and redness of the skin caused by leakage of fluid and plasma proteins from small vessels into the dermis during an immediate hypersensitivity reaction.

V gene segments DNA sequence that encodes the variable domain of an Ig heavy chain or light chain or a TCR α, β, γ, or δ chain. Each antigen receptor locus contains many different V gene segments, any one of which may recombine with downstream D or J segments during lymphocyte maturation to form functional antigen receptor genes.

VDJ recombinase The complex of RAG-1 and RAG-2 proteins that catalyzes lymphocyte antigen receptor gene recombination.

Vaccine A preparation of microbial antigen, often combined with adjuvants, which is administered to individuals to induce protective immunity against microbial infections. The antigen may be in the form of live but avirulent microorganisms, killed microorganisms, purified macromolecular components of a microorganism, or a plasmid that contains a complementary DNA encoding a microbial antigen.

Variable region The extracellular, N-terminal region of an Ig heavy or light chain or a TCR α, β, γ, or δ chain that contains variable amino acid sequences that differ between every clone of lymphocytes and that are responsible for the specificity for antigen. The antigen-binding variable sequences are localized to extended loop structures or hypervariable segments.

Virus Primitive obligate intracellular parasitic organism or infectious particle that consists of a simple nucleic acid genome packaged in a protein capsid, sometimes surrounded by a membrane envelope. Many pathogenic animal viruses cause a wide range of diseases. Humoral immune responses to viruses can be effective in blocking infection of cells, and NK cells and CTLs are necessary to kill cells already infected.

Western blot Immunologic technique to determine the presence of a protein in a biologic sample. The method involves separation of proteins in the sample by electrophoresis, transfer of the protein array from the electrophoresis gel to a support membrane by capillary action (blotting), and finally detection of the protein by binding of an enzymatically or radioactively labeled antibody specific for that protein.

Wheal and flare reaction Local swelling and redness in the skin at a site of an immediate hypersensitivity reaction. The wheal reflects increased vascular permeability, and the flare results from increased local blood flow, both changes resulting from mediators such as histamine released from activated dermal mast cells.

White pulp Part of the spleen that is composed predominantly of lymphocytes, arranged in periarteriolar lymphoid sheaths, and follicles and other leukocytes. The remainder of the spleen contains sinusoids lined with phagocytic cells and filled with blood, called the *red pulp*.

Wiskott-Aldrich syndrome X-linked disease characterized by eczema, thrombocytopenia (reduced blood platelets), and immunodeficiency manifested as susceptibility to bacterial infections. The defective gene encodes a cytosolic protein involved in signaling cascades and regulation of the actin cytoskeleton.

Xenoantigen Antigen on a graft from another species.

Xenograft Organ or tissue graft derived from a species different from the recipient. Transplantation of xenogeneic grafts (e.g., from a pig) to humans is not yet practical because of special problems related to immunologic rejection. Also called xenogeneic graft.

Xenoreactive Describing a T cell or antibody that recognizes and responds to an antigen on a graft from another species (a xenoantigen). The T cell may recognize an intact xenogeneic MHC molecule or a peptide derived from a xenogeneic protein bound to a self MHC molecule.

X-linked agammaglobulinemia Immunodeficiency disease, also called Bruton's agammaglobulinemia, characterized by a block in early B cell maturation and absence of serum Ig. Patients have pyogenic bacterial infections. The disease is caused by mutations or deletions in the gene encoding Btk, an enzyme involved in signal transduction in developing B cells.

X-linked hyper-IgM syndrome Rare immunodeficiency disease caused by mutations in the

CD40 ligand gene and characterized by failure of B cell heavy-chain isotype switching and cell-mediated immunity. Patients have both pyogenic bacterial and protozoal infections.

Zeta (ζ) chain Transmembrane protein expressed in T cells as part of the TCR complex that contains ITAMs in its cytoplasmic tail and binds the ZAP-70 protein tyrosine kinase during T cell activation.

Zeta-associated protein of 70 kD (ZAP-70) Cytoplasmic protein tyrosine kinase, similar to Syk in B cells, that is critical for early signaling steps in antigen-induced T cell activation. ZAP-70 binds to phosphorylated tyrosines in the cytoplasmic tails of the ζ chain and CD3 chains of the TCR complex and in turn phosphorylates adaptor proteins that recruit other components of the signaling cascade.

Major Cytokines

This table includes cytokines with well-defined functions in innate or adaptive immune responses. Other cytokines that have less important or poorly understood roles are not included. The table is organized into families of cytokines based on shared structural homologies. Members of each family bind to receptors that are also homologous to one another and use similar signaling pathways to activate cellular responses.

Cytokine; Subunits	Principal Cell Source	Cytokine Receptor; Subunits*	Principal Cellular Targets and Biologic Effects
Type 1 Cytokine Family Members			
Interleukin-2 (IL-2)	T cells	CD25 (IL2Rα) CD122 (IL2Rβ) CD132 (γc)	T cells: proliferation and differentiation into effector and memory cells; promotes regulatory T cell development, survival, and function NK cells: proliferation, activation
Interleukin-3 (IL-3)	T cells	CD123 (IL-3Rα) CD131 (βc)	Immature hematopoietic progenitors: induced maturation of all hematopoietic lineages
Interleukin-4 (IL-4)	CD4+ T cells (TH2), mast cells	CD124 (IL-4Rα) CD132 (γc)	B cells: isotype switching to IgE T cells: TH2 differentiation Macrophages: alternative activation and inhibition of IFN-γ-mediated classical activation
Interleukin-5 (IL-5)	CD4+ T cells (TH2)	CD125 (IL-5Rα) CD131 (βc)	Eosinophils: activation, increased generation B cells: IgA production
Interleukin-6 (IL-6)	Macrophages, endothelial cells, T cells	CD126 (IL-6Rα) CD130 (gp130)	Liver: synthesis of acute-phase proteins B cells: proliferation of antibody-producing cells
Interleukin-7 (IL-7)	Fibroblasts, bone marrow stromal cells	CD127 (IL7R) CD132 (γc)	Immature lymphoid progenitors: proliferation of early T and B cell progenitors T lymphocytes: survival of naive and memory cells

Continued

Cytokine; Subunits	Principal Cell Source	Cytokine Receptor; Subunits*	Principal Cellular Targets and Biologic Effects
Interleukin-9 (IL-9)	CD4+ T cells	CD129 (IL-9R) CD132 (γ_c)	Mast cells, B cells, T cells, and tissue cells: survival and activation
Interleukin-12 (IL-12) IL-12A (p35) IL-12B (p40)	Macrophages, dendritic cells	CD212 (IL-12Rβ1) IL-12Rβ2	CD4+ T cells: T_H1 differentiation NK cells and CD8+ T cells: IFN-γ synthesis, increased cytotoxic activity
Interleukin-13 (IL-13)	CD4+ T cells (T_H2), NKT cells, mast cells	CD213 α1 (IL-13Rα1) CD213 α2 (IL-13Rα2) CD132 (γ_c)	B cells: isotype switching to IgE Epithelial cells: increased mucus production Fibroblasts: increased collagen synthesis Macrophages: alternative activation
Interleukin-15 (IL-15)	Macrophages, others	IL-15Rα CD122 (IL2Rβ) CD132 (γ_c)	NK cells: proliferation T cells: survival and proliferation of memory CD8+ cells
Interleukin-17A (IL-17A) Interleukin-17F (IL-17F)	T cells, other cells	CD217 (IL-17RA)	Endothelial cells: increased chemokine production Macrophages: increased chemokine and cytokine production Epithelial cells: increased defensin GM-CSF and G-CSF production
Interleukin-21 (IL-21)	T cells	IL-21R CD132 (γ_c)	B cells: activation, proliferation, differentiation T_H17 cells: increased generation T_{FH} cells: development
Interleukin-23 (IL-23) IL-23A (p19) IL-12B (p40)	Macrophages, dendritic cells	IL-23R CD212 (IL-12Rβ1)	T cells: increased stability and inflammatory activity of IL-17 producing T cells
Interleukin-27 (IL-27) IL-27-p28 EBI3 (IL-27B)	Macrophages, dendritic cells	IL-27Rβα CD130 (gp130)	T cells: inhibition of T_H1 cells NK cells: IFN-γ synthesis
Stem cell factor (c-Kit ligand)	Bone marrow stromal cells	CD117 (c-KIT)	Pluripotent hematopoietic stem cells: induced maturation of all hematopoietic lineages
Granulocyte-monocyte CSF (GM-CSF)	T cells, macrophages, endothelial cells, fibroblasts	CD116 (GM-CSFRa) CD131 (β_c)	Immature and committed progenitors, mature macrophages: induced maturation of granulocytes and monocytes, macrophage activation
Monocyte CSF (M-CSF, CSF1)	Macrophages, endothelial cells, bone marrow cells, fibroblasts	CD115 (CSF1R)	Committed hematopoietic progenitors: induced maturation of monocytes
Granulocyte CSF (G-CSF, CSF3)	Macrophages, fibroblasts, endothelial cells	CD114 (CSF3R)	Committed hematopoietic progenitors: induced maturation of granulocytes
Type 2 Cytokine Family Members			
IFN-α (multiple proteins)	Plasmacytoid dendritic cells, macrophages	IFNAR1 CD118 (IFNAR2)	All cells: antiviral state, increased class I MHC expression NK cells: activation
IFN-β	Fibroblasts, plasmacytoid dendritic cells	IFNAR1 CD118 (IFNAR2)	All cells: antiviral state, increased class I MHC expression NK cells: activation

Cytokine; Subunits	Principal Cell Source	Cytokine Receptor; Subunits*	Principal Cellular Targets and Biologic Effects
Interferon-γ (IFN-γ)	T cells (T$_H$1, CD8$^+$ T cells), NK cells	CD119 (IFNGR1) IFNGR2	Macrophages: classical activation (increased microbicidal functions) B cells: isotype switching to opsonizing and complement-fixing IgG subclasses (best established in mice) T cells: T$_H$1 differentiation Various cells: increased expression of class I and class II MHC molecules, increased antigen processing and presentation to T cells
Interleukin-10 (IL-10)	Macrophages, T cells (mainly regulatory T cells)	CD210 (IL-10R1) CD210B (IL-10R2)	Macrophages, dendritic cells: inhibition of expression of IL-12, costimulators and class II MHC
Interleukin-22 (IL-22)	T$_H$17 cells	IL-22R1 CD210B (IL-10R2) *or* IL22BP CD210B (IL-10R2)	Epithelial cells: production of defensins, increased barrier function Hepatocytes: survival
TNF Superfamily Cytokines†			
Tumor necrosis factor (TNF, TNFSF2, TNF-α)	Macrophages, NK cells, T cells	CD120a (TNFRSF1); *or* CD120b (TNFRSF2)	Endothelial cells: activation (promotes inflammation, coagulation) Neutrophils: activation Hypothalamus: fever Liver: synthesis of acute-phase proteins Muscle, fat: catabolism (cachexia)
Lymphotoxin-α (LTα, TNFSF1, TNF-β)	T cells, B cells	CD120a (TNFRSF1) *or* CD120b (TNFRSF2)	Same as TNF
Lymphotoxin-β (LTβ)	T cells, NK cells, follicular B cells, lymphoid inducer cells	LTβR *or* HVEM	Lymphoid tissue stromal cells and FDCs: chemokine expression and lymphoid organogenesis
BAFF (CD257, TNFSF13B)	B cells, dendritic cells, monocytes, follicular dendritic cells	BAFF-R (TNFRSF13C) *or* TACI (TNFRSF13B) *or* BCMA (TNFRSF17)	B cells: survival, proliferation
APRIL	T cells, dendritic cells, monocytes, follicular dendritic cells	TACI (TNFRSF13B) *or* BCMA (TNFRSF17)	B cells: survival, proliferation
IL-1 Family Cytokines			
Interleukin-1α (IL-1α)	Macrophages, dendritic cells, fibroblasts, endothelial cells, keratinocytes, hepatocytes	CD121a (IL-1R1) IL-1RAP *or* CD121b (IL-1R2)	Endothelial cells: activation (promotes inflammation, coagulation) Hypothalamus: fever Liver: synthesis of acute phase proteins

Continued

Cytokine; Subunits	Principal Cell Source	Cytokine Receptor; Subunits*	Principal Cellular Targets and Biologic Effects
Interleukin-1β (IL-1β)	Macrophages, dendritic cells, fibroblasts, endothelial cells, keratinocytes, hepatocytes	CD121a (IL-1R1) IL-1RAP *or* CD121b (IL-1R2)	Endothelial cells: activation (promotes inflammation, coagulation) Hypothalamus: fever Liver: synthesis of acute-phase proteins
Interleukin-1 receptor antagonist (IL-1RA)	Macrophages	CD121a (IL-1R1) IL-1RAP	Various cells: competitive antagonist of IL-1
Interleukin-18 (IL-18)	Monocytes, macrophages, dendritic cells, Kupffer cells, keratinocytes, chondrocytes, synovial fibroblasts, osteoblasts	CD218a (IL-18R1) CD218b (IL-18RAP)	NK cells and T cells: IFN-γ synthesis Monocytes: expression of GM-CSF, TNF, IL-1β Neutrophils: activation, cytokine release
Interleukin-33 (IL-33)	Epithelial cells, endothelial cells	IL-1RL1 IL-1RAP	T cells: IL-5, IL-13 expression B1B cells: IgM production Mast cells: activation Eosinophils: activation
Other Cytokines			
Transforming growth factor beta (TGF-β)	T cells (mainly Tregs), macrophages, other cell types		T cells: inhibition of proliferation and effector functions; differentiation of T_H17 and Treg B cells: inhibition of proliferation; IgA production Macrophages: inhibition of activation; stimulation of angiogenic factors Fibroblasts: increased collagen synthesis

Abbreviations: APRIL, a proliferation-inducing ligand; IFN, interferon; MHC, major histocompatibility complex; NK, natural killer. BAFF, B cell–activating factor belonging to TNF family; BCMA, B cell maturation protein; CSF, colony-stimulating factor; HVEM, herpesvirus entry mediator; NK cell, natural killer cell; TACI, transmembrane activator and calcium modulator and cyclophilin ligand interactor; TNF, tumor necrosis factor; TNSF, TNF super family; TNFRSF, TNF receptor superfamily.

*Most cytokine receptors are dimers or trimers composed of different polypeptide chains, some of which are shared between receptors for different cytokines. The set of polypeptides that comprise a functional receptor (cytokine binding plus signaling) for each cytokine are listed. The functions of each subunit polypeptide are not listed.

[†]All TNF superfamily (TNFSF) members are expressed as cell surface transmembrane proteins, but only the subset that are predominantly active as proteolytically released soluble cytokines are listed in the table. Other TNSF members, which function predominantly in the membrane-bound form and are not, strictly speaking, cytokines, are not listed in the table.

Principal Features of Select CD Molecules

The following list includes select CD molecules that are referred to in the text. Many cytokines and cytokine receptors have been assigned CD numbers, but we refer to these by the more descriptive cytokine designation. A complete and up-to-date listing of CD molecules may be found at http://www.hlda8.org.

CD Number* (Other Names)	Molecular Structure, Family	Main Cellular Expression	Known or Proposed Function(s)
CD1a-d	49 kD; class I MHC–like Ig superfamily; β_2-microglobulin associated	Thymocytes, dendritic cells (including Langerhans cells)	Presentation of nonpeptide (lipid and glycolipid) antigens to some T cells
CD1e	28 kD; class I MHC–like; β_2-microglobulin associated	Dendritic cells	Same as CD1a
CD2 (LFA-2)	50 kD; Ig superfamily	T cells, NK cells	Adhesion molecule (binds CD58); T cell activation; CTL- and NK cell–mediated lysis
CD3γ	25-28 kD; associated with CD3δ and CD3ε in TCR complex; Ig superfamily; ITAM in cytoplasmic tail	T cells	Cell surface expression of and signal transduction by the T cell antigen receptor
CD3δ	20 kD; associated with CD3δ and CD3ε in TCR complex; Ig superfamily; ITAM in cytoplasmic tail	T cells	Cell surface expression of and signal transduction by the T cell antigen receptor
CD3ε	20 kD; associated with CD3δ and CD3ε in TCR complex; Ig superfamily; ITAM in cytoplasmic tail	T cells	Required for cell surface expression of and signal transduction by the T cell antigen receptor

Continued

CD Number* (Other Names)	Molecular Structure, Family	Main Cellular Expression	Known or Proposed Function(s)
CD4	55 kD; Ig superfamily	Class II MHC–restricted T cells; some macrophages	Coreceptor in class II MHC–restricted antigen-induced T cell activation (binds to class II MHC molecules); thymocyte development; receptor for HIV
CD5	67 kD; scavenger receptor family	T cells; B-1 B cell subset	Signaling molecule; binds CD72
CD8α	34 kD; expressed as homodimer or heterodimer with CD8β	Class I MHC–restricted T cells	Coreceptor in class I MHC–restricted antigen-induced T cell activation (binds to class I MHC molecules); thymocyte development
CD8β	34 kD; expressed as heterodimer with CD8α; Ig superfamily	Same as CD8α	Same as CD8α
CD10	100 kD; type II membrane protein	Immature and some mature B cells; lymphoid progenitors, granulocytes	Metalloproteinase; unknown function in immune system
CD11a (LFA-1 α chain)	180 kD; noncovalently linked to CD18 to form LFA-1 integrin	Leukocytes	Cell-cell adhesion; binds to ICAM-1 (CD54), ICAM-2 (CD102), and ICAM-3 (CD50)
CD11b (Mac-1; CR3)	165 kD; noncovalently linked to CD18 to form Mac-1 integrin	Granulocytes, monocytes-macrophages, dendritic cells, NK cells	Phagocytosis of iC3b-coated particles; neutrophil and monocyte adhesion to endothelium (binds CD54) and extracellular matrix proteins
CD11c (p150,95; CR4 α chain)	145 kD; noncovalently linked to CD18 to form p150,95 integrin	Monocytes-macrophages, granulocytes, NK cells	Similar functions as CD11b
CD14	53 kD; GPI linked	Dendritic cells, monocytes, macrophages, granulocytes	Binds complex of LPS and LPS-binding protein and displays LPS to TLR4; required for LPS-induced activation of macrophages and dendritic cells
CD16a (FcγRIIIA)	50-70 kD; transmembrane protein; Ig superfamily	NK cells, macrophages	Binds Fc region of IgG; phagocytosis and antibody-dependent cellular cytotoxicity
CD16b (FcγRIIIB)	50-70 kD; GPI linked; Ig superfamily	Neutrophils	Binds Fc region of IgG; synergy with FcγRII in immune complex–mediated neutrophil activation
CD18	95 kD; noncovalently linked to CD11a, CD11b, or CD11c to form β₂ integrins	Leukocytes	See CD11a, CD11b, CD11c

CD Number* (Other Names)	Molecular Structure, Family	Main Cellular Expression	Known or Proposed Function(s)
CD19	95 kD; Ig superfamily	Most B cells	B cell activation; forms a coreceptor complex with CD21 and CD81 that delivers signals that synergize with signals from B cell antigen receptor complex
CD20	35-37 kD; tetraspan (TM4SF) family	B cells	?Role in B cell activation or regulation; calcium ion channel
CD21 (CR2; C3d receptor)	145 kD; regulators of complement activation	Mature B cells, follicular dendritic cells	Receptor for complement fragment C3d; forms a coreceptor complex with CD21 and CD81 that delivers activating signals in B cells; receptor for Epstein-Barr virus
CD22	130-140 kD; Ig superfamily; sialadhesin family; ITIM in cytoplasmic tail	B cells	Regulation of B cell activation; adhesion molecule
CD23 (FcεRIIB)	45 kD; C-type lectin	Activated B cells, monocytes, macrophages	Low-affinity Fcε receptor, induced by IL-4; function unclear
CD25 (IL-2 receptor α chain)	55 kD; noncovalently associates with IL-2Rβ (CD122) and IL-2Rγ (CD132) chains to form high-affinity IL-2 receptor	Activated T and B cells, regulatory T cells (Treg)	Binds IL-2 and promotes responses to low concentrations of IL-2
CD28	Homodimer of 44-kD chains; Ig superfamily	T cells (all CD4$^+$ and >50% of CD8$^+$ cells in humans; all mature T cells in mice)	T cell receptor for costimulatory molecules CD80 (B7-1) and CD86 (B7-2)
CD29	130 kD; noncovalently linked with CD49a-d chains to form VLA (β$_1$) integrins	T cells, B cells, monocytes, granulocytes	Leukocyte adhesion to extracellular matrix proteins and endothelium (see CD49)
CD30	120 kD; TNFR superfamily	Activated T and B cells, NK cells, monocytes, Reed-Sternberg cells in Hodgkin's disease	Not established
CD31 (platelet/endothelial cell adhesion molecule 1, PECAM-1)	130-140 kD; Ig superfamily	Platelets; monocytes, granulocytes, B cells, endothelial cells	Adhesion molecule involved in leukocyte transmigration through endothelium
CD32 (FcγRII)	40 kD; Ig superfamily; ITIM in cytoplasmic tail; A, B, and C forms are products of different but homologous genes	B cells, macrophages, dendritic cells, granulocytes	Fc receptor for aggregated IgG; acts as inhibitory receptor that blocks activation signals in B cells and other cells

Continued

CD Number* (Other Names)	Molecular Structure, Family	Main Cellular Expression	Known or Proposed Function(s)
CD34	105-120 kD; sialomucin	Precursors of hematopoietic cells, endothelial cells in high endothelial venules	?Role in cell-cell adhesion
CD35 (type 1 complement receptor, CR1)	190-285 kD (four products of polymorphic alleles); regulator of complement activation family	Granulocytes, monocytes, erythrocytes, B cells, follicular dendritic cells, some T cells	Binds C3b and C4b; promotes phagocytosis of C3b- or C4b-coated particles and immune complexes; regulates complement activation
CD36	85-90 kD	Platelets, monocytes and macrophages, endothelial cells	Scavenger receptor for oxidized low-density lipoprotein; platelet adhesion; phagocytosis of apoptotic cells
CD40	Homodimer of 44- to 48-kD chains; TNFR superfamily	B cells, macrophages, dendritic cells, endothelial cells	Binds CD154 (CD40 ligand); role in T cell–mediated activation of B cells, macrophages, and dendritic cells
CD43	95-135 kD; sialomucin	Leukocytes (except circulating B cells)	?Role in cell-cell adhesion
CD44	80 to >100 kD, highly glycosylated	Leukocytes, erythrocytes	Binds hyaluronan; involved in leukocyte adhesion to endothelial cells and extracellular matrix
CD45 (leukocyte common antigen, LCA)	Multiple isoforms, 180-220 kD (see CD45R); protein tyrosine phosphatase receptor family; fibronectin type III family	Hematopoietic cells	Tyrosine phosphatase that regulates T and B cell activation
CD45R	CD45RO:180 kD CD45RA: 220 kD CD45RB: 190-, 205-, and 220-kD isoforms	CD45RO: memory T cells, subset of B cells, monocytes, macrophages CD45RA: naive T cells, B cells, monocytes CD45RB: B cells, subset of T cells	See CD45
CD46 (membrane cofactor protein, MCP)	52-58 kD; regulators of complement activation family	Leukocytes, epithelial cells, fibroblasts	Regulation of complement activation
CD47	47-52 kD; Ig superfamily	All hematopoietic cells, epithelial cells, endothelial cells, fibroblasts	Leukocyte adhesion, migration, activation; "Don't eat me" signal to phagocytes
CD49d	150 kD; noncovalently linked to CD29 to form VLA-4 ($\alpha_4\beta_1$ integrin)	T cells, monocytes, B cells, NK cells, eosinophils, dendritic cells, thymocytes	Leukocyte adhesion to endothelium and extracellular matrix; binds to VCAM-1 and MadCAM-1; binds fibronectin and collagens

CD Number* (Other Names)	Molecular Structure, Family	Main Cellular Expression	Known or Proposed Function(s)
CD54 (ICAM-1)	75-114 kD; Ig superfamily	T cells, B cells, monocytes, endothelial cells (cytokine inducible)	Cell-cell adhesion; ligand for CD11aCD18 (LFA-1) and CD11bCD18 (Mac-1); receptor for rhinovirus
CD55 (decay-accelerating factor, DAF)	55-70 kD; GPI linked; regulators of complement activation family	Broad	Regulation of complement activation
CD58 (leukocyte function–associated antigen 3, LFA-3)	55-70 kD; GPI-linked or integral membrane protein	Broad	Leukocyte adhesion; binds CD2
CD59	18-20 kD; GPI linked	Broad	Binds C9; inhibits formation of complement membrane attack complex
CD62E (E-selectin)	115 kD; selectin family	Endothelial cells	Leukocyte-endothelial adhesion
CD62L (L-selectin)	74-95 kD; selectin family	B cells, T cells, monocytes, granulocytes, some NK cells	Leukocyte-endothelial adhesion; homing of naive T cells to peripheral lymph nodes
CD62P (P-selectin)	140 kD; selectin family	Platelets, endothelial cells (present in granules, translocated to cell surface on activation)	Leukocyte adhesion to endothelium, platelets; binds CD162 (PSGL-1)
CD64 (FcγRI)	72 kD; Ig superfamily; noncovalently associated with the FcR common γ chain	Monocytes, macrophages, activated neutrophils	High-affinity Fcγ receptor; role in phagocytosis, ADCC, macrophage activation
CD66e (carcino-embryonic antigen, CEA)	180-220 kD; Ig superfamily; CEA family	Colonic and other epithelial cells	?Adhesion; clinical marker of carcinoma burden
CD69	23 kD; C-type lectin	Activated B cells, T cells, NK cells, neutrophils	Reduces surface expression of S1PR1 and egress of recently activated lymphocytes from lymphoid tissues; ?other roles in T cell activation
CD74 (class II MHC invariant chain, I_i)	33-, 35-, and 41-kD isoforms	B cells, dendritic cells, monocytes, macrophages; other class II MHC–expressing cells	Binds to and directs intracellular sorting of newly synthesized class II MHC molecules
CD79a (Igα)	33, 45 kD; forms dimer with CD79b; Ig superfamily; ITAM in cytoplasmic tail	Mature B cells	Required for cell surface expression of and signal transduction by B cell antigen receptor complex
CD79b (Igβ)	37-39 kD; forms dimer with CD79a; Ig superfamily; ITAM in cytoplasmic tail	Mature B cells	Required for cell surface expression of and signal transduction by B cell antigen receptor complex

Continued

CD Number* (Other Names)	Molecular Structure, Family	Main Cellular Expression	Known or Proposed Function(s)
CD80 (B7-1)	60 kD; Ig superfamily	Dendritic cells, activated B cells and macrophages	Costimulator for T lymphocyte activation; ligand for CD28 and CD152 (CTLA-4)
CD81 (target for anti-proliferative antigen 1, TAPA-1)	26 kD; tetraspan (TM4SF)	T cells, B cells, NK cells, dendritic cells, thymocytes, endothelium	B cell activation; forms a co-receptor complex with CD19 and CD21 that delivers signals that synergize with signals from B cell antigen receptor complex
CD86 (B7-2)	80 kD; Ig superfamily	B cells, monocytes, dendritic cells; some T cells	Costimulator for T lymphocyte activation; ligand for CD28 and CD152 (CTLA-4)
CD88 (C5a receptor)	43 kD; G protein–coupled, 7 membrane–spanning receptor family	Granulocytes, monocytes, dendritic cells, mast cells	Receptor for C5a complement fragment; role in complement-induced inflammation
CD89 (Fcα receptor, FcαR)	55-75 kD; Ig superfamily; noncovalently associated with the common FcRγ chain	Granulocytes, monocytes, macrophages, T cell subset, B cell subset	Binds IgA; mediates IgA-dependent cellular cytotoxicity
CD90 (Thy-1)	25-35 kD; GPI linked; Ig superfamily	Thymocytes, peripheral T cells (mice), CD34⁺ hematopoietic progenitor cells, neurons	Marker for T cells; unknown function
CD94	43 kD; C-type lectin; on NK cells, covalently assembles with other C-type lectin molecules (NKG2)	NK cells; subset of CD8⁺ T cells	CD94/NKG2 complex functions as an NK cell inhibitory receptor; binds HLA-E class I MHC molecules; *is it only an inhibitory receptor?*
CD95 (Fas)	Homotrimer of 45-kD chains; TNFR superfamily	Broad	Binds Fas ligand; delivers signals leading to apoptotic death
CD103 (α_E integrin subunit)	Dimer of 150- and 25-kD subunits; noncovalently linked to β_7 integrin subunit to form $\alpha_E\beta_7$ integrin	Intraepithelial lymphocytes, other cell types	Role in T cell homing to and retention in mucosa; binds E-cadherin
CD106 (vascular cell adhesion molecule 1, VCAM-1)	100-110 kD; Ig superfamily	Endothelial cells, macrophages, follicular dendritic cells, marrow stromal cells	Adhesion of cells to endothelium; receptor for CD49dCD29 (VLA-4) integrin; role in lymphocyte trafficking, activation
CD150 (signaling lymphocyte activation molecule, SLAM)	37 kD; Ig superfamily	Thymocytes, activated lymphocytes, dendritic cells, endothelial cells	Regulation of B cell–T cell interactions and lymphocyte activation
CD152 (cytotoxic T lymphocyte–associated protein 4, CTLA-4)	33, 50 kD; Ig superfamily	Activated T lymphocytes, regulatory T cells	Mediates suppressive function of regulatory T cells; inhibits T cell responses; binds CD80 (B7-1) and CD86 (B7-2) on antigen-presenting cells

CD Number* (Other Names)	Molecular Structure, Family	Main Cellular Expression	Known or Proposed Function(s)
CD154 (CD40 ligand, CD40L)	Homotrimer of 32- to 39-kD chains; TNFR superfamily	Activated CD4+ T cells	Activates B cells, macrophages, and endothelial cells; ligand for CD40
CD158 (killer Ig-like receptor, KIR)	50, 58 kD; Ig superfamily; KIR family; ITIMs or ITAMs in cytoplasmic tail	NK cells, T cell subset	Inhibition or activation of NK cells on interaction with appropriate class I HLA molecules
CD159a (NKG2A)	43 kD; C-type lectin; forms heterodimer with CD94	NK cells, T cell subset	Inhibition or activation of NK cell on interaction with class I HLA molecules
CD159c (NKG2C)	40 kD; C-type lectin; forms heterodimer with CD94	NK cells	Activation of NK cell on interaction with appropriate class I HLA molecules
CD162 (P-selectin glycoprotein ligand 1 [PSGL-1])	Homodimer of 120-kD chains; sialomucin	T cells, monocytes, granulocytes, some B cells	Ligand for selectins (CD62P, CD62L); adhesion of leukocytes to endothelium
CD178 (Fas ligand, FasL)	Homotrimer of 31-kD subunits; TNF superfamily	Activated T cells	Ligand for CD95 (Fas); triggers apoptotic death
CD206 (mannose receptor)	166 kD; C-type lectin	Macrophages	Binds high-mannose–containing glycoproteins on pathogens; mediates macrophage endocytosis of glycoproteins and phagocytosis of bacteria, fungi, and other pathogens
CD247 (TCR complex ζ chain)	18 kD; ITAMs in cytoplasmic tail	T cells; NK cells	Signaling chain of TCR and NK cell activating receptors
CD252 (OX40 ligand)	21 kD; TNF superfamily	Dendritic cells, macrophages, B cells	Ligand for CD134 (OX40,TNFRSF4); costimulates T cells
CD267 (TACI)	31 kD; TNFR superfamily	B cells	Receptor for cytokines BAFF and APRIL; mediates B cell survival
CD268 (BAFF receptor)	19 kD; TNFR superfamily	B cells	Receptor for BAFF; mediates B cell survival
CD269 (B cell maturation antigen, BCMA)	20 kD; TNFR superfamily	B cells	Receptor for BAFF and APRIL; mediates B cell survival
CD273 (PD-L2)	25 kD; Ig superfamily; structurally homologous to B7	Dendritic cells, monocytes, macrophages	Ligand for PD-1; inhibition of T cell activation
CD274 (PD-L1)	33 kD; Ig superfamily; structurally homologous to B7	Leukocytes, other cells	Ligand for PD-1; inhibition of T cell activation
CD275 (ICOS ligand)	60 kD; Ig superfamily; structurally homologous to B7	B cells, dendritic cells, monocytes	Binds ICOS (CD278); T cell costimulation
CD278 (inducible costimulator, ICOS)	55-60 kD; Ig superfamily; structurally homologous to CD28	Activated T cells	Binds ICOS-L (CD275); T cell costimulation

Continued

CD Number* (Other Names)	Molecular Structure, Family	Main Cellular Expression	Known or Proposed Function(s)
CD279 (PD1)	55 kD; Ig superfamily; structurally homologous to CD28	Activated T cells, activated B cells	Binds PD-L1 and PD-L2; inhibits T cell activation
CD314 (NKG2D)	42 kD; C-type lectin	NK cells, activated CD8$^+$ T cells, NK-T cells, some myeloid cells	Binds MHC class I and class I–like molecules MIC-A, MIC-B, Rae1, and ULBP4; role in NK cell and CTL activation
CD357 (GITR)	26 kD; TNFR superfamily	CD4$^+$ and CD8$^+$ T cells, Treg	?Role in T cell tolerance or Treg function
CD363 (S1PR1, type 1 sphingosine-1-phosphate receptor 1)	42.8 kD; G protein–coupled, 7 membrane–spanning receptor family	Lymphocytes, endothelial cells	Binds sphingosine-1-phosphate and mediates chemotaxis of lymphocytes out of lymphoid organs

Abbreviations: ADCC, Antibody-dependent cellular cytotoxicity; APRIL, a proliferation-inducing ligand; BAFF, B cell–activating factor belonging to the TNF family; CTL, cytotoxic T lymphocyte; gp, glycoprotein; GPI, glycophosphatidylinositol; HIV, human immunodeficiency virus; ICAM, intercellular adhesion molecule; Ig, immunoglobulin; IL, interleukin; ITAM, immunoreceptor tyrosine-based activation motif; ITIM, immunoreceptor tyrosine-based inhibition motif; LFA, lymphocyte function–associated antigen; LPS, lipopolysaccharide; MadCAM, mucosal addressin cell adhesion molecule; MHC, major histocompatibility complex; NK cells, natural killer cells; PAMPs, pathogen-associated molecular patterns; TACI, transmembrane activator and CAML interactor; TCR, T cell receptor; TNF, tumor necrosis factor; TNFR, TNF receptor; VCAM, vascular cell adhesion molecule; VLA, very late activation.

*The lowercase letters affixed to some CD numbers refer to CD molecules that are encoded by multiple genes or that belong to families of structurally related proteins.

Clinical Cases

This appendix presents five clinical cases illustrating various diseases involving the immune system. These cases are not meant to teach clinical skills but rather show how the basic science of immunology contributes to our understanding of human diseases. Each case illustrates typical ways in which a disease manifests, what tests are used in diagnosis, and common modes of treatment. The appendix was compiled with the assistance of Dr. Richard Mitchell and Dr. Jon Aster, Department of Pathology, Brigham and Women's Hospital, Boston; Dr. George Tsokos, Department of Medicine, Beth Israel-Deaconess Hospital, Boston; Dr. David Erle, Department of Medicine, University of California, San Francisco; and Dr. James Faix, Department of Pathology, Stanford University School of Medicine, Palo Alto.

CASE 1: LYMPHOMA

E.B. was a 58-year-old chemical engineer who had been well all his life. One morning, he noticed a lump in his left groin while showering. It was not tender, and the overlying skin appeared normal. After a few weeks, he began to worry about it because it did not go away, and he finally made an appointment with a physician after 2 months. On physical examination, the physician noted a subcutaneous firm, movable nodule, about 3 cm in diameter, in the left inguinal region. The physician asked E.B. if

he had recently noticed any infections of his left foot or leg; E.B. had not. E.B. did complain that he had been waking up frequently at night drenched in perspiration. The physician also found some slightly enlarged lymph nodes in E.B.'s right neck. Otherwise, the physical examination findings were normal. The physician explained that the inguinal mass probably was a lymph node that was enlarged as a result of a reaction to some infection. However, he drew some blood for tests and referred E.B. to a surgeon, who performed a fine-needle aspiration of cells from the lymph node. Examination of smears prepared from aspirated cells revealed mainly small, irregular lymphocytes. Flow cytometric evaluation of these cells showed a 10-fold excess of cells expressing λ immunoglobulin (Ig) light chain compared with cells expressing κ Ig light chain.

Because of the suspicion of B cell lymphoma, the surgeon elected to remove the entire lymph node. Histologic examination revealed an expansion of the node by follicular structures composed of monotonous collections of mainly small to intermediate-sized lymphocytes with irregular or cleaved nuclear contours mixed with smaller numbers of large lymphocytes with prominent nucleoli (Fig. A-1). Flow cytometric analysis of these cells showed a predominant population of B cells expressing IgM, λ light chain, CD10 and CD20, and immunohistochemical stains performed on slides showed strong cytoplasmic staining for BCL-2. On this basis, the diagnosis

FIGURE A–1 Lymph node biopsy with follicular lymphoma. The microscopic appearance of the patient's inguinal lymph node is shown. The follicular structures are abnormal, composed of a monotonous collection of neoplastic cells. By contrast, a lymph node with reactive hyperplasia would have follicles with germinal center formation, containing a heterogeneous mixture of cells.

of follicular lymphoma of low histologic grade was made.

1. Why does the presence of a B cell population in which a large majority of the cells express λ light chain indicate a neoplasm rather than a response to an infection?

2. If the lymph node cells were analyzed by PCR to assess Ig heavy-chain rearrangements, what abnormal finding would you expect?

E.B.'s blood tests indicated he was anemic (low red blood cell count). He underwent staging tests to determine the extent of his lymphoma. Positron emission tomography (PET) and computed tomography (CT) scanning showed enlarged hilar and mediastinal lymph nodes, splenomegaly, and hepatic lesions. A bone marrow biopsy showed presence of lymphoma as well. E.B. was treated with injections of a mouse/human chimeric monoclonal IgG antibody called rituximab, which is specific for human CD20. Imaging studies performed 6 months after the rituximab treatment was begun showed regression in the size of lesions, and E.B. felt well enough to continue working.

3. By what mechanisms would the anti-CD20 antibody help this patient?

4. What are the advantages of using a "humanized" antibody, such as rituxan, as a drug, instead of a mouse antibody?

Answers to Questions for Case 1

1. Each clone of B cells has a unique rearrangement of its Ig heavy-chain and light-chain genes, which encode a unique Ig protein composed of two identical heavy chains and two identical κ or λ light chains (see Chapter 4). In an infection, many different clones of lymphocytes are activated. More than one clone may be specific for the same microbial antigen, and different clones may be responding to different antigens produced by the microbe. Furthermore, even in a lymph node draining a site of infection, there are many clones of normal B cells not specific for the microbe. Thus, immune reactions in a lymph node draining a site of infection contain polyclonal mixtures of B cells that on average include about equal numbers of cells expressing either κ or λ light chains, which can be stained with specific antibodies. B cell tumors such as follicular lymphoma arise from a single transformed cell, the progeny of which share the same set of rearranged Ig genes and express the same immunoglobulin as the cell of origin. Because E.B.'s lymph node was filled with B cells all derived from a single clone, the cells produce and all stain positive for the same Ig light chain, in this case λ light chain, indicating that this is a monoclonal (e.g., neoplastic) proliferation.

2. As explained above, B cell lymphomas are monoclonal, being composed of cells that all contain the same Ig heavy-chain and light-chain gene rearrangements. B cells can be stained with antibodies specific for different types of Ig heavy chains (e.g., IgG, IgM), but it is not possible to distinguish reactive polyclonal proliferations and monoclonal B cell tumors reliably by this method. A different approach that is effective in doing so involves the use of polymerase chain reaction (PCR) amplification of rearranged Ig heavy-chain (IgH) gene segments. This method uses consensus PCR primers that hybridize with virtually all IgH variable (V) gene segments and joining (J) gene segments. These primers are used with the PCR to amplify essentially all the heavy-chain gene rearrangements in a sample (e.g., DNA prepared from enlarged lymph node). The size of the amplified products is then analyzed by capillary electrophoresis, which can separate PCR products that

differ in size by as little as a single nucleotide. You will recall that when the V, D, and J segments of IgH genes (as well as other antigen receptor genes) are joined during antigen receptor rearrangement in pre-B cells, the rearranged segments are of differing length due to the action of enzymes that remove (nucleases) and add (a specialized DNA polymerase called terminal deoxyribonucleotide transferase [TdT]). Within a normal population of B cells, many PCR products of different sizes are generated, and these appear as a broad distribution of fragments of differing size. In the case of a B cell lymphoma, all the B cells have the same VDJ rearrangement, and the PCR product is of one size, appearing as a single, sharp peak.

3. CD20 is expressed on most mature B cells and is also uniformly expressed by all the tumor cells in follicular lymphomas. Injected rituximab (rituxan) will therefore bind to the lymphoma cells and facilitate their destruction, likely through similar mechanisms by which antibodies normally destroy microbes. These mechanisms involve binding of the Fc portion of rituximab to different proteins in the patient, including Fc receptors on macrophages leading to phagocytic clearance of the lymphoma cells, and binding of the Fc portion to complement proteins leading to complement-mediated killing of the lymphoma cells (see Chapter 8). Many normal B cell, will also be destroyed by rituximab, although antibody-secreting plasma cells, which do not express CD20, are not affected.

4. Monoclonal antibodies (mAbs) derived from nonhuman B cells (e.g., mouse) will appear foreign to the human immune system. When injected multiple times with these mAbs, humans will mount humoral immune responses and produce antibodies specific for the injected foreign mAb. These anti-antibody responses will promote clearance of the mAb from the circulation and therefore reduce the therapeutic benefits of the mAb. Furthermore, the Fc regions of human IgG bind better than mouse IgG to human Fc receptors and complement proteins, both of which are important for the effectiveness of mAb drugs (see Answer 3). For these reasons, most recently developed mAbs used as drugs have been genetically engineered to contain mainly or all human Ig amino acid sequences.

Patients will be tolerant to these drugs, just as they are tolerant to their own antibodies. Rituximab is a chimeric mAb, with the CD20-binding variable regions originating from mouse IgG, while the remainder of the antibody including the Fc region originating from human IgG. The small amount of mouse sequences in rituximab do not appear to induce anti-antibody responses in patients, perhaps because potentially responding B cells are destroyed by the drug.

CASE 2: HEART TRANSPLANTATION COMPLICATED BY ALLOGRAFT REJECTION

C.M., a computer software salesman, was 48 years old when he came to his primary care physician because of fatigue and shortness of breath. He had not seen a doctor on a regular basis before this visit and felt well up until 1 year ago, when he began experiencing difficulty climbing stairs or playing basketball with his children. Over the past 6 months he had had trouble breathing when he lay down in bed. He did not remember ever experiencing significant chest pain and had no family history of heart disease. He did recall that about 18 months ago he had to take 2 days off from work because of a severe flulike illness.

On examination, he had a pulse of 105 beats per minute, a respiratory rate of 32 breaths per minute, a blood pressure of 100/60 mm Hg, and was afebrile. His physician heard rales (evidence of abnormal fluid accumulation) in the bases of both lungs. His feet and ankles were swollen. A chest x-ray film showed pulmonary edema and pleural effusions and a significantly enlarged left ventricle. C.M. was admitted to the cardiology service of the University Hospital. On the basis of further tests, including coronary angiography and echocardiography, a diagnosis of dilated cardiomyopathy was made. His physicians told him he would benefit from aggressive medical management, including inotropic agents, afterload reduction, and diuretics, but if his underlying heart disease continued to progress, the best long-term option would be to receive a heart transplant. Unfortunately, despite optimal medical management, his symptoms of congestive heart failure continued to worsen until he was no longer able to manage even routine activities of daily living, and he was listed for heart transplantation.

A panel-reactive antibody (PRA) test was performed on C.M.'s serum to determine whether he had been previously sensitized to alloantigens. This test showed the patient had no circulating antibodies against human leukocyte antigens (HLA), and no further immunologic testing was performed. Two weeks later in a nearby city, a donor heart was removed from a victim of a construction-site accident. The donor had the same ABO blood group type as C.M. The transplant surgery, performed 4 hours after the donor heart was removed, went well, and the allograft was functioning properly postoperatively.

1. What problems might arise if the transplant recipient and the donor have different blood types, or if the recipient has high levels of anti-HLA antibodies?

C.M. was placed on immunosuppressive therapy the day after transplantation, which included daily doses of cyclosporine, mycophenolic acid, and prednisone. Endomyocardial biopsy was performed 1 week after surgery and showed no evidence of myocardial injury or inflammatory cells. He was sent home 10 days after surgery, and within a month he was able to do light exercise without problems. A routinely scheduled endomyocardial biopsy performed within the first 3 months after transplantation was normal, but a biopsy performed 14 weeks after surgery showed the presence of numerous lymphocytes within the myocardium and a few apoptotic muscle fibers (Fig. A-2). The findings were interpreted as evidence of acute allograft rejection.

2. What was the patient's immune system responding to, and what were the effector mechanisms in the acute rejection episode?

C.M.'s serum creatinine level, an indicator of renal function, was high (2.2 mg/dL; normal, <1.5 mg/dL). His physicians therefore did not want to increase his cyclosporine dose because this drug can be toxic to the kidneys. He was given three additional doses of a steroid drug over 18 hours, and a repeat endomyocardial biopsy 1 week later showed only a few scattered macrophages and a small focus of healing tissue. C.M. went home feeling well, and he was able to live a relatively normal life, taking cyclosporine, mycophenolic acid, and prednisone daily.

FIGURE A–2 Endomyocardial biopsy showing acute cellular rejection. The heart muscle is infiltrated by lymphocytes, and necrotic muscle fibers are present. *(Courtesy Dr. Richard Mitchell, Department of Pathology, Brigham and Women's Hospital, Boston.)*

3. What is the goal of the immunosuppressive drug therapy?

Coronary angiograms performed yearly since the transplant showed a gradual narrowing of the lumens of the coronary arteries. In the sixth year after transplantation, C.M. began experiencing some shortness of breath after mild exercise and showed some left ventricular dilation on radiographic examination. An intravascular ultrasound examination demonstrated significant thickening of the walls and narrowing of the lumen of the coronary arteries (Fig. A-3). An endomyocardial biopsy showed areas of ischemic necrosis. C.M. and his physicians are now considering the possibility of a second cardiac transplant.

4. What process has led to failure of the graft after 6 years?

Answers to Questions for Case 2

1. If the recipient and the heart donor had different blood types, or if the recipient had high levels of anti-HLA antibodies, hyperacute rejection might occur after transplantation (see Chapter 10). People with type A, B, or O blood have circulating IgM antibodies against the antigens they do not possess (B, A, or both, respectively). People who have received previous blood transfusions or transplants, or were previously pregnant, may have circulating anti-HLA antibodies. Blood group

FIGURE A–3 Coronary artery with transplant-associated arteriosclerosis. This histologic section was taken from a coronary artery of a cardiac allograft that was removed from a patient 5 years after transplantation because of graft failure. The lumen is greatly narrowed by the presence of intimal smooth muscle cells. *(Courtesy Dr. Richard Mitchell, Department of Pathology, Brigham and Women's Hospital, Boston.)*

antigens and HLA antigens are present on endothelial cells. Preformed antibodies, already present in the recipient at transplantation, can bind to these antigens on graft endothelial cells, causing complement activation, leukocyte recruitment, and thrombosis. As a result, the graft blood supply becomes impaired, and the organ can rapidly undergo ischemic necrosis. The PRA test typically is performed to determine whether a patient needing a transplant has preexisting antibodies specific for a broad panel of HLA antigens. The test is performed by mixing the patient's serum with a collection of HLA-coated microbeads; antibody binding is detected by flow cytometry of the beads, after addition of fluorescence-labeled antibodies directed against human immunoglobulin. The results are expressed as a percentage (0-100%) of the various HLA-coated beads that have bound to the patient's serum antibodies. The higher the PRA value obtained, the greater is the chance that the recipient will have an antibody that can potentially react with a graft and cause hyperacute rejection.

2. In the acute rejection episode, the patient's immune system is responding to alloantigens in the graft. These antigens are likely to include donor major histocompatibility complex (MHC) molecules encoded by alleles not shared by the recipient, as well as unshared allelic variants of other proteins (minor histocompatibility antigens). These alloantigens may be expressed on the graft endothelial cells, leukocytes, and parenchymal cells within the donor heart. The effector mechanisms in the acute rejection episode include both cell-mediated and humoral immune responses. Recipient CD4+ T cells secrete cytokines that promote macrophage activation and inflammation, and can cause myocyte or endothelial cell injury and dysfunction, as well as CD8+ cytotoxic T lymphocytes that can directly kill graft cells. Recipient antibodies, produced in response to the graft antigens, bind to graft cells, leading to complement activation and leukocyte recruitment.

3. The goal of the immunosuppressive drug therapy is to impair the recipient's immune response to alloantigens present in the graft, thereby preventing rejection. The drugs work by blocking T cell activation (cyclosporine), lymphocyte proliferation (mycophenolic acid), and inflammatory cytokine production (prednisone). An attempt is made to preserve some immune function to combat infections.

4. The graft has failed as a result of chronic rejection manifested as a thickening of the walls and narrowing of the lumens of the graft arteries (see Chapter 10). This vascular change, called graft arteriosclerosis or transplant-associated arteriosclerosis, leads to ischemic damage to the heart and is the most frequent reason for long-term graft failure. It may be caused by a chronic T cell–mediated inflammatory reaction against vessel wall alloantigens, resulting in cytokine-stimulated smooth muscle cell migration into the intima and proliferation of the smooth muscle cells.

CASE 3: ALLERGIC ASTHMA

Ten-year-old I.E. was brought to her pediatrician's office in November because of frequent coughing for the past 2 days, wheezing, and a feeling of tightness in her chest. Her symptoms had been especially severe at night. In addition to her routine checkups, she had visited the physician in the past for occasional ear and upper respiratory tract infections but had not previously experienced wheezing or chest tightness. She had eczema, but otherwise, she was in good health and was developmentally normal. Her immunizations were up to date. She lived at home with her mother, father, and two sisters, ages 12 and 4, and a pet cat. Both her parents smoked cigarettes, her father suffered from hay fever, and her older sister had a history of sinus infections.

At the time of her examination, I.E. had a temperature of 37° C (98.6° F), blood pressure of 105/65 mm Hg, and a respiratory rate of 28 breaths per minute. She did not appear short of breath. There were no signs of ear infection or pharyngitis. Auscultation of the chest revealed diffuse wheezing in both lungs without signs of congestive heart failure (rales). There was no evidence of pneumonia. The physician made a presumptive diagnosis of bronchospasm and referred I.E. to a pediatric allergist-immunologist. In the meantime, the patient was given a prescription for a short-acting β_2-adrenergic agonist bronchodilator inhaler, and the child was instructed to administer the drug every 6 hours to relieve symptoms. This drug binds to β_2-adrenergic receptors on bronchial smooth muscle cells and causes them to relax, resulting in dilation of the bronchioles.

1. Asthma is usually an *atopic* disease. What are the different ways in which atopy may manifest clinically?

One week later, I.E. was seen by the allergist. He auscultated her lungs and confirmed the presence of wheezing. I.E. was instructed to blow into a flowmeter, and the physician determined that her peak expiratory flow rate was 65% of normal, indicating airway obstruction. The physician then administered a nebulized bronchodilator, and 10 minutes later performed the test again. The repeat flow rate was 85% of normal, indicating reversibility of the airway obstruction. Blood was drawn and sent for total and differential blood cell count and determination of IgE levels. In addition, a skin test was performed to determine hypersensitivity to various antigens and showed a positive result for cat dander and house dust (Fig. A-4). The patient was instructed to begin using an inhaled corticosteroid and to use her bronchodilator only as needed for respiratory symptoms. Her parents were instructed to make a return appointment 2 weeks later for reevaluation of I.E. and discussion of blood test results.

2. What is the immunologic basis for a positive skin test?

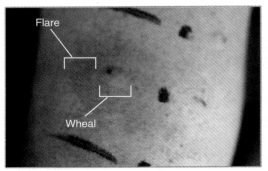

FIGURE A–4 Positive result on skin testing for environmental antigens. Small doses of the antigens are injected intradermally. If mast cells are present with bound IgE specific for the test antigen, the antigen will cross-link the Fc receptors to which the IgE is bound. This induces degranulation of the mast cells and the release of mediators that cause the wheal and flare reaction.

At I.E.'s return appointment 2 weeks later, laboratory tests revealed that she had a serum IgE level of 1200 IU/mL (normal range, 0-180) and a total white blood cell count of 7000/mm³ (normal, 4300-10,800/mm³) with 3% eosinophils (normal, <0.5%). When she returned to the allergist's office 1 week later, her respiratory status on physical examination was significantly improved, with no audible wheezing. I.E.'s peak expiratory airflow had improved to 90% of predicted. The family was told that I.E. had reversible airway obstruction, possibly triggered by a viral illness and possibly related to cat and dust allergies. The physician advised that the cat should at least be kept out of I.E.'s bedroom. The mother was told that smoking in the house probably was contributing to I.E.'s symptoms. The physician recommended that I.E. continue to use the short-acting inhaler for acute episodes of wheezing or shortness of breath. I.E. was asked to return in 3 months, or sooner if she used the inhaler more than twice per month.

3. What is the mechanism for the increased IgE levels seen in patients who have allergic symptoms?

The family cat was given to a neighbor, and I.E. did well on the therapy for about 6 months, experiencing only mild wheezing a few times. The next spring, she began to have more frequent episodes of coughing and wheezing. During a soccer game one Saturday, she became very short of breath, and her parents brought her to the emergency department (ED) of the local hospital. After confirming that she was wheezing and showed signs of accessory respiratory muscle use, the ED physician treated her with a nebulized β_2-agonist bronchodilator and an oral corticosteroid. After 6 hours, her symptoms resolved, and she was sent home. The following week, I.E. was brought to her allergist, who increased her maintenance dose of the inhaled corticosteroid. She has subsequently been well, with occasional mild attacks that are cleared by the bronchodilator inhaler.

    4. What are the therapeutic approaches to allergic asthma?

Answers to Questions for Case 3

1. Atopic reactions to essentially harmless antigens are mediated by IgE on mast cells but may manifest in a variety of ways (see Chapter 11). The signs and symptoms usually reflect the site of entry of the allergen. Hay fever (allergic rhinitis) and asthma usually are responses to inhaled allergens, whereas urticaria and eczema more often occur with skin exposure. Food allergies may cause gastrointestinal symptoms in small children but usually also provoke systemic urticaria in adults. The most dramatic presentation of allergies to insect venom, foods, or drugs is anaphylaxis, an allergic reaction characterized by systemic vasodilation, increased vascular permeability, and bronchoconstriction. Patients with anaphylaxis may progress to asphyxia and cardiovascular collapse.

2. Immediate release of histamine from triggered mast cells produces a central wheal of edema (from leakage of plasma) and the surrounding flare of vascular congestion (from vessel dilation). However, in the subsequent late-phase reaction, there are infiltrates of inflammatory cells in the tissues affected by allergic reactions (see Chapter 11). The allergy skin test should not be confused with the skin test used to assess prior sensitization to certain infectious agents, such as *Mycobacterium tuberculosis*. A positive tuberculosis skin test is an example of a delayed-type hypersensitivity (DTH) reaction, mediated by antigen-stimulated helper T cells, which release cytokines such as interferon-γ, leading to macrophage activation and inflammation (see Chapter 6).

3. For unknown reasons, patients with atopy mount helper T cell responses of the T_H2 type

to a variety of essentially harmless protein antigens, and the T_H2 cells produce interleukin-4 (IL-4) and IL-5. IL-4 induces IgE synthesis by B cells, and IL-5 promotes eosinophil production and activation (see Chapters 5 and 11). Atopy appears to run in families, and genetic susceptibility is clearly involved. Attention has been focused especially on genes on the long arm of chromosome 5 (5q) that encode several T_H2 cytokines and on 11q, where the gene for a chain of the IgE receptor is located.

4. A major therapeutic approach for allergies is prevention by avoidance of precipitating allergens, if known. Although pharmacologic therapy previously has been focused on treating the symptoms of bronchoconstriction by elevating intracellular cyclic adenosine monophosphate (cAMP) levels (using β_2-adrenergic agents and inhibitors of cAMP degradation), the balance of therapy has shifted to use of antiinflammatory agents. These include corticosteroids (which block cytokine release) and receptor antagonists for lipid mediators (e.g., leukotrienes). A newer treatment that is also approved for asthma is anti-IgE antibody.

CASE 4: SYSTEMIC LUPUS ERYTHEMATOSUS

N.Z., a 25-year-old woman, presented to her primary care physician with complaints of joint pain involving her wrists, fingers, and ankles. When seen in the physician's office, N.Z. had normal body temperature, heart rate, blood pressure, and respiratory rate. There was a noticeable red rash on her cheeks, most marked around her nose, sparing the nasolabial folds, and on questioning she said the redness worsened after being in the sun for 1 or 2 hours. The joints of her hands and her wrists were swollen and tender. The other physical examination findings were unremarkable.

Her physician took a blood sample for various tests. Her hematocrit was 35% (normal, 37%-48%). The total white blood cell count was 9800/mm^3 (within normal range) with a normal differential count. The erythrocyte sedimentation rate (ESR) was 40 mm per hour (normal, 1-20). Her serum antinuclear antibody (ANA) test was positive at 1:256 dilution (normally, negative at 1:8 dilution). Other laboratory findings were unremarkable. On the basis of these findings, a

Granular deposits of immunoglobulin
and complement in the basement membrane

FIGURE A–5 Glomerulonephritis with immune complex deposition in systemic lupus erythematosus. A, Light micrograph of a renal biopsy specimen in which neutrophilic infiltration in a glomerulus can be seen. **B,** Immunofluorescence micrograph showing granular deposits of immunoglobulin G (IgG) along the basement membrane. (In this technique, called immunofluorescence microscopy, a frozen section of the kidney is incubated with a fluorescein-conjugated antibody against IgG, and the site of deposition of the IgG is defined by determining where the fluorescence is located.) **C,** Electron micrograph of the same tissue revealing immune complex deposition. *(Courtesy Dr. Helmut Rennke, Department of Pathology, Brigham and Women's Hospital, Boston.)*

diagnosis of systemic lupus erythematosus (SLE) was made. N.Z.'s physician prescribed oral prednisone, a corticosteroid, and with this treatment, her joint pain subsided.

1. What is the significance of the positive result for the ANA test?

Three months later, N.Z. began feeling unusually tired and thought that she had the flu. For about a week she had noticed that her ankles were swollen, and she had difficulty putting on her shoes. She returned to her primary care physician. Her ankles and feet showed severe edema (swollen as a result of extra fluid in the tissue). Her abdomen appeared slightly distended, with a mild shifting dullness to percussion (a sign of an abnormally high amount of fluid in the peritoneal cavity). Her physician ordered several laboratory tests. Her ANA test result was still positive, with a titer of 1:256, and her ESR was 120 mm per hour. Serum albumin was 0.8 g/dL (normal, 3.5-5.0). Measurement of serum complement proteins revealed a C3 of 42 mg/dL (normal, 80-180) and a C4 of 5 mg/dL (normal, 15-45). Urinalysis showed 4+ proteinuria, both red and white blood cells, and numerous hyaline and granular casts. A 24-hour urine sample contained 4 g of protein.

2. What is the likely reason for the decreased complement levels and the abnormalities in blood and urinary proteins?

Because of the abnormal urinalysis findings, the physician recommended a renal biopsy,

which was performed 1 week later. The biopsy specimen was examined by routine histologic methods, immunofluorescence, and electron microscopy (Fig. A-5).

3. What is the explanation for the pathologic changes seen in the kidney?

The physician made the diagnosis of proliferative lupus glomerulonephritis, prescribed a higher dose of prednisone, and recommended treatment with a cytotoxic drug (mycophenolate). N.Z.'s proteinuria and edema subsided over a 2-week period, and serum C3 levels returned to normal. Her corticosteroid dose was tapered to a lower amount. Over the next few years, she has had intermittent flare-ups of her disease, with joint pain and tissue swelling and laboratory tests indicating depressed C3 levels and proteinuria. These have been effectively managed with corticosteroids, and N.Z. has been able to lead an active life.

Answers to Questions for Case 4

1. A positive ANA test reveals the presence of serum antibodies that bind to components of cellular nuclei. The test is performed by placing different dilutions of the patient's serum on top of a monolayer of human cells on a glass slide. A second fluorescently labeled anti-Ig is then added, and the cells are examined with a fluorescent microscope to detect if any serum antibodies bound to the nuclei.

The ANA titer is the maximum dilution of the serum that still produces detectable nuclear staining. Patients with SLE usually (98%) have ANAs, which may be specific for histones, other nuclear proteins, or double-stranded DNA. These are autoantibodies, and their production is evidence of autoimmunity. Autoantibodies may also be produced against various cell membrane protein antigens. Autoantibodies may be present for 5 years or more before the formal establishment of the diagnosis of SLE. Titers of autoantibodies do not reflect disease activity and should not be used to adjust treatment.

2. Some of the autoantibodies form circulating immune complexes by binding to antigens in the blood. Nuclear antigens may be increased in the circulation of patients with SLE because of increased apoptosis of several cell types (e.g., white blood cells, keratinocytes) and defective clearance of apoptotic cells. When these immune complexes deposit in the basement membranes of vessel walls, they may activate the classical pathway of complement, leading to inflammation and depletion of complement proteins through consumption. Inflammation caused by the immune complexes in the kidney leads to leakage of protein and red blood cells into the urine. The loss of protein in the urine results in reduced plasma albumin, reduction of osmotic pressure of the plasma, and fluid loss into the tissues. This explains the edema of the feet and abdominal distention.

3. The pathologic changes in the kidney result from the deposition of circulating immune complexes in the basement membranes of renal glomeruli. In addition, autoantibodies may bind directly to tissue antigens and form in situ immune complexes. These deposits can be seen by immunofluorescence (indicating type of antibody deposited) and electron microscopy (showing exact localization). The immune complexes activate complement, and leukocytes are recruited by complement by-products (C3a, C5a) and by binding of leukocyte Fc receptors to the IgG molecules in the complexes. These leukocytes become activated, and they produce reactive oxygen species and lysosomal enzymes that damage the glomerular basement membrane. These findings are characteristic of immune complex–mediated tissue injury, and complexes may deposit in joints and small blood vessels anywhere in the body, as well as in the kidney. SLE is a prototype of an immune complex disease (see Chapter 11).

CASE 5: HUMAN IMMUNODEFICIENCY VIRUS INFECTION AND ACQUIRED IMMUNODEFICIENCY SYNDROME

J.C. was a 28-year-old assistant carpenter with a history of intravenous heroin use and human immunodeficiency virus (HIV) infection. During admission to the city hospital 7 years earlier because of a drug overdose, he had tested positive for both anti-HIV and anti–hepatitis B virus antibodies by enzyme-linked immunosorbent assay (ELISA). On discharge from the hospital, he was referred to an HIV clinic, where Western blot testing confirmed the presence of anti-HIV antibodies. A reverse-transcriptase PCR test for viral RNA in the blood revealed 15,000 copies/mL of viral genome. His CD4$^+$ T cell count was 800/mm^3 (normal, 500-1500/mm^3). There was no evidence of opportunistic infections at that time. He was also referred to a drug abuse rehabilitation program.

1. What was this patient's major risk factor for acquiring HIV infection? What are other risk factors for HIV infection?

J.C. was prescribed anti-HIV medications after his diagnosis of HIV infection, including two nucleoside reverse-transcriptase inhibitors and one viral protease inhibitor (antiretroviral [ART] therapy). One year after starting triple-drug therapy, J.C.'s CD4$^+$ T cell count remained about 800/mm^3, and a viral load test indicated less than 100 copies/mL. At about this time, J.C. returned to using heroin on multiple occasions, and he did not reliably take his medications. Over the next several years, his CD4$^+$ T cell count gradually declined to 300/mm^3. His physicians changed his medications to different reverse-transcriptase inhibitors three times and to a different protease inhibitor once, in an attempt to stop the decline in his CD4$^+$ count. J.C. was also started on antibiotic prophylaxis for *Pneumocystis jiroveci* pneumonia. The only sign of his HIV disease over this time was multiple enlarged lymph nodes.

2. What caused the gradual decline in the CD4$^+$ T cell count?

After 6 years from the time of initial diagnosis of HIV infection, J.C. began to lose weight. At a

Normal individual   HIV-infected patient

1395 CD4$^+$ T cells/mm^3 66 CD4$^+$ T cells/mm^3

FIGURE A–6 Flow cytometry analysis of CD4$^+$ and CD8$^+$ T cells in blood of patient with human immunodeficiency virus (HIV) infection. A suspension of the patient's white blood cells was incubated with monoclonal antibodies specific for CD4 and CD8. The anti-CD4 antibody was labeled with the fluorochrome allophycocyanin (APC), and the anti-CD8 antibody was labeled with the fluorochrome phycoerythrin (PE). These two fluorochromes emit light of different colors when excited by the appropriate wavelengths. The cell suspensions were analyzed in a flow cytometer, which can enumerate the number of cells stained by each of the differently labeled antibodies. In this way, the number of CD4$^+$ and CD8$^+$ T cells can be determined. Shown here are two-color plots of a control blood sample **(A)** and that of the patient **(B)**. The CD4$^+$ T cells are shown in orange (upper left quadrant), and the CD8$^+$ T cells are shown in green (lower right quadrant). (Note that these are not the colors of light emitted by the APC and PE fluorochromes.)

clinic visit at this time, he complained of a sore throat and had white plaque lesions in his mouth. Flow cytometry indicated a CD4$^+$ count of 64/mm^3 (Fig. A-6), and the viral load was more than 500,000 copies/mL. A diagnosis of acquired immunodeficiency syndrome (AIDS) was made.

3. What is the likely reason for why the anti-HIV drugs given to this patient became ineffective over time?

Six months later, J.C. came to the emergency department with a temperature of 39° C (102.2° F), blood pressure of 160/55 mm Hg, and shallow respirations, with a respiratory rate of 40 breaths per minute. He had lost 10 kg (22 lb) of body weight since his last clinic visit. Several red skin nodules were present on his chest and arms. A chest radiograph showed a diffuse pneumonia. Intravenous antibiotics were administered for presumed *P. jiroveci* pneumonia, and the patient was admitted to the infectious disease service.

That night, a sputum sample was collected, and the following day, skin biopsy specimens were taken from J.C.'s chest. Staining of the sputum sample revealed numerous *P. jiroveci* organisms. The skin biopsy specimens showed Kaposi's sarcoma. Despite intensive care, J.C.'s pneumonia progressed, and he died 3 days later.

4. Why are patients with AIDS at high risk for developing opportunistic infections such as *Pneumocystis jiroveci* and malignancies such as Kaposi's sarcoma?

Answers to Questions for Case 5

1. Intravenous drug use is the major risk factor for HIV infection in this patient. Shared needles among drug addicts transmit blood-borne viral particles from one infected person to others. Other major risk factors for HIV infection include sexual intercourse with an infected person, transfusion of contaminated blood products, and birth from an infected mother (see Chapter 12).

2. After initial infection, the HIV rapidly enters various types of cells in the body, including CD4$^+$ T lymphocytes, dendritic cells, mononuclear phagocytes, and others. Once in an intracellular location, the virus is safe from antibody neutralization. The gradual decline in CD4$^+$ T cells in this patient was caused by repetitive cycles of HIV infection of CD4$^+$ T cells in lymphoid organs, leading to their death. The symptoms of AIDS do not usually occur until the blood count of CD4$^+$ T cells is

below 200/mm^3, reflecting a severe depletion of T cells in the lymphoid organs.

3. HIV has a very high mutation rate. Mutations in the reverse-transcriptase gene that render the enzyme resistant to nucleoside inhibitors occur frequently in patients receiving these drugs. Resistance to protease inhibitors may come about by similar mechanisms. Triple-drug therapy greatly reduces the chances of viral drug resistance, but poor compliance, as in this patient, permits the emergence of mutant strains resistant to several drugs.

4. The deficiencies in T cell–mediated immunity in patients with AIDS lead to impaired immunity to viruses, fungi, and protozoa, which otherwise are easily controlled by a normal immune system. *Pneumocystis jiroveci* is a fungal organism that usually is eradicated by the action of activated CD4$^+$ T cells. Many of the common malignancies in patients with AIDS are caused by oncogenic viruses to which patients are more susceptible because of the immune defects. For example, Kaposi's sarcoma is associated with human herpesvirus-8 infection. Many of the lymphomas that occur in patients with AIDS are associated with the Epstein-Barr virus, and many of the skin and cervical carcinomas that occur in these patients are caused by human papillomavirus.

INDEX